CARDIAC SURGERY

Current Issues 2

CARDIAC SURGERY

Current Issues   2

Edited by

Aurel C. Cernaianu
and
Anthony J. DelRossi

University of Medicine and Dentistry of New Jersey
Robert Wood Johnson Medical School at Camden
Camden, New Jersey

SPRINGER SCIENCE+BUSINESS MEDIA, LLC

Proceedings of a symposium entitled Cardiac Surgery: 1993,
held November 11–14, 1993, in St. Thomas, U.S. Virgin Islands

ISSN 1072-9798

ISBN 978-0-306-44671-9   ISBN 978-1-4615-2423-6 (eBook)
DOI 10.1007/978-1-4615-2423-6

© 1994 Springer Science+Business Media New York
Originally published by Plenum Press New York in 1994

PREFACE

The topics in this book represent the presentations given at the Fifth Annual Meeting entitled "Cardiac Surgery: Current Issues" held at the Frenchman's Reef Beach Resort, St. Thomas, U.S. Virgin Islands, November 11–14, 1992.

This symposium was sponsored by the Division of Cardiothoracic Surgery, the School of Cardiovascular Perfusion and the Department of Nursing Education and Quality Assurance of Cooper Hospital/University Medical Center, the University of Medicine and Dentistry of New Jersey, Robert Wood Johnson Medical School, Camden, New Jersey, as well as the Academy of Medicine of New Jersey.

Chapter authors were charged with the task of writing brief overviews of major issues related to the field of cardiac surgery. The book is specifically tailored to the needs of cardiothoracic surgeons, cardiovascular perfusionists, allied health professionals and nursing personnel involved in all phases of caring for the cardiac surgical patient.

Although intended as a reference source with emphasis on up-dated approaches applied in cardiac surgery, it is hoped that the discussion of these topics will compliment other texts and manuscripts. Obviously, a book of this length cannot cover the whole multidisciplinary and complex field of cardiac surgery. However, co-editors are certain that the annual appearance of this text will highlight comprehensive, new and interesting approaches to the field of cardiac surgery.

The co-editors are greatly thankful to the contributors for their efforts in providing comprehensive chapters. Without their expertise this work would not have been possible. We would also like to thank Ms. Mary Safford and the staff at Plenum Publishing Corporation for their tremendous help in completing this work.

Aurel C. Cernaianu, M.D.
Anthony J. DelRossi, M.D.

CONTENTS

TRANSPLANTATION OF THE HEART AND HEART-LUNGS

Norman E. Shumway, M.D.

Stanford University School of Medicine
Stanford, California

HISTORY OF HEART TRANSPLANTATION

The history of heart transplantation goes back to the turn of this century. At that time, Alexis Carrel and Charles Guthrie, then at the University of Chicago, placed puppy hearts into the necks of adult mongrel dogs.{1} Suture materials were primitive and these heterotopic hearts would beat for only a few hours. Not much further work was done in the field until the mid 1950's when Demikhov and Sinitisin in Russia placed the donor heart in the chest, still in a heterotopic locus.{2} Perhaps some work of the circulation was provided by this preparation but nothing could be quantitated physiologically.

When we first considered orthotopic transplantation of the heart in 1958, there were three obvious problems. First, a successful surgical technique had never been developed. Second, physiological performance of an orthotopically transplanted heart was totally unknown. As it turned out, of course, the heart is the only striated muscle in the body which when separated from the central nervous system does not wither and die. Third, the pattern of homograft rejection with respect to the heart had never been studied, and its control posed substantial problems.

The surgical method was easy to develop and it amounted to leaving behind segments of either atrium to facilitate implantation of the donor heart.{3} Numerous venous connections were simply combined into a long arterial suture line, and the outflow tracts consisting of aorta and pulmonary artery were then easily anastomosed. Performance of the heart was better studied in the autotransplanted preparation which, of course, was free of any immunologic challenge. The denervated heart supported the circulation effectively, and heart rate actually would increase with exercise but over a slightly longer time frame. There appeared to be a humoral substitute for the effect of denervation.{4} The third problem of homograft rejection, of course, remains to this day a threat to the survival of any transplanted organ. At the outset, we thought the dog would be wise enough not to reject something as important to his survival as an orthotopically transplanted heart. The usual laws of immunology with respect to transplanted tissue prevailed, however, and survival of the transplant and the animal ranged from three days to three weeks, depending on the chance matching or mismatching of donor-recipient pairs. Chemical immunosuppression became available in the early 1960's so we adopted similar protocols to obtain long-term survival of the orthotopic heart transplant recipient.[5] With the clinical success of kidney and liver transplantation in the late 1960's, we felt prepared for heart transplantation in patients. The necessary laboratory experience had been accumulated and on January 6, 1968, the first of 734 heart transplants was performed at the Stanford University Hospital.

Worldwide there was great enthusiasm for heart transplantation, but by the mid-1970's, most centers had stopped heart transplantation owing to almost universal loss of the patients. In fact, during the 1970's, Stanford alone could report results from an ongoing clinical heart transplant program. Further advances in the laboratory were mainly responsible for the improved clinical results at Stanford. Rabbit antithymocyte globulin was found useful in providing better immunosuppression than could be afforded through the protocol of azathioprine and prednisone alone. Philip Caves and Margaret Billingham combined their talents in 1972 to develop percutaneous, trans-venous, endomyocardial biopsy of the heart transplant.[6]

This technique has been applied at Stanford more than 10,000 times without mortality and only a very rare complication, such as a pneumothorax. Cardiac biopsy remains today the gold standard for assaying the immunologic health of the heart transplant. Prior to the introduction of rabbit antithymocyte globulin and cardiac biopsy, the five year survival for heart transplantation was no better than 25 percent. With these two then new modalities, five year survival reached slightly more than 40 percent. In December 1980, Stanford was privileged to introduce cyclosporine A into the immunosuppressive protocol for heart transplantation. One year survival improved immediately from 66 to 80 percent. Cyclosporine was first used in renal transplantation by Sir Roy Calne in Cambridge, England. Not until cyclosporine became available in heart transplantation was the severe renal toxic effect of the molecule completely elucidated. Protocols which began with cyclosporine and prednisone were then modified by smaller dosages of cyclosporine and the addition of azathioprine. The age of triple drug maintenance therapy was begun. The nephrotoxicity associated with cyclosporine could be mitigated through the use of lower dosages and the combination of azathioprine and prednisone. Five-year survival for patients on triple drug therapy, this is cyclosporine based immunosuppression, advanced to between 66 and 70 percent. Today, there are a number of new immunosuppressive molecules under investigation which might further improve survival statistics after organ transplantation, but only FK-506, developed by the Fugisawa Pharmaceutical Company of Japan has been used clinically. Early results from the Pittsburgh group are encouraging, and there is at least a suggestion that FK-506 is not as toxic to the kidneys as cyclosporine. It will be interesting during the last years of this century to see if more specific and less toxic immunosuppression will further benefit patients after heart transplantation.

TRANSPLANTATION IN CHILDREN AND NEONATES

Early in the cyclosporine era, a patient was sent to Stanford in extremis from the Kansas City area with blood pressure maintained at shock levels only through use of the intra-aortic balloon pump. Since the situation was of such an emergency nature, we transplanted the heart from a twelve year old female donor into the so-called "piggyback" or heterotopic locus. We were convinced that the heart was too small for orthotopic placement so the transplant was done in such a way as to take over as much of the systemic output as possible. To our amazement, one year later when routine annual studies were done, the entire systemic output was assumed by the transplant, and the aortic valve of the recipient never opened. Obviously, this is one of the reasons that orthotopic transplants are much preferred over the "piggyback" procedure, but in this patient, the immunologic balance was so perfect that we maintained the status quo but with great attention to anticoagulation. This clinical experiment, coupled with the steroid-sparing properties of cyclosporine, convinced us that the time had arrived to consider heart transplantation in younger patients. We were certain that the donor heart would grow and develop not only because of its genetic makeup but also because the donor heart would respond to the increasing physiologic demand. At the present time, more than 83 heart transplants have been performed at Stanford in patients from three days of age to under 14 years. Five-year survival in this patient population would appear to be somewhat better than for patients in the older age group. We have found no evidence that neonates or children are less likely to reject the transplanted heart. As a matter of fact, we lost a neonate two weeks after transplantation from irreversible rejection. This patient was nine days old at the time of the original procedure. Preservation of the immature donor heart provides longer periods of safe extracorporeal residence than is the case with adult donor hearts. At Stanford, the longest duration of a donor heart between donor and recipient was eight hours. This heart was removed some 2,000 miles from the Stanford Hospital and not implanted into a five months old recipient until eight hours later. This patient continues to do well now some six years post-transplant.

DEVELOPMENTS IN THE ARTIFICIAL HEART

Studies in the developmental of an artificial heart have been underway at Stanford for the past 19 years.[7] It has been our feeling that an electromechanical device would be much more practical than any of the various artificial hearts driven by intermittent pneumatic pressure. The ultimate goal obviously would be to implant the device totally without the need for tubes to exit the skin and thereby to avoid an avenue for infectious complications. We also felt that utilization of any artificial heart on a temporary basis, as a bridge to transplantation, could only be justified if there were some promise that the device ultimately could be totally implanted. The Jarvik total artificial heart had a most dismal clinical history owing to bleeding and thromboembolic complications when the apparatus was used in a few patients for permanent implantation. Later, the Jarvik total artificial heart became a prominent player in the bridging concept to transplantation. Our feeling all along has been that any device used as a bridge merely intensifies an already critical donor shortage because such a patient would immediately rise to the top of the recipient list.

The Novacor left ventricular substitute has been applied in 20 patients at Stanford for periods up to six weeks. The Federal Drug Administration (FDA) has approved the Novacor only as a temporary device for patients awaiting transplantation. We have participated in the bridging program only because experimental work indicates that the Novacor may become a permanent substitute for the left ventricle, and these clinical studies were essential in looking at that ultimate application. Experiments in sheep have indicated that it is possible to transmit sufficient energy through the intact skin to a receptor belt placed subcutaneously to drive the left ventricular substitute. As a matter of fact, in the next few years, the FDA has approved the Novacor for so-called permanent implantation at two medical centers on a highly selective and limited basis. The Jarvik device, of course, has been taken completely off the market. In the presence of normal pulmonary vascular resistance, and since there are no valves in the pulmonary venous system, a left heart substitute would appear to suffice to drive the circulation rather than any need for a biventricular substitute. The Fontan operation, in which the right ventricle is completely bypassed, lends credence to this proposition. Accordingly, at Stanford all efforts in the artificial heart developmental area have been directed to the replacement of the systemic ventricle.

CORONARY ARTERY DISEASE IN THE HEART TRANSPLANT PATIENT

At Stanford, 54 patients have undergone retransplantation for coronary artery disease in the transplanted heart. Also, of course, many patients have succumbed as a result of coronary artery disease in the donor heart. We think this intimal proliferation and often serious luminal obstruction is the result of insidious, chronic, antibody-mediated rejection of the transplant. Probably one third of all patients two years after heart transplantation will exhibit some degree of coronary artery disease. The only factor that seems to correlate with the incidence of coronary artery disease in the graft is the number and severity of rejection episodes. Cardiac biopsy, of course, does not delineate this problem unless by chance a tiny capillary is biopsied. Accordingly, annual coronary arteriography is essential in all patients to follow closely the possible development of coronary occlusive disease in the graft.

TRANSPLANTATION OF THE HEART AND BOTH LUNGS

At Stanford, some 103 heart-lung transplants have been performed on 99 patients since the first successful procedure in March, 1981.[8] Five-year survival is not as good as with heart transplantation alone, but at the present time, approximately 50 percent of the patients can be expected to live five years. At the outset, the principal indication for heart-lung transplantation was severe pulmonary vascular disease either of a primary nature or secondary to cardiac disease, the Eisenmenger complex. More recently, it has been possible to do single lung transplants in patients with Eisenmenger's syndrome along with closure of the patent ductus or septal defect if cardiac function remains satisfactory. A certain number of patients, however, with the Eisenmenger complex or severe pulmonary vascular disease or some other kind of complex congenital heart disease, will require heart-lung transplantation. Transplantation of the heart and both lungs has also proved useful for patients with cystic fibrosis. In some of these cases, it is possible to utilize the heart of the heart-lung recipient for an individual who needs only a heart transplant, the so-called domino donor phenomenon.

Only two double lung transplants have been performed at Stanford but in each case, bilateral bronchial anastomoses were utilized. Since there is no blood supply from the donor set of organs in a double lung transplant, it is much preferred to construct individual bronchial anastomoses rather than a single tracheal anastomosis. Experience elsewhere with the tracheal anastomosis in a double lung transplant has been fraught with complications. In heart-lung transplantation, there is collateral blood flow from the coronary arteries into the bronchial circulation all the way up to the tracheal anastomosis so that healing is ensured. When the heart is not in the circuit and a double lung transplant is performed, there is no such collateral circulation and the tracheal connection can easily disrupt or become stenotic. In our experience, both patients with double lung transplants have done well.

Nineteen single lung transplants have been carried out at the Stanford University Hospital, and to date, there has been no problem with healing of the bronchial connection. It is clear than an omental wrap is unnecessary for the bronchial anastomosis. Polypropylene sutures always should be used for the bronchial or tracheal anastomosis.

In an effort again to widen the potential donor pool, Vaughn A. Starnes, then at Stanford and now Chairman of Cardiothoracic Surgery at the University of Southern California, transplanted a living related right upper lobe of a 46 year old mother into the pneumonectomized right chest of her 12 year old daughter suffering from bronchopulmonary dysplasia secondary to prolonged oxygen ventilation in the neonatal period. The right upper lobe of the mother was a perfect fit for the entire right chest of the recipient, and this type of accommodation between a donor and recipient may very well prove useful to increase the pool of potential donors. Lungs are much better suited to lobar dissection and transplantation than is the liver, and of course, a long experience with living related kidney transplantation also supports this new concept.

Since the first clinical heart transplant at Stanford in January 1968, 734 heart transplants have been performed on 681 patients. The longest survivor died a few weeks short of 22 years due to infectious complications. The five-year survival of all patients is 66 percent. One hundred-two heart-lung transplants have been performed on 98 patients with the five year survival at 40 percent. Single lung transplants have been effective and 11 of 18 patients are living and well. Only two double lung transplants are in the series but both patients are out of the hospital leading full lives. The use of a living related pulmonary lobe donor is now being explored as a possible solution to the critical shortage of lung donors.

With new drugs on the horizon, more specifically directed to the homograft rejection process, it is important that every effort be made to utilize as many donors as possible, whether it be for heart, heart-lung or lung transplantation.

REFERENCES

1. Carrel A, Guthrie CC: The transplantation of veins and organs. Am J Med 1905;10:1101.

2. Demikhov VP: Experimental transplantation of vital organs. New York, Consultants and Bureau, 1962.

3. Lower RR, Shumway NE: Studies on the orthotopic homotransplantation of the canine heart. Surg Forum 1960;11:18.

4. Angell WW, Shumway NE: Resuscitation storage of the cadaver heart transplant. Surg Forum 1966;17:224.

5. Lower RR, Dong E, Shumway NE: Long-term survival of cardiac homografts. Surgery 1965;58:110.

6. Caves PK, Stinson EB, Billingham ME et al: Percutaneous endomyocardial biopsy in human heart recipients. Ann Thorac Surg 1973;16:325.

7. Portner PM, Oyer PE, McGregor CG et al: First human use of an electrically powered implantable ventricular assist system. Artif Organs 1985;9(A):3.

8. Reitz BA, Wallwork JL, Hunt SA et al: Heart-lung transplantation: Successful therapy for patients with pulmonary vascular disease. N Engl J Med 1982;306:557.

PHYSIOLOGIC PRINCIPLES AND CLINICAL USE OF HYPOTHERMIA

Laurie K. Davies, M.D. and Richard F. Davis, M.D.*

University of Florida College of Medicine
Gainesville, Florida

*Oregon Health Sciences University
Portland Department of Veterans Affairs Medical Center
Portland, Oregon

INTRODUCTION

Hypothermia has been used to treat a wide variety of diseases for centuries. Lowered body temperature has been used to combat cancer, infections, trauma, central nervous system diseases and as a regional method to produce anesthesia for amputation.[1,2] Although Bigelow demonstrated in 1950 that tolerance to inflow occlusion in hypothermic animals was longer than in their normothermic counterparts, the first clinical application of hypothermia in cardiac surgery was reported by Lewis and Taufic who used surface cooling to 28°C with 5.5 minutes of inflow occlusion to facilitate successful closure of an atrial septal defect in a 5 year old child.[3,4] Despite the introduction of the pump oxygenator in clinical practice by Gibbon in 1954 it was not until 1958 that hypothermia was used in conjunction with the cardiopulmonary bypass circuit for intracardiac repairs.[5,6] The use of the pump oxygenator and hypothermia has allowed the repair of more and more complex cardiac lesions with remarkably low mortality. A better understanding of the underlying physiologic principles of hypothermia will increase its safe clinical application.

PHYSIOLOGY OF HYPOTHERMIA

Humans are homeothermic and have evolved very effective mechanisms that maintain body temperature at 37°C independent of environmental temperature. Thermoreceptors in the skin sense cold, and afferent impulses from these sensors to the hypothalamus where sympathetic nervous stimulation is initiated. Vasoconstriction occurs in skin vessels to conserve heat while there is vasodilation of the skeletal muscle vasculature to support

Cardiac Surgery: Current Issues 2, Edited by A. C. Cernaianu and A. J. DelRossi,
Plenum Press, New York, 1994

augmented muscular activity (increased tension and shivering) that produces heat. Oxygen consumption is increased and heart rate, cardiac output, and blood pressure are elevated. Because of the efficiency of thermoregulatory mechanisms in man, there is not a natural hypothermic state for study.{7}

Therefore, one must extrapolate from animal studies, biochemical reactions, accidental hypothermia survivors, and normal organ temperature gradients to understand the clinical pathophysiology of hypothermia.

Rationale for Use of Hypothermia

The major advantage to the clinical use of hypothermia is a reduction in metabolic rate and oxygen consumption. The mechanism for this reduction is quite complex and not entirely understood. At a biochemical level, hypothermia changes the reaction rate of all biochemical processes, especially enzymatic reactions. This temperature dependence of reaction rates is quantitated as the change reaction rate per 10°C temperature change (Q_{10}). For instance a process with a Q_{10} of 2 will double its reaction rate with a 10°C increase in temperature or halve it with a drop of 10°C. Most reactions, including whole body oxygen consumption, have a Q_{10} of 2 to 3.7

Some biochemical processes, especially those localized to cell membranes, show a step change in reaction rates at certain critical temperatures. This has been termed a phase transition and is thought to be a result of a change in the cell membrane from a fluid to a gel.{8} In mammalian tissues, phase transitions often occur at about 25°C to 28°C, and may cause disturbed cell homeostasis.

Biophysical processes such as osmosis and water diffusion are affected by temperature to a lesser extent. For example, a linear change of about 3 percent per 10°C is seen for diffusion. However, osmolar effects become

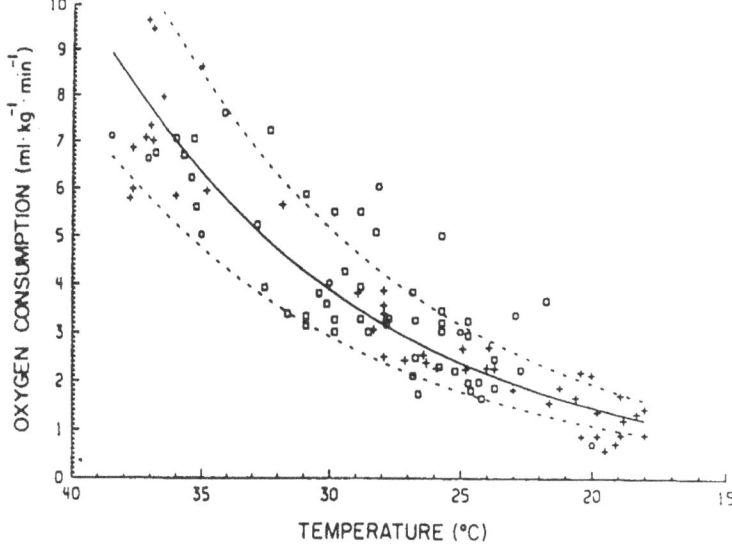

Figure 1. Whole body oxygen consumption (O_2) as a function of body temperature in dogs made hypothermic by surface cooling. (Reprinted with permission from Kirklin JW. Hypothermia, circulatory arrest, and cardiopulmonary bypass. In: Cardiac Surgery, Kirklin JW, Barratt-Boyes BG, eds. John Wiley and Sons, New York 1986:30-82.)

pronounced as the freezing point of water is approached. Ice formation in tissue concentrates solutes in the residual non-frozen cytosol, causing marked fluid shifts and membrane disruption. For this reason the freezing point of water is the physical limit to the beneficial effects of hypothermia. Mammalian tissue will not regain function upon thawing from a frozen state with the exception of some very simple systems, red blood cells for example.

In cardiac surgery, systemic hypothermia is used in conjunction with cardiopulmonary bypass to allow lower pump flows, facilitate myocardial protection, lessen blood trauma and promote organ protection.{9} Oxygen consumption predictably falls with lowered temperature, which allows lowered bypass blood flows while still providing adequate perfusion as assessed by mixed venous oxygen tension and return of organ function following bypass (Figure 1). Hickey et al. have shown in humans that a reduction in flow rate from 2.1 L/min/m^2 to 1.2 L/min/m^2 at 25°C did not alter O_2.{10} Using moderate hypothermia and hemodilution low flow, low pressure bypass does not correlate with postoperative renal or central nervous system dysfunction.{11} Because lower bypass flow will decrease return flow from bronchial, pulmonary, and non-coronary collateral vessels, flow that tends to warm the heart, hypothermia by permitting a lower flow bypass may facilitate myocardial protection. Blood trauma is decreased by the use of lower pump flows. Because most central nervous system damage on bypass is embolic in origin and because lower bypass flows may decrease the mechanical production of gaseous or particulate emboli, hypothermia may indirectly contribute to a reduction of central nervous system (CNS) damage. Finally, systemic hypothermia also provides some margin of safety for organ protection if equipment failure occurs or transient circulatory arrest must be employed.

Acid-Base Management

One of the often discussed aspects of clinical hypothermia is appropriate acid-base management. In this regard, it is helpful to consider the behavior of blood in vitro, in exercising muscle, and in poikilothermic animals.

The "normality" of a pH of 7.40 and a $PaCO_2$ of 40 mmHg exists only at 37°C in blood. Because gas solubility in liquid increases with decreased temperature, O_2 and CO_2 become more soluble at lower temperatures and both PaO_2 and $PaCO_2$ will decrease if the total content of each is constant. The $\Delta pH/°C$ change in temperature is quite constant at about –0.015.{12} The slope of this relationship is remarkable in its similarity to the slope of the neutral pH (pN) of water ($\Delta pH/°C = -0.017$) Figure 2. The buffer system primarily responsible for this constant relationship of blood pH to pN with temperature changes is the imidazole moiety of protein-bound histidine. This buffer system promotes a constant ratio of $[OH^-]/[H^+]$ in blood averaging about 16:1 over a wide range of temperatures. Thus, a constant relative alkalinity with reference to the neutrality of water is preserved and no change in acid-base equilibrium occurs with this system even though the pH and PCO_2 values change remarkably with temperature. The physiologically important parameter is a constant amount of H^+ *relative* to OH^-, rather than a constant amount of H^+.

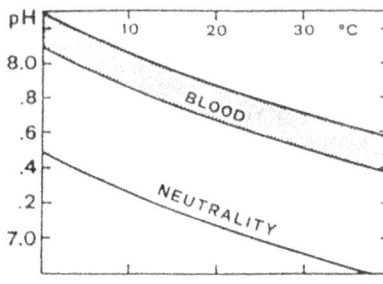

Figure 2. Blood pH and the pN_{H_2O} as a function of body temperature. (Reprinted with permission from Rahn H. Body temperature and acid-base regulation. Pneumonologie 1974;151:87–94.)

The temperature of different tissues in man can vary considerably. For example, the skin may be at about 25°C on a cold day, while exercising muscle can achieve a temperature of 40°C to 41°C. The arterial blood coming from the heart at 37°C is pumped to these tissues and behaves very much like blood in vitro as it is cooled or warmed. Total CO_2 content remains constant. Therefore, in the skin the pH is 7.60 while in the muscles it is 7.35 (Figure 3). Acid-base equilibrium and a constant $[OH^-]/[H^+]$ are maintained at widely different temperatures.

In cold-blooded vertebrates, the blood pH-temperature curve also runs parallel to the pN of water. Intracellular pH has also been measured in various animals and shows identical changes with temperature.{13} The intracellular pH parallels the slope of the pN and blood pH temperature regression and differs from the extracellular pH by a constant but species-specific factor of about –0.6 to –0.8 pH units. Thus, at 37°C intracellular pH is about 6.8 to 6.9 with a 1:1 $[OH^-]/[H^+]$ ratio.

As mentioned this constant ratio of $[OH^-]$ to $[H^+]$ is accomplished predominantly by the buffering capacity of the imidazole group of histidine. As temperature changes this imidazole protein buffer changes its pK, in parallel with the pN of water. The fraction of unprotonated histidine imidazole groups, in the alpha position, remains constant, total CO_2 remains constant, and pH changes as temperature changes. The term "alpha-stat" refers to maintenance of this constant net charge on proteins during temperature changes by keeping total CO_2 stores constant. It has come to signify a pH management technique that allows pH and $PaCO_2$ to follow their requisite course with temperature change. The alternative method of acid-base strategy is termed pH-stat. With this method, pH is maintained constant over varying temperatures. Obviously, as blood is cooled, CO_2 must be added to maintain a $PaCO_2$ of 40 mmHg and a pH of 7.40. Extracellular and intracellular $[OH^-]/[H^+]$ are altered and total CO_2 stores are elevated.

During the first two decades of hypothermic bypass, pH stat management with addition of 5 percent CO_2 to the oxygenator gas flow was predominant. Appreciation of the expected changes in pH with temperature seemed to be lacking and CO_2 was thought to be beneficial for cerebral vasodilation and maintenance of cerebral blood flow. Improved understanding of the physiology of hypothermia over the past 15 to 20 years has produced questioning of this practice. On a theoretical basis, alpha-stat management may be preferable. Maintenance of constant intracellular electrochemical neutrality appears to be essential for normal cellular function.{14} Intracellular depletion of the metabolic intermediates of high-energy phosphate production occurs

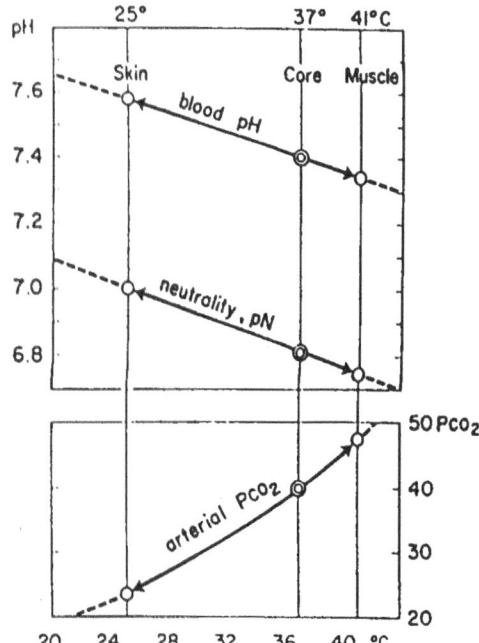

Figure 3. Changes in arterial pH and PCO_2 as 37°C blood arrives at the skin or exercising muscle at temperatures of 25°C and 41°C, respectively. Neutrality of water, pN, changes in parallel with the changes in blood pH. Thus the relative alkalinity of the blood or the ratio between [OH⁻] and [H⁺] ion remains constant. (Reprinted with permission from Rahn H. Body temperature and acid-base regulation. Pneumonologie 1974;151:87–94.)

if the intracellular pH changes and these metabolites lose their charged state making them free to diffuse across lipid membranes. Most enzyme systems are dependent on optimal pH for their function. Electrochemical neutrality is also important in maintaining the Donnan equilibrium across cellular membranes, allowing normal intracellular anion concentrations and water content.{15}

Poikilothermic animals, whose tissues must function optimally despite wide variations in temperature, follow the alpha-stat acid-base scheme. But, hibernating mammals tend to maintain a pH-stat strategy with hypoventilation, increased CO_2 stores, and development of intracellular acidosis in most tissues.{14} This acidotic state causes a further depression of metabolism that, teleologically, may be useful in tissues requiring less energy during hibernation, such as skeletal muscle, gastrointestinal tract, and higher brain centers. Importantly, however, active tissues such as heart and liver actively extruding H⁺ across their cell membranes to maintain intracellular pH at or near alpha-stat values. Thus hibernating mammals are able to vary their intracellular-extracellular pH gradient in different tissues, thereby allowing a tissue specific type of acid-base regulation. At the onset of arousal from hibernation, the first noticeable change is hyperventilation. This depletes CO_2 stores, raises intracellular pH, and increases the overall metabolic rate. Thus, hibernating mammals change to alpha-stat pH control during awakening to allow tissues to regain optimal function.The practical clinical question of how acid-base status should be regulated during hypothermic CPB in man remains. Animal studies suggest that alpha-stat acid-base management is beneficial in terms of myocardial protection. McConnell demonstrated significant elevations in coronary blood flow, left ventricular oxygen consumption, lactate utilization, and peak developed pressure that occurred with maintenance of pH 7.7 at 28°C (alpha-stat) compared to a pH of 7.4 (pH-stat).{16} Poole-Wilson has shown greater contractility in hypothermic perfused papillary muscle when the pH of the perfusate is more alkaline than 7.4.{17} They have also demonstrated a rapid fall in myocardial tension development as well as changes in Ca^{2+} flux by increasing the CO_2 content of the perfusate.{18} One the other hand, Sinet found no effect of pH on isolated rat heart performance.{19} Alkalinization of the blood before ischemia has been shown to decrease the development of acidosis in coronary sinus blood and improve contractility on reperfusion.{20} The pH of the blood during reperfusion may be critical to recovery of ventricular performance. Becker demonstrated improved myocardial performance after one hour of circulatory arrest and cardioplegia with moderate further alkalinization compared to alpha-stat.{21} The electrical stability of the heart is improved (less spontaneous ventricular fibrillation) using alpha-stat pH regulation compared to pH-stat.{22} Kroncke found a 40 percent incidence of ventricular fibrillation in patients cooled to 24°C using pH-stat management compared to a 20 percent incidence in those following alpha-stat.{23}

Cerebral blood flow and cerebral metabolic rate decrease significantly with hypothermia, but the response of the cerebral circulation to changes in $PaCO_2$ is preserved.{24} Alpha-stat management therefore, results in lower cerebral blood flows than does pH-stat strategy at temperatures from 21°C to 29°C.{25} Murkin showed that coupling of cerebral blood flow and metabolism was maintained independent of cerebral perfusion pressure over the range of 20 to 100 mm Hg when alpha-stat management was employed.{26} In contrast, pressure-flow autoregulation was abolished and the coupling of flow to metabolic rate was lost when pH-stat strategy was used Figure 4.

During anoxic perfusion there is a decrease in the extent and magnitude of brain lesions when the perfusate has a higher pH, while an acidic perfusate enhanced the extent of the lesions.{27} The cerebral blood flow during pH-stat hypothermia actually is in excess of metabolic need and unnecessarily high blood flows may put the brain at risk for damage due to microemboli, or high intracranial pressure, and may actually predispose to an adverse redistribution of blood flow ("steal") away from marginally perfused areas in patients with cerebrovascular disease.

A recent clinical study examined the influence of pH management on outcome in 86 patients undergoing mild hypothermic bypass and found no differences in cardiac or neuropsychologic outcome regardless of acid-base management.{28} However, the degree of hypothermia was not very profound (30.1°C), so the difference in $PaCO_2$ between groups was not great (40.2 vs 47.3, uncorrected values). Also, the analysis examined differences in mean group performances rather than and change of individual patient performance, a methodology that may have decreased the sensitivity of the study to detect any existing difference. Although this study provides a welcome clinical addition to this controversial area, further work must be done, particularly during deeper hypothermia, to determine the influence, if any, of pH management on clinical outcome after CPB.

Alterations in Organ Function

Hypothermia generally results in a decrease in blood flow to all organs of the body by virtue of a decrease in metabolic rate. Skeletal muscle and the extremities have the greatest reduction in flow, followed by the kidneys,

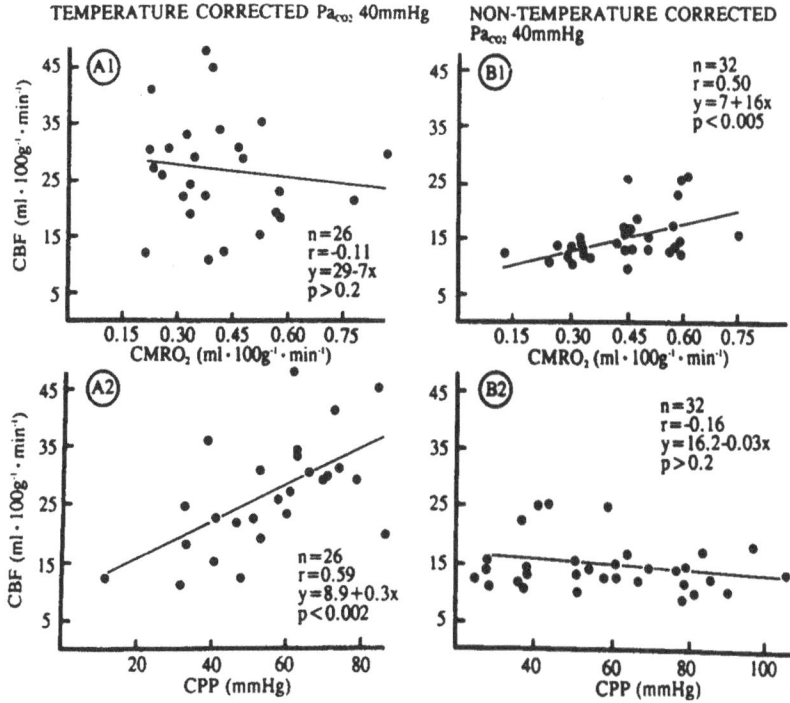

Figure 4. Simple linear regression of cerebral blood flow (CBF) versus cerebral perfusion pressure (CPP) or cerebral oxygen consumption (CMRO$_2$) for temperature-corrected and non-temperature corrected groups. Upper panel: There is no significant correlation between CBF and CMRO$_2$ in the temperature-corrected group (A1), whereas CBF significantly correlates with CMRO$_2$ in the non-temperature corrected group (B1). Lower panel: CBF is significantly correlated with CPP in the temperature corrected group (A2), whereas CBF is independent of CPP in the non-temperature corrected group (B2). (Reprinted with permission from Murkin JM, Farrar JK, Tweed WA, McKenzie FN, Guiraudon G. Cerebral autoregulation and flow/metabolism coupling during cardiopulmonary bypass: the influence of PaCO$_2$. Anes Analg 1987;66:825–32.)

splanchnic bed, heart and brain. Despite these decreases in flow, arteriovenous oxygen content differences either decrease or are not changed, implying that oxygen supply is adequate to meet the regional metabolic requirements.

With cooling, heart rate decreases, contractility remains stable, and arrhythmias become more frequent, the latter including nodal rhythm, premature ventricular beats, AV block, atrial and ventricular fibrillation, and asystole progressively as temperature decreases. The mechanism of this arrhythmogenic effect is unknown but may involve disruption of normal coordination of depolarization and repolarization, uneven cooling, and autonomic nervous system imbalance. Since coronary blood flow is well preserved during hypothermia it is unlikely that myocardial hypoxia plays a role in the genesis of these arrhythmias.

The pulmonary system is characterized by a progressive decrease in ventilation as the temperature is lowered. Physiologic and anatomic dead space increase, but overall the gas exchange (ventilation/perfusion balance) is largely unaffected.

Hypothermia increases renal vascular resistance, with decreased outer and inner cortex blood flow and oxygen delivery. Tubular transport of electrolytes and water are decreased leading to decreased concentrating ability; urine flow may be increased with hypothermia, but this effect may be masked by the stress induced release of arginine vasopression, antidiuretic hormone. The ability of the hypothermic kidney to handle glucose is impaired and glucose often appears in the urine.

In general, significant hepatic injury with hypothermic CPB cardiopulmonary bypass is rare. Hepatic arterial blood flow is reduced in proportion to the fall in cardiac output. The most significant effect of hypothermia is the decrease in metabolic and excretory function of the liver. Obviously, drug actions and requirements will be modified by this change in liver function. With rewarming, hepatic efficiency reverts to normal.

Hypothermia causes marked changes in the peripheral circulation. Systemic and pulmonary vascular resistance typically rise with cooling below 26°C.{29} This increase in vascular resistance relates to increases in blood viscosity and catecholamines, hemoconcentration, and other factors. In addition, arteriovenous shunts appear at low temperatures,{30} and may cause a diminution in tissue oxygen delivery. These circulatory changes can be somewhat ameliorated by adequate (stress response obtunding) anesthesia, hemodilution, heparinization and the use of vasodilators.

The hormonal response to hypothermia is somewhat dependent on the level of anesthesia. Non-anesthetized subjects demonstrate a marked sympathetic stimulation in response to cold. This response can be almost ablated if deep anesthesia is used. After deep hypothermia and total circulatory arrest, a massive release of catecholamines occurs,{31} which may contribute to the impaired cerebral perfusion found by Greely and colleagues.{32} Corticosteroid release is suppressed with long-term hypothermia below 28°C but appears to be normal with short periods of hypothermia.{33} Hypothermia, hemodilution, and heparin reduce complement activation during bypass and may protect patients from harmful sequelae. Circulating bradykinin increases during hypothermia and cardiopulmonary bypass and may contribute to altered vascular permeability and circulatory instability.{34}

CLINICAL USE OF HYPOTHERMIA

Currently, hypothermia is used most commonly in cardiac surgery, although its use has also been described for major vascular procedures, intracranial surgery, and for removal of hepatic and renal tumors. For most cardiac procedures, mild to moderate systemic hypothermia (above 25°C) is used for its protective effects previously described. More profound selective myocardial hypothermia is also often used during aortic cross-clamping to aid in preservation of ischemic myocardium.

The most dramatic application demonstrating the protective effects of hypothermia is in deep hypothermia and circulatory arrest. Systemic temperatures of 20°C to 22°C or less are used to allow circulatory arrest for periods up to 40 to 60 minutes, often without detectable organ injury,[7] in a variety of situations. For example, in pediatric cardiac surgical patients (particularly those less than 8 kg to 10 kg) repair of complex congenital cardiac lesions is often facilitated by the asanguinous surgical field provided with circulatory arrest. Also, surgical procedures requiring occlusion of multiple cerebral vessels, particularly aortic arch aneurysms often necessitate circulatory arrest.

The brain is the organ at most risk for injury and limits the duration of "safe" arrest time. Cerebral metabolic activity is decreased with temperature but never ceases altogether, even at temperatures approaching 0°C. The protective effect of hypothermia may involve more than just a reduction in cerebral metabolic rate. A Q_{10} of 2.7 would predict a "safe" arrest time of only about 15 minutes at 20°C. Clinical and experimental evidence indicate that 30 to 45 minutes is well tolerated while other factors such as extracellular pH may play a role, cerebral oxygen consumption decreases in non-linear fashion with profound hypothermia. Michenfelder and Milde showed a change in Q_{10} from 2.23 between 37°C and 27°C to 4.53 between 27°C and 14°C.[35] They postulated that this marked drop in oxygen consumption at lower temperatures could be explained by a primary effect of hypothermia on integrated neuronal function (as shown by suppression of the EEG).

The rate of cooling also appears to be important in the production of brain injury. Wide gradients between body and perfusate temperature in dogs correlated with brain cell necrosis and death.[36] The optimal site for temperature monitoring is controversial, but it must be remembered that gradients exist among the different regions.[37] Monitoring multiple sites to assure uniform cooling prior to arrest is advisable. Some authors suggest using EEG monitoring to determine ideal depth of cooling for safe circulatory arrest because no peripheral body temperature consistently predicted electral silence.[38]

The question of whether hypothermic bypass with or without circulatory arrest has an effect on later intellectual development remains unanswered. There is some evidence of a decreased intelligence quotient and developmental capacity related to the duration of circulatory arrest,[39–41] but most studies have not been able to demonstrate an adverse effect on intellectual capacity and development when circulatory arrest times are less than 60 minutes at nasopharyngeal temperatures of about 20°C.[42–44] It is difficult to interpret many of these studies because of difficulty in defining an appropriate control group. Blackwood and colleagues used each child as his own control and found no difference between preoperative and postoperative scores with arrest intervals as long as 74 minutes.[45] Choreoathetosis and postoperative seizures are occasionally seen following deep hypothermia.[7] The incidence ranges from 1 to 10 percent and may relate to uneven brain cooling, uneven brain reperfusion, air or particle embolization and excessive glycolysis. Both problems are more common following circulatory arrest but can be seen with continuous hypothermic perfusion. Choreoathetosis usually lessens in severity with time but may persist. Seizures are usually transient and do not general imply permanent brain dysfunction.

Thus, the question of "safe" circulatory arrest time is complex and cannot be answered with certainty. Hypothermia can delay but not prevent the appearance of metabolic and structural changes that occur during ischemia and lead to functional neurologic impairment. Cardiac surgery has advanced remarkably over the last 30 years. Hypothermia has contributed substantially toward improving patient outcome. Current efforts must be directed toward defining methods of maximizing cerebral protection and refining critical techniques.

REFERENCES

1. Fay T: Observations on prolonged human refrigeration. NY State J Med 1940;40:1351–1354.

2. Crossman LW, Ruggiero WF, Hurley V, Allen FM: Reduced temperatures in surgery. II. Amputations for peripheral vascular disease. Arch Surg 1942;44:139–156.

3. Bigelow WG, Callaghan JC, Hopps JA: General hypothermia for experimental intracardiac surgery. Ann Surg 1950;132:531–539.

4. Lewis FJ, Taufic M: Closure of atrial septal defects with the aid of hypothermia; experimental accomplishments and the report of one successful case. Surgery 1953;33:52–59.

5. Gibbon JH: Application of a mechanical heart and lung apparatus to cardiac surgery. Minn Med 1954;37:171–180.

6. Sealy WC, Brown IW Jr, Young WG Jr: A report on the use of both extracorporeal circulation and hypothermia for open heart surgery. Ann Surg 1958;147:603–613.

7. Kirklin JW: Hypothermia, circulatory arrest, and cardiopulmonary bypass. In: Cardiac Surgery, Kirklin JW, Barratt-Boyes BG, eds. John Wiley & Sons, New York 1986:30-82.

8. Hearse DJ, Braimbridge MV, Jynge P: Protection of the ischemic myocardium: cardioplegia. Raven Press, New York 1981.

9. Cameron DE, Gardner TJ: Principles of clinical hypothermia. Cardiac Surgery: State of the Art Reviews 1988;2:13–25.

10. Hickey RF, Hoar PF: Whole body oxygen consumption during low-flow hypothermic cardiopulmonary bypass. J Thorac Cardiovasc Surg 1983;86:903–906.

11. Slogoff S, Reul GJ, Keats AS, et al: Role of perfusion pressure and flow in major organ dysfunction after cardiopulmonary bypass. Ann Thorac Surg 1990;50:911–918.

12. Rahn H: Body temperature and acid-base regulation. Pneumonologie 1974;151:87–94.

13. Malan A, Wilson TL, Reeves RB: Intracellular pH in cold-blooded vertebrates as a function of body temperature. Respir Physiol 1976;28:29–47.

14. Hickey PR, Hansen DD: Temperature and blood gases: the clinical dilemma of acid-base management for hypothermic cardiopulmonary bypass. In: Cardiopulmonary Bypass: Current Concepts and Controversies, Tinker JH, ed. WB Saunders, Philadelphia 1989:1–20.

15. Reeves RB: Temperature-induced changes in blood acid-base status: Donnan r_{cl} and red cell volume. J Appl Physiol 1976;40:762–767.

16. McConnell DH, White F, Nelson RL, et al: Importance of alkalosis in maintenance of "ideal" blood pH during hypothermia. Surg Forum 1975;26:263-265.

17. Poole-Wilson PA, Langer GA: Effect of pH on ionic exchange and function in rat and rabbit myocardium. Am J Physiol 1975;229:570-581.

18. Poole-Wilson PA, Langer GA: Effects of acidosis on mechanical function and Ca^{2+} exchange in rabbit myocardium. Am J Physiol 1979;236:H525-H533.

19. Sinet M, Muffat-Joly M, Bendaace T, Pocidalo JJ: Maintaining blood pH at 7.4 during hypothermia has no significant effect on work of the isolated rate heart. Anesthesiology 1985;62:582–587.

20. Austen WG: Experimental studies on the effects of acidosis and alkalosis on myocardial function after aortic occlusion. J Surg Res 1965;5:191–194.

21. Becker H, Vinten-Johansen J, Buckberg G, et al: Myocardial damage caused by keeping pH 7.40 during systemic deep hypothermia. J Thorac Cardiovasc Surg 1981;82:810-820.

22. Swain JA, White FN, Peters RM: The effect of pH on the hypothermic ventricular fibrillation threshold. J Thorac Cardiovasc Surg 1984;87:445–451.

23. Kroncke GM, Nichols RD, Mendenhall JT, Myerowitz PD, Starling JR: Ectothermic philosophy of acid-base balance to prevent fibrillation during hypothermia. Arch Surg 1986;121:303–304.

24. Prough DS, Stump DA, Roy RC, et al: Response of cerebral blood flow to changes in carbon dioxide during hypothermic cardiopulmonary bypass. Anesthesiology 1986;64:576–581.

25. Govier AV, Reves JG, McKay RD, et al: Factors and their influence on regional cerebral blood flow during nonpulsatile cardiopulmonary bypass. Ann Thorac Surg 1984;38:592–600.

26. Murkin JM, Farrar JK, Tweed WA, McKenzie FN, Guiraudon G: Cerebral autoregulation and flow/metabolism coupling during cardiopulmonary bypass: the influence of $PaCO_2$. Anesth Analg 1987;66:825–832.

27. Norwood WI, Norwood CR, Castaneda AR: Cerebral anoxia: effect of deep hypothermia and pH. Surgery 1979;86:203–209.

28. Bashein G, Townes BD, Nessly ML, et al: A randomized study of carbon dioxide management during hypothermic cardiopulmonary bypass. Anesthesiology 1990;72:7-15.

29. Cooper KE: The circulation in hypothermia. Br Med Bull 1961;17:48–51.

30. Suzuki M, Penn I: A reappraisal of the microcirculation during general hypothermia. Surgery 1965;58:1049–1060.

31. Wood M, Shand DG, Wood AJJ: The sympathetic response to profound hypothermia and circulatory arrest in infants. Ann Anaesth Soc J 1980;27:125-132.

32. Greeley WJ, Ungerleider RM, Smith LR, Reves JG: The effects of deep hypothermic cardiopulmonary bypass and total circulatory arrest on cerebral blood flow in infants and children. J Thorac Cardiovasc Surg 1989;97:737–745.

33. Blair E. Clinical hypothermia. McGraw-Hill, New York 1964.

34. Pang LM, Stalcup SA, Lipset JS, Hayes CJ, Bowman OF, Mellins RB: Increased circulating bradykinin during hypothermia and cardiopulmonary bypass in children. Circulation 1979;60:1503–1507.

35. Michenfelder JD, Milde JH: The relationship among canine brain temperature, metabolism, and function during hypothermia. Anesthesiology 1991;75:130-136.

36. Almond CH, Jones JC, Snyder HM, Grant SM, Meyer BW: Cooling gradients and brain damage with deep hypothermia. J Thorac Cardiovasc Surg 1964;48:890-897.

37. Stefaniszyn HJ, Novick RJ, Keith FM, Salerno TA: Is the brain adequately cooled during deep hypothermic cardiopulmonary bypass? Curr Surg 1983;40:294–297.

38. Coselli JS, Crawford ES, Beall AC Jr, Mizrahi EM, Hess KR, Patel VM: Determination of brain temperatures for safe circulatory arrest during cardiovascular operation. Ann Thorac Surg 1988;45:638–642.

39. Wells FC, Coghill S, Caplan HL, Lincoln C: Duration of circulatory arrest does influence the psychological development of children after cardiac operation in early life. J Thorac Cardiovasc Surg 1983;86:823–831.

40. Wright JS, Hicks RG, Newman DC: Deep hypothermic arrest: observations on later development in children. J Thorac Cardiovasc Surg 1979;77:466–468.

41. Settergren G, Öhqvist G, Lundberg S, Henze A, Björk VO, Persson B: Cerebral blood flow and cerebral metabolism in children following cardiac surgery with deep hypother-

mia and circulatory arrest. Clinical course and follow-up of psychomotor development. Scand J Thorac Cardiovasc Surg 1982;16:209–215.

42. Dickinson DF, Sambrooks JE: Intellectual performance in children after circulatory arrest with profound hypothermia in infancy. Arch Dis Child 1979;54:1–6.

43. Clarkson PM, MacArthur BA, Barratt-Boyes BG, Whitlock RM, Neutze JM: Developmental progress after cardiac surgery in infancy using hypothermia and circulatory arrest. Circulation 1980;62:855–861.

44. Messmer BJ, Schallberger U, Gattiker R, Senning A: Psychomotor and intellectual development after deep hypothermia and circulatory arrest in early infancy. J Thorac Cardiovasc Surg 1976;72:495–502.

45. Blackwood MJA, Haka-Ikse K, Steward DJ: Developmental outcome in children undergoing surgery with profound hypothermia. Anesthesiology 1986;65:437–440.

ANESTHETIC EVALUATION AND MANAGEMENT IN BLOODLESS SURGERY

N. Simon Faithfull, M.D., Ph.D.

Alliance Pharmaceutical Corp.
San Diego, California

One of the more difficult problems that occur during treatment of the surgical patient concerns the assessment of blood loss and deciding when a blood transfusion is really necessary. This has become especially so recently with the heightened awareness both in the lay and medical communities of the dangers of allogenic transfusion. Problems range from minor side effects, such as fever, chills and urticaria to life threatening diseases, such as viral hepatitis and the currently universally fatal HIV infection. The latter, though only occurring in the United States following about 1 in 150,000 allogenic transfusions, is very much in the public awareness and is one factor driving the increased use of autologous blood and other "bloodless" techniques in surgery.

It was previously thought that allogenic blood transfusion was a valuable and worthwhile treatment. However, the American College of Physicians has recently published a paper entitled "Practice Strategies for Elective Red Cell Transfusions" in which a physician contemplating giving transfusions is urged to discuss risks and benefits with the patient, anticipate the need for autologous blood and "regard elective transfusion with allogenic blood as an outcome to be avoided."[1]

When considering the need for a blood transfusion a number of important physiological points should be born in mind. Firstly the relationships between arterial oxygen tension (PaO_2), saturation (SaO_2) and content (CaO_2) should be realized; then the effect of cardiac output must be factored into the clinicians assessment of the adequacy of oxygen delivery (DO_2) to the tissues.

CaO_2 depends primarily on the hemoglobin (Hb) concentration and the SaO_2. Under ambient conditions (PaO_2 of 100 mm Hg) the oxygen dissolved in plasma contributes little to overall CaO_2 due to the low solubility for oxygen (0.3 mL/100 mL). When a patient with a normal Hb concentration of 14 g/dL breaths air, plasma dissolved oxygen accounts for only about 1.6 percent of total CaO_2.

When blood passes through the tissues, oxygen is extracted and its partial pressure decreases as the capillary is transited. Different amounts of oxygen extraction occur in different tissues. Though it is impractical to monitor the partial pressure of oxygen in veins exiting from various organs the partial pressure of the mixed venous blood (PvO$_2$) as it passes through the pulmonary artery is often measured. Though it is often taken as a measurement of the level of tissue oxygenation, it should be stressed that PvO$_2$ is no more than it's name states, i.e., the mixed or mean oxygen partial pressure of all blood exiting from all tissues of the body.

An anesthetized patient will have an oxygen consumption (VO$_2$) of about 3 mL/kg/min. At a PaO$_2$ of 100 mm Hg, 22.6 percent of CaO$_2$ will be extracted as blood passes through the tissues; PvO$_2$ will be 41.4 mm Hg. Twenty-two percent of Hb bound oxygen will be extracted, whereas almost 60 percent of plasma dissolved oxygen will be utilized. This is because unlike the sigmoid relationship between SaO$_2$ and PaO$_2$, the oxygen content of plasma is directly proportional to the oxygen partial pressure (Henry's law). This concept is very important and explains the greater percentage extraction of oxygen from plasma than from Hb.

A healthy anesthetized patient breathing 100 percent oxygen the will have a PaO$_2$ of approximately 500 mm Hg. Plasma dissolved oxygen accounts for 7.4 percent of CaO$_2$ and for 32.1 percent of VO$_2$. PvO$_2$ will rise from 41.4 mm Hg to 49.5 mm Hg and "the tissues" will be at a potentially higher level of oxygenation.

During surgery, blood volume is maintained by the infusion of crystalloid or colloid solutions to replace blood loss. Hb concentration decreases and whole blood viscosity will fall. Less pressure is required to cause flow of a less viscous fluid through a tube and hence the resistance to flow is decreased. Physiologically, homeostatic mechanisms (baroreceptor reflexes) will be necessary to prevent a decrease in systemic blood pressure under these circumstances. The result of the activation of baroreceptor reflexes is therefore maintenance of blood pressure and an increase in cardiac output. Figure 1

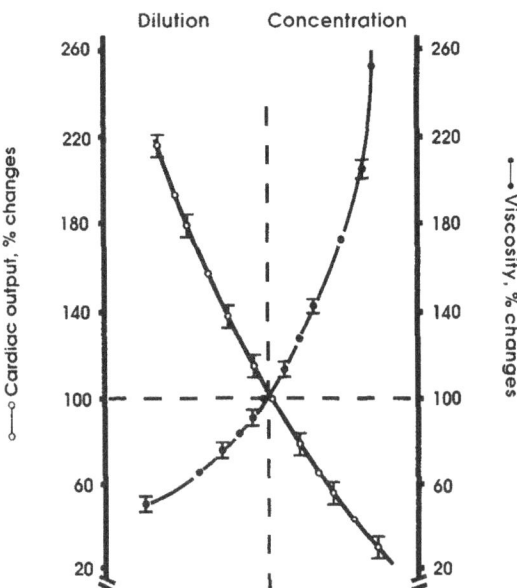

Figure 1. The relationship between cardiac output, whole blood viscosity and hematocrit during progressive hemodilution in dogs. Reproduced with permission from Messmer et al. [3]

shows the relationship between cardiac output, blood viscosity and hematocrit (Hct) during both hemodilution and hemoconcentration. A virtually straight line relationship exists between Hct and cardiac output over a wide range of Hcts.

It is important to realize that not all subjects will increase their cardiac output to the same extent for the same degree of hemodilution. Total peripheral resistance is made up of a vascular resistance component and a blood viscosity component. The relative importance of these two components will vary from patient to patient. Thus, a patient with arteriosclerotic hypertension and increased vascular resistance will not have such a dramatic response to the decrease of the blood viscosity component. Hence cardiac output will not increase as much as in a normal healthy patient. Additionally, patients with obstruction to vascular flow such as aortic stenosis or peripheral vascular disease may have reduced cardiac output response to hemodilution and less than optimal improvements in flow distal to the obstruction. The latter point is of course important when patients with coronary artery disease are hemodiluted. [2]

Let us now look at the situation of a patient who has been hemodiluted to a Hb concentration of 9 g/dL, either intentionally as part of an autologous transfusion program or following surgical bleeding. Let us assume that he is reasonably fit and can increase his cardiac output by 0.5 L/min for each 1 g/dL decrease in Hb.

While breathing air his CaO_2 will be 12.36 mL/dL, 2.2 percent of which will be contributed by plasma dissolved oxygen. Cardiac output will have increased from 5 L/min at 14 g/dL Hb to 7.5 L/min at a Hb of 9 g/dL. Total oxygen delivery (DO_2) will be 927 mL/min, which is only marginally lower than the 953 mL/min at a Hb of 14 g/dL. This, to some, surprising fact is of course due to raised cardiac output compensating for decreases in CaO_2. When this patient respires 100 percent oxygen, PvO_2 increases from 41.2 mm Hg to 53.7 mm Hg. Plasma dissolved oxygen contributes 47.9 percent of oxygen consumption (VO_2).

The relationship between Hb concentration (g/dL) and cardiac output, arterial oxygen tension (PaO_2), PvO_2 and the percentage contribution to VO_2 of oxygen carried in the plasma phase of blood (percentage VO_2 from plasma) should be discussed.

The above calculations which are presented in Table 1, demonstrate the importance of cardiac output and PaO_2 when Hb levels are decreased. Increased PaO_2 can increase "tissue" oxygenation and can very significantly increase the contribution to oxygen consumption from the plasma phase of

Table 1.

Hb (g/dL)	CaO₂ (mL/dL)	CO (L/min)	PaO₂ (mm Hg)	PvO₂ (mm Hg)	VO₂ from Plasma (%)
14	18.6	5.0	100	41.4	4.3
14	20.2	5.0	500	49.5	32.1
9	11.8	7.5	100	41.2	6.4
9	13.6	7.5	500	53.7	47.9

Hb=hemoglobin; CaO₂= arterial oxygen content; CO= cardiac output; PaO₂= arterial oxygen partial pressure; PvO₂= venous oxygen partial pressure.

the blood. Though there is little change in PvO_2 following hemodilution in this example there is experimental evidence that (Figure 2), tissue oxygen tensions may actually rise following hemodilution to levels in the range of 8–9 g/dL. [3]

There are a number of therapeutic maneuvers available to the clinician to improve oxygen supply apart from allowing the patient to breathe 100 percent oxygen. Meticulous attention to ventilatory technique will ensure that there is good distribution of gases in the alveoli and that alveolar-arterial oxygen tension differences are minimized. PaO_2 can sometimes be increased by hyperventilation and thus raising alveolar tensions of oxygen, though this technique may be undesirable as it lowers arterial partial pressure of carbon dioxide and causes vasoconstriction of the cerebral circulation. This will increase cerebral vascular resistance and lead to decrease in blood flow. Additionally hyperventilation shifts the oxyhemoglobin dissociation curve to the left and may impair oxygen offloading in the tissues.

Optimal cardiac output is determined by the Starling curve and it is important to realize that the relationship between cardiac output and pulmonary artery occlusive pressure may vary from patient to patient. A process of titration may be necessary to maximize cardiac output. The choice of anesthetic agents may also be of importance in determining optimal cardiac output responses to hemodilution as myocardial depression may deleteriously affect the response. Vasodilation with attention to normovolemia may increase cardiac output; spinal or epidural anesthesia may be helpful in this respect.

Oxygen extraction from the blood depends on the relationship between oxygen delivery and oxygen consumption. The higher the consumption, the higher will be the extraction for a given level of oxygen delivery. As extraction from Hb increases, PvO_2 will fall and hence tissue oxygen tensions will decrease. Certain tissues, notably the myocardium, extract a higher proportion of CaO_2 than other less oxygen demanding organs such as the skin and kidneys. As a result, mean oxygen tensions will be lower in the myocardium than in the other two organs. For every organ there is probably a critical PvO_2 below which metabolism begins to switch from aerobic oxidative phosphory-

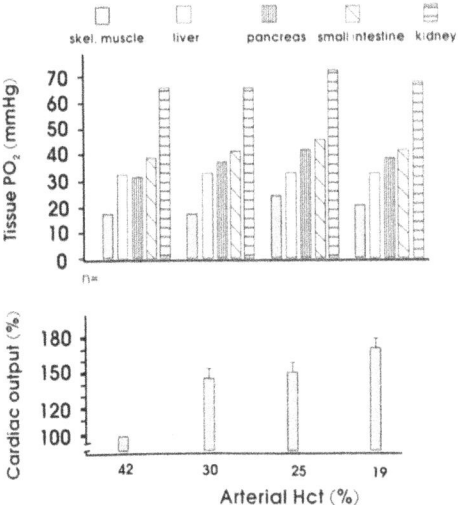

Figure 2. Surface tissue oxygen tensions in various organs during progressive hemodilution in dogs. Reproduced with permission from Messmer et al. [3].

lation to anaerobic glycolysis. The myocardium, due to it's high oxygen utilization is probably the first organ to fail during progressive hemodilution. The onset of anaerobic glycolysis can be experimentally detected by monitoring lactate efflux from the coronary sinus. The onset of disordered ventricular wall motion can be detected clinically be the use of transesophageal echocardiography (TEE).

As the limits of Hb oxygen extraction are reached and oxidative metabolism begins to fail, VO_2 will start to decrease. At this critical level of oxygen delivery, PvO_2 is about 32 mm Hg in hemodiluted dogs. [4] In patients prior to cardiopulmonary bypass, it is in the region of 37 mm Hg. [5] It is important to prevent increases in VO_2 as critical delivery levels are approached. Oxygen consumption can be reduced by general anesthesia and muscular paralysis. Mechanical ventilation will reduce the oxygen demands of the muscles of respiration. In the case of patients refusing blood transfusions on religious grounds it may be justified to induce mild hypothermia which will lower metabolism and oxygen demand. It should not however be forgotten that VO_2 will increase in the postoperative patient and this may then lead to supply/demand imbalance in the myocardium. [6]

Having seen from the above examples the benefit of hemodilution and oxygen breathing on the extraction of oxygen from Hb, it is logical to ask if it is possible to further increase oxygen content in the plasma phase of blood to further increase this "sparing" effect on Hb. Perfluorochemicals (PFCs) are metabolically inert chemicals that have a very high solubility for respiratory gases. Though they are virtually insoluble in water they can be made into stable oil in water emulsions for intravenous administration. As with plasma, there is a straight line relationship between oxygen content and the oxygen partial. Thus, when PFC emulsions are introduced into the circulation they effectively increase the plasma solubility for oxygen.

A highly concentrated emulsion of perflubron (perfluorooctyl bromide [PFOB]) is currently being tested. A 90 percent (w/v) emulsion, known as under the trade name of *Oxygent*™ *HT* (Alliance Pharmaceutical Corp., San Diego, CA) and can carry 25 mL of oxygen/dL when equilibrated at 760 mm Hg. Early clinical trials are taking place using this product which is destined for use in autologous blood transfusion techniques.

It is anticipated that *Oxygent*™ *HT* will be given at the point at which blood transfusion would normally be given. This would cause a rise in PvO_2 and allow further blood loss to occur before autologous blood is given. In this way the need for allogenic blood may be reduced or eliminated.

REFERENCES

1. American College of Physicians, Practice strategies for elective red blood cell transfusion. Ann Intern Med 1992; 116(5):403–406.

2. Christopherson R, Frank S, Norris E, Rock P, Gottlieb S, Beattie C: Low postoperative hematocrit is associated with cardiac ischemia in high-risk patients. Anesthesiology 1991; 75(3A):A99.

3. Messmer K, Sunder-Plassman L, Jesch F, Fornandt L, Sinagowitz E, Kessler M, Pfeiffer R, Horn E, Hoper J, Joachimsmeier K: Oxygen supply to the tissues during limited normovolemic hemodilution. Res Exp Med 1973; 159:152–166.

4. Faithfull NS, Cain SM: Critical levels of oxygen extraction following hemodilution with dextran or Fluosol-DA. J Crit Care 1988; 3:14–18.

5. Shibutani K, Komatsu TJ, Kubal K, Sanchala V, Kumar V, Bizzarri DV: Critical level of oxygen delivery in anesthetized man. Crit Care Med 1983; 11(8):640–643.

6. Nelson AH, Fleisher LA, Rosenbaum SH: The relationship between postoperative anemia and cardiac morbidity in high risk vascular patients in the ICU. 1991; 20(4):S71.

NORMOTHERMIC MYOCARDIAL PRESERVATION

An Optimal Approach for Myocardial Protection during All Forms of Open-Heart Surgery

Richard M. Engelman, M.D., John A. Rousou, M.D.,
Joseph E. Flack III, M.D., David W. Deaton, M.D.,
A. Bernard Pleet, M.D., and Dipak K. Das, Ph.D. *

Baystate Medical Center
Springfield, Massachusetts

*The University of Connecticut School of Medicine
Farmington, Connecticut

INTRODUCTION

Dennis Melrose and his colleagues[1] in 1955 published the initial work in *Lancet* on "elective cardiac arrest" using potassium ion in the form of potassium citrate administered through the coronary arteries to effect "cardioplegic arrest." The authors, far in advance of their time, postulated that this approach could be used to permit cardiac procedures to be carried out in the arrested, quiescent heart, permitting reestablishment of normal cardiac function after correction of the intracardiac defect. This report was initially accepted and used in the clinical setting, albeit in a limited fashion since "open-heart surgery" was not widely utilized in the 1950's. It rapidly became apparent that significant myocardial necrosis was associated with this technique and the approach was abandoned. [2] In fact, it was not until a number of years later that the deficiencies of the Melrose approach were found to be the relatively high concentration of citrate which was toxic and not the technique of potassium cardioplegia itself. [3]

In the 1960's, the concept of myocardial preservation, predominantly for valve replacement, was that of continuous coronary perfusion, often with the fibrillating heart. [4,5] Studies[4,5] were written supporting this approach with relatively low mortality and with most surgeons accepting the method as that of "optimal preservation." In fact, numerous cannulae were developed[5,6] to provide a means of safe cannulation of the coronary ostia. Despite this, intimal hyperplasia and coronary stenoses remains a complication of direct coronary cannulation, [7] and continuous ventricular fibrillation has been shown to lead to subendocardial ischemia, particularly in association with left ventricular hypertrophy. [8]

Cardiac Surgery: Current Issues 2. Edited by A. C. Cernaianu and A. J. DelRossi,
Plenum Press, New York, 1994

To obviate problems noted in the fibrillating heart, induced myocardial ischemia was proposed as a method permitting operative procedures in a quiescent heart. {9} During induced myocardial ischemia, often at or near normothermia, a condition termed "stone heart" was noted which was associated with very severe hemorrhagic necrosis. {10} This generally fatal outcome was manifested by a firm, contracted heart unable to beat effectively during reperfusion. The pathophysiology of this injury was clearly shown to be a consequence of massive calcium influx into the cell during reperfusion. {10}

With the development and acceptance of ischemic arrest as a method for accomplishing a quiet, bloodless operative field, Shumway and associates{11} explored the use of deep cardiac hypothermia. This work derived from successful studies utilizing deep hypothermia for organ preservation, particularly kidneys, and the initials results at Stanford were outstanding. The rationale for cardiac hypothermia is based upon the marked decrease in myocardial oxygen demand with a decrease in myocardial temperature down to the range of 5–10°C. This is illustrated in Figure 1.

With the general acceptance of myocardial hypothermia in the late 1960's, the stage was set for a significant improvement in myocardial preservation in the 1970's. The rejuvenation of chemical cardioplegia occurred initially in Germany in 1970 with the development of a solution based on an intracellular milieu, abolishing a transcellular sodium gradient and interrupting sarcolemmal function. {12} Because of significant inconvenience attendant in the use of an intracellular infusate, and the variability of solution content and volumes required, this approach has never assumed general acceptance in the United States. {12}

At about the same time that Kalmar{13} and Bretschneider{14} were working on one approach to clinical cardioplegia, Gay and Ebert{15} in New York City were exploring the use of hyperkalemic, hypothermic crystalloid cardioplegia to accomplish both cardiac hypothermia and rapid cardioplegic arrest. Their goal was to use cardioplegia for inducing hypothermia and immediate arrest, not to provide nutrients to the myocardium. {15} The demands of this approach involved the use of potassium to produce asystole by diastolic arrest without necessitating systemic potassium overload. The most effective concentration of potassium was found to be from 20–35 mEq/L of potassium chloride. The crystalloid cardioplegic solution was routinely cooled to 4°C resulting in myocardial temperatures of 10–20°C from intermittent cardioplegic administration in an antegrade fashion. By manipulating potassium concentration in the extracellular fluid, the fast phase of membrane depolarization is interrupted and cardiac arrest ensues. Utilizing the approach proposed by Gay and Ebert and further perfected by St. Thomas' Hospital in London, {16} this cardioplegic formulation is extracellular-based containing a high sodium and high potassium concentration, leading to diastolic depolarization. The antegrade crystalloid cardioplegic administration of a cold solution with systemic hypothermia became generally accepted in the latter half of the 1970's as the best method of optimal preservation. It was immediately associated with extremely gratifying results, and became the standard for all aspects of cardiac surgery. Only hemodilution and disposable oxygenators have had such a positive effect on cardiac surgery in reducing morbidity and mortality.

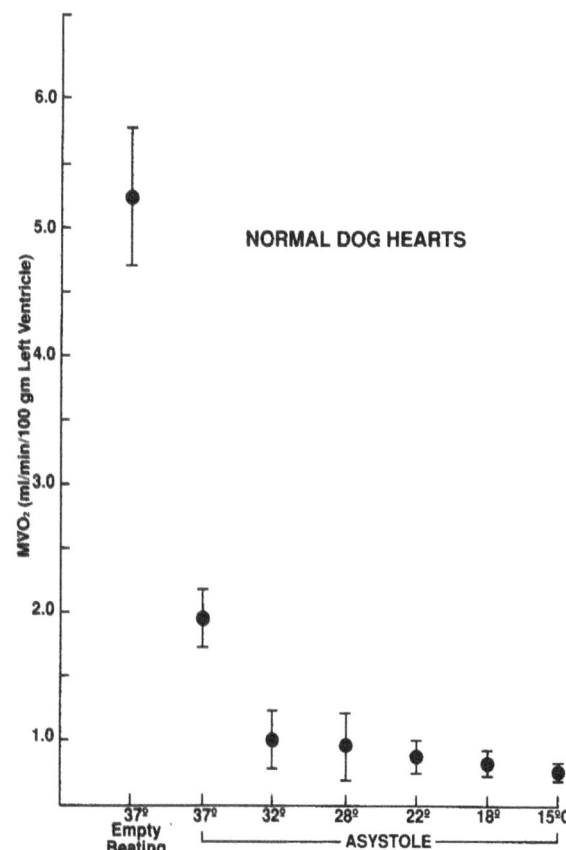

Figure 1. The decrease in myocardial oxygen consumption with induced cardioplegic arrest is dramatic and significant at normothermia. There is an additional decrease in MVO_2 with decreasing myocardial temperature as is evident on the above graph.

Further improvements in myocardial preservation were generated by Gerald Buckberg[17] who developed and perfected the concept of hypothermic blood cardioplegia making the administration of blood cardioplegia relatively easy to perform. This approach was designed to optimize oxygen, substrate and buffer administration, none of which is readily available with crystalloid cardioplegia. The 1980's have seen a further maturing of myocardial preservation with the development and sophistication of retrograde cardioplegia using any of numerous catheters permitting placement through an intact atrial wall. Additionally, the concept of normothermic preservation of the arrested heart was developed and popularized at the University of Toronto and since then has become a standard of practice in 10 to 20 percent of cardiac centers worldwide. [18] The following will discuss the rationale and our "optimal" approach to normothermic myocardial preservation.

METHODS AND RATIONALE

Warm heart surgery is the concept of cardioplegic arrest in the normothermic heart. To facilitate this process, we use normothermic perfusion and normothermic blood cardioplegia with continuous or near continuous cardioplegic administration initially via the antegrade route followed by retrograde cardioplegic administration. Systemic hypothermia is avoided because: a) rewarming the patient post-pump is associated with shivering and peripheral vasoconstriction; b) operations may be more expeditiously performed because rewarming is no longer necessary; c) hypothermia induces platelet dysfunction contributing to bleeding; [19] and d) hypothermia may be associated with increased neurologic dysfunction, a feature of so-called rewarming injury. [20] Studies we have previously reported have shown how myocardial preservation is improved in the normothermic heart. Specifically, we have documented reduced creatine kinase (CK) production in normothermic versus hypothermic patients; [21,22] reduced postoperative aortic balloon pump use (8.5 percent in 1989 to 6.3 percent in 1991); reduced intraventricular conduction disturbance as a consequence of coronary revascularization; [22] and reduced inotrope use. [23]

We believe that warm blood cardioplegia supports aerobic metabolism in the arrested heart. Basically, by utilizing retrograde cardioplegia, we are able to maintain arrest while reducing myocardial oxygen demand and supporting adequate distribution of retrograde perfusion to maintain oxygen need. It is well known that oxygen delivery is adversely affected by hypothermia with a shift of the oxyhemoglobin dissociation curve to the left as illustrated in Figure 2. Myocardial oxygen demand is markedly reduced in the arrested heart from a level of more than 8 mL O_2/min/100 g left ventricle in the working heart, to 5.6 mL in the beating non-working heart on bypass and to 1.1 mL in the arrested normothermic heart. While the subsequent reduction in oxygen demand with hypothermia is proportional to the decrease in the temperature, the oxygen demand simply cannot decrease to zero. Furthermore, myocardial temperatures can rarely be reduced below 10°C except in the presence of topical slush, which is really contraindicated as an approach for myocardial

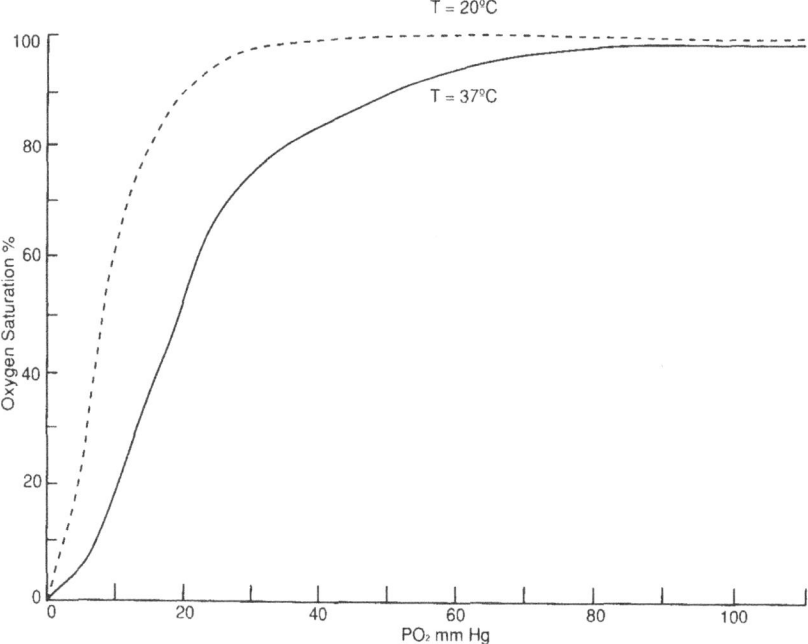

Figure 2. The leftward shift of the oxyhemoglobin dissociation curve is illustrated above with the decrease in temperature to 20°C. The further leftward shift with decreasing temperature prevents the dissociation of oxygen from arterial blood at hypothermic temperatures.

hypothermia because of the high incidence of phrenic paresis associated with this approach. {24}

The number and extent of coronary collaterals between venous and arterial conduits in the coronary drainage system in the heart is illustrated in Figure 3. Generally, approximately one-quarter of the coronary arterial perfusate drains directly into the ventricular chambers via arterio-sinusoidal and Thebesian channels, the former draining into the left ventricle and the latter into the right ventricle. The major circulation of the heart exists from the coronary arteries through arterioles into capillaries and subsequently into epicardial veins and finally, into the coronary sinus.

Coronary sinus retroperfusion is, in fact, not a new procedure. Pratt{25} in 1898 used coronary sinus retroperfusion in the isolated cat heart for maintaining contractility for several minutes and Blanco and associates{26} in 1956 used retrograde perfusion of the canine heart for more than seven minutes supporting continued contractility. The clinical use of retrograde perfusion for valvular surgery was first employed by Dr. Lillihei and his associates{27} who successfully used retrograde perfusion of warm oxygenated blood for direct vision aortic valve surgery in January, 1956. This case was reported in *Surgery, Gynecology and Obstetrics* in 1957. {27}

The coronary microcirculation, while providing a plethora of collaterals between venous and arterial channels, must clearly represent a wide spec-

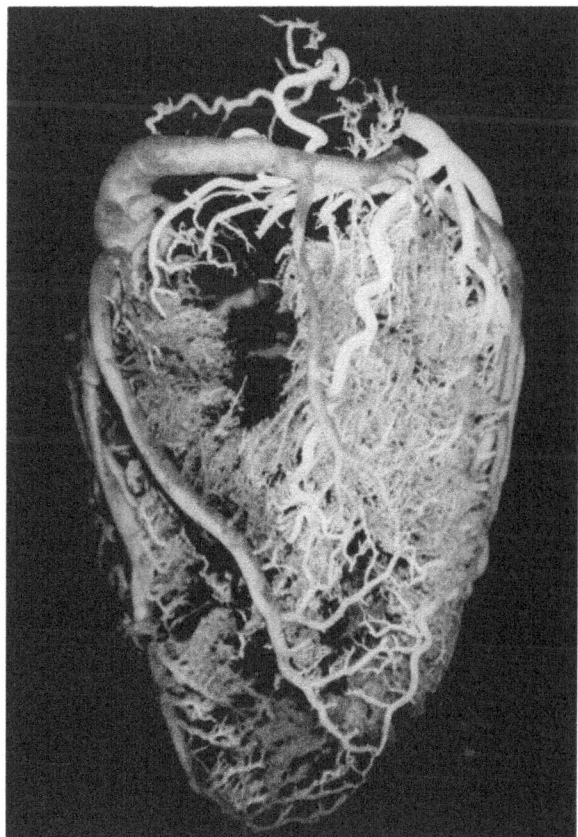

Figure 3. A photograph of the coronary arterial and venous circulation in a plastic mold is illustrated above. The large extent of coronary collaterals between venous and arterial conduits is evident.

trum of variability. The critical issue which is constantly being discussed relates to the adequacy of right ventricular perfusion using only retrograde coronary sinus perfusion. As can be seen in a picture of an adult opened coronary sinus (Figure 4), with a balloon-tipped retroperfusion catheter lying in the sinus, there are clearly numerous right ventricular coronary venous conduits (note probe in Figure 4) entering the coronary sinus beyond or distal to the inflated balloon. These veins would therefore not receive any retrograde perfusion with the catheter in its normal location, within the body of the coronary sinus. In fact, the venous drainage channels are so close to the ostium of the coronary sinus that it would not be possible to have a catheter to support all of these coronary veins with retrograde perfusion. In fact, it is our empiric observation that right ventricular preservation is adequate with retroperfusion using a coronary sinus indwelling balloon catheter placed well into the coronary sinus. The companies manufacturing coronary sinus catheters which we use are DLP (#94115, Grand Rapids, MI 49501) and Research Medical (#RC014, Salt Lake City, UT 84047). A recent report describes the amount of nutrient flow to the human right ventricle using coronary sinus retroperfusion to be between 5 to 10 percent of the flow to the left ventricle. [28] In the presence of induced cardioplegic arrest with optimal oxygen transport at normothermia, it is our opinion that this amount of blood flow is sufficient to support right ventricular oxygen demand. Clearly the right ventricle is a lower-pressured ventricle not requiring the same degree of muscular tone or contractility that is necessary for left ventricular function.

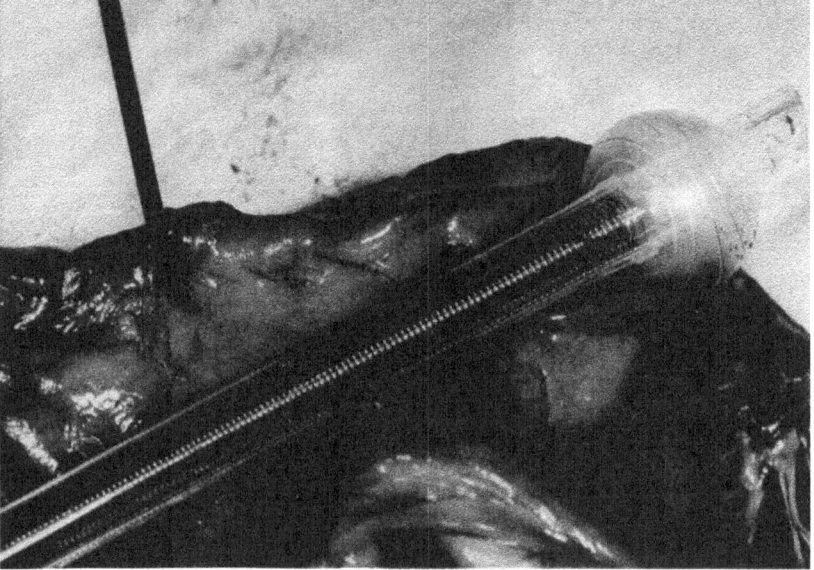

Figure 4. A photograph of a coronary sinus with an indwelling, inflated balloon-tipped retroperfusion catheter is illustrated above. A probe is placed in a coronary vein, which opens into the coronary sinus near its ostium at the right atrium, clearly excluded from any retrograde circulation through the coronary sinus retroperfusion catheter. This illustration documents how the venous channels of the right ventricle are not all available for retroperfusion utilizing an indwelling coronary sinus catheter.

The oxygen demand to the right ventricle is certainly decreased from that of the left.

The approach used in our group is to provide maximal oxygenated blood delivery to the myocardium during cardioplegic arrest. The blood cardioplegia contains our crystalloid cardioplegic composition (Table 1) which is mixed with blood from the oxygenator in a ratio of 4:1. This cardioplegic composition has maintained the arrest of the myocardium in a manner which is consistent with performing the operation without leading to significant hyperkalemia in the vast majority of operations lasting between 60 and 120 minutes of total cardioplegic arrest. When cardioplegic arrest exceeds 120 minutes, hyperkalemia is easily controlled with glucose and insulin administration. It has never presented a serious problem in potassium management.

In addition, it is our opinion that maximal oxygen delivery to the ischemic myocardium is advantageous. Accordingly our approach involves the use of the octopus infusion catheter which permits simultaneous infusion into completed saphenous vein grafts and the coronary sinus (Figure 5). Each vein graft is opened to the infusion of antegrade blood cardioplegia at the same time that the octopus is attached to the coronary sinus catheter providing for retrograde cardioplegic infusion. The octopus adaptor is marketed by DLP (#14007, Grand Rapids, MI 49501) and Research Medical (#CDS004, Salt Lake City, UT 84047).

Pressure monitoring in the coronary sinus is considered essential. We have found that the pressure measurement is best used to be certain that the coronary sinus catheter is functioning normally. Indeed, the upper limit of pressure measured in the coronary sinus during infusion is variable

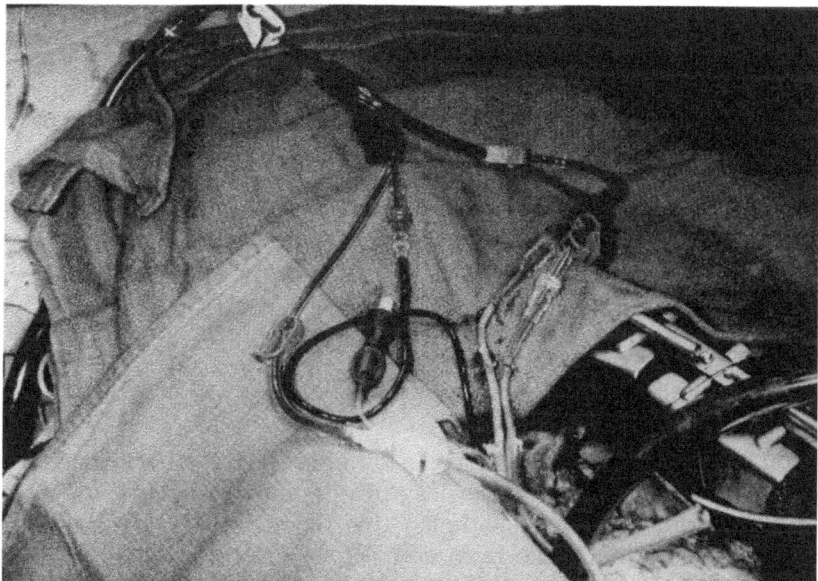

Figure 5. The approach used in our institution is to achieve maximal delivery of normothermic oxygenated blood cardioplegia to the distal coronary circulation. This is accomplished by simultaneous infusion utilizing the octopus adapter as illustrated above, permitting simultaneous infusion into the coronary sinus and into each completed vein graft in turn.

Table 1. Baystate Blood Cardioplegia Solution

CPD	50 mL/L
Tham	100 mL/L
High K (Induction)	40 mL/L (80 mEq)
Low K (Maintenance)	20 mL/L (40 mEq)
Glucose (50 percent)	10 mL/L (5 g)
Normal Saline	820 mL/L
Total Volume	1020 mL/L (High K)
	1000 mL/L (Low K)
High K	19 mEq/L
Low K	10–12 mEq/L

Blood:Crystalloid = 4:1.

depending upon the position of the myocardium vis-a-vis retraction for grafts. Indeed, with retraction for grafts, we have allowed coronary sinus perfusion pressures to reach 60–80 mm Hg without concern. Normally, however, coronary sinus perfusion pressure is in the range of 20–40 mm Hg and is not allowed to proceed any higher. We primarily utilize coronary sinus blood flow as a guide to adequacy of perfusion, and employ a minimum of 150 cc/min, and a maximum of 300 cc/min, depending upon the bulk of the left ventricular myocardium and the circumstances of the operation. In instances in which the operation is an aortic valve replacement with significant left ventricular hypertrophy, 300 cc/min is a commonly utilized blood flow. In the setting of coronary revascularization, 150 cc/min is our most frequently used retroperfusion blood flow.

One of the principles of blood cardioplegia as addressed by Dr. Buckberg deals with the importance of hyperglycemia. {29} Unfortunately, when using constant or near constant coronary sinus perfusion, and using a Buckberg-type cardioplegic formulation, serum glucose levels have reached more than 1,000 mg/dL in the diabetic patient. Because this prohibitive level of hyperglycemia is not acceptable, we have modified our cardioplegic infusion as described in Table 1. We now use only 5 g of dextrose per liter of infusate in the crystalloid portion of the cardioplegia, thereby administering only one-fifth of that amount of glucose per liter when the cardioplegia is mixed 4:1::blood:crystalloid. This has avoided the adverse influence of severe hyperglycemia when using either the Buckberg or Fremes solutions.

RESULTS OF CARDIOPLEGIC INFUSION

When incising a coronary artery in a patient receiving retrograde perfusion in the warm arrested state, dark desaturated venous blood exits from the incised arteriotomy. We have sampled this blood for pH, hematocrit, PO_2, potassium, glucose, lactate and ionized calcium and compared it with arterial blood sampled at the same time. The results are shown in Table 2. It is evident that pH is maintained alkalotic. The hematocrit varies dependent upon the underlying hemodilution of the cardiopulmonary bypass perfusate. The coronary effluent PO_2 is markedly reduced, but not desaturated so severely that it is unable to deliver additional oxygen if necessary. Indeed, it could have an even lower oxygen if oxygen demand increased for any reason. The myocardium absorbs potassium as expected. Glucose levels are in the 200 range, a level which is certainly acceptable both in diabetic and non-diabetic patients. Lactate is not produced to any significant degree. Ionized calcium is maintained at a low level. We feel this is an appropriate metabolic response to warm cardioplegic arrest. Warm retrograde cardioplegia has been used at the Baystate Medical Center since September, 1990, and we have an experience in excess of 1,500 patients. When we first studied this approach, we evaluated warm heart surgery in a prospective randomized trial. This was presented by Dr. Rousou at the 1991 Surgical Forum[21] and was published in the book *A Textbook of Cardioplegia for Difficult Clinical Problems* which was published in 1992. [23] The gist of the study found that the cold retrograde crystalloid cardioplegia group had worse myocardial preservation as compared to the warm or cold blood cardioplegia group. In fact, this clearly elucidated the deficiencies of cold crystalloid cardioplegia. Associated with the poorer preservation, as monitored by CK generation, was an increased use of inotropes and the greater requirement for intra-aortic balloon pump insertion following surgery.

Another finding in our series was reported by Dr. Flack at the American Heart Association Annual Meeting in 1991. [22] In that study, cold blood cardioplegia was found to be associated with a significant increase in the development of intraventricular conduction defects. These were permanent defects and were usually new right bundle branch blocks, both complete and incomplete (Figure 6). In correlating these new conduction defects with the release of postoperative CK-MB, Dr. Flack was able to show that a greater release of CK-MB was correlated with a higher incidence of intraventricular conduction disturbance. This would imply by chi-square analysis that the development of a conduction disturbance was associated with increased myocardial necrosis, as measured by CK-MB release. In addition, it is important to point out that, in both the prospective randomized trial and the conduction disturbance study, there were no differences noted between warm and cold preservation in the incidence of atrial tachyarrhythmias. These two studies have concluded that warm cardioplegia provides excellent myocardial preservation, superior to that of both cold crystalloid and blood cardioplegic preservation.

Finally, a prospective randomized trial was performed to evaluate the neurologic function of patients with warm versus cold blood preservation. This study, as yet unreported, incorporated only 28 patients with 16 in the

Table 2. Coronary Sinus and Arterial Metabolic Studies with Optimal Warm Cardioplegia

	Inflow (venous)	Outflow (arterial)
pH	7.61	7.59
Hct (%)	12–20	12–20
PO_2 (torr)	160–340	44–96
K^+ (mEq/L)	12–18	12–17
Glucose (mg/dL)	242	232
Lactate (mmol/L)	1.6	2.2
Calcium (mg/dL)	0.5	0.5

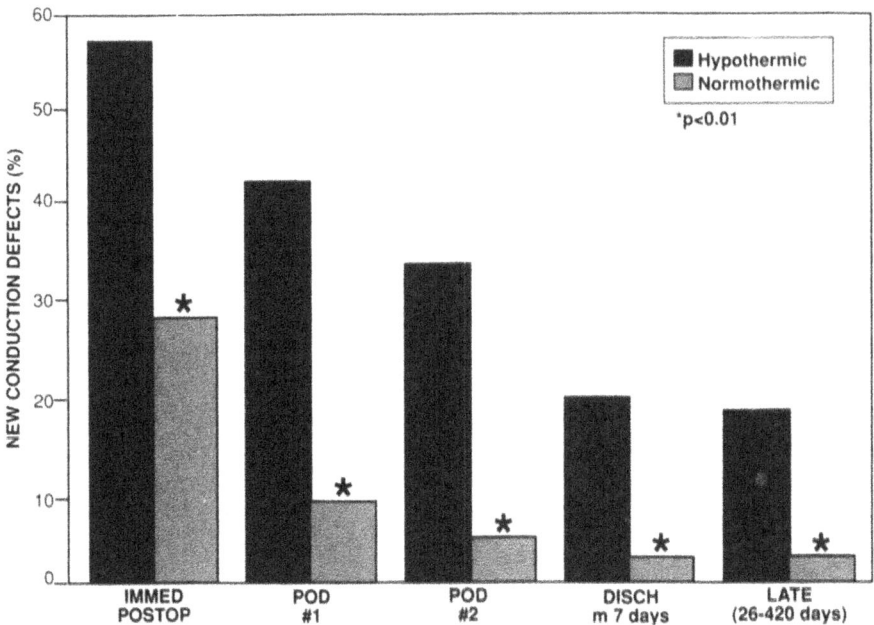

Figure 6. The effect of cardioplegia temperature, normothermic versus hypothermic, on the development of new conduction defects following revascularization is illustrated above. There is an apparent marked decrease in the incidence of new conduction defects associated with normothermic preservation rather than hypothermic.

warm group, and 12 in the cold group. On the fourth postoperative day, significantly more "cold" than "warm" patients had new neurologic defects: 75% cold versus 37.5% warm (P < 0.05). By the one month follow-up, this difference was no longer apparent. Fifty percent of "cold" patients and 46% of "warm" patients exhibited a decline in the neurologic testing scale called the Mathew score, relative to the preoperative value. Stroke occurred with equal frequency in both groups, approximately 20% in both warm and cold groups. This early prospective randomized trial supports the use of warm preservation and warm cardiopulmonary bypass perfusion.

PITFALL OF WARM PRESERVATION

One of the issues that is often raised is how to maintain cardioplegic arrest. Indeed, using our cardioplegic solution we rarely have cardiac activity initiate once arrest has started. If that should happen, we would increase the level of potassium for a short while and the activity abates. When cardioplegic arrest runs for two or more hours, there is potential risk of hyperkalemia and potassium levels are generally above 8 mEq/L. Levels above 7 may not be prohibitively high; however, those above 8, should be treated with insulin (12.5 to 25 units intravenously) and glucose (12.5 to 25 g intravenously). This will enable a reduction in the potassium to levels which are commensurate with cardiac activity. Potassium rapidly returns to normal range in the presence of adequate renal function.

There is some question about the possibility of volume overload. One must remember that cardioplegia is administered in a 4:1 ratio of blood to crystalloid and therefore, if one uses 5 L of cardioplegia, only 1 L is crystalloid. A hemoconcentrator is routinely employed during cardiopulmonary bypass and whatever excess crystalloid is administered is rapidly removed. In our experience, excess fluid administration has not been a problem.

The issue of heparin management is obviously critical. During normothermic perfusion, heparin is metabolized more rapidly and heparin levels must be checked during perfusion at 15 to 30 minute intervals. Further, with the warm state, heparin is absorbed into adipose tissue more readily and heparin rebound is to be expected postoperatively. For this reason, heparin reversal must take place in the Intensive Care Unit following the completion of surgery.

As mentioned previously, visualization of the operative field is occasionally difficult with blood emanating from the opened arteriotomy during coronary bypass or blood accumulating in the aortic root or the left atrium with valvular procedures. With short intervals of interruption of the cardioplegic infusion, lasting from 5 to 10 minutes at a time, we have not found myocardial ischemia to be a problem. The heart being metabolically active during the arrest phase rapidly reverses whatever minimal ischemia accumulates during the 5 to 10 minute anoxic interval and, indeed, appears to not suffer from any untoward ischemia related to this short term of anoxic stress. In fact, this short term ischemia followed by reperfusion may be beneficial in performing ischemic preconditioning of the myocardium, leading to an increase in resistance to subsequent ischemia. [30] This last proposition has not been satisfactorily shown to be the case in the clinical setting but indeed, short periods of ischemic stress followed by reperfusion in the animal model have led to preconditioning and an increased resistance to ischemic injury with subsequent ischemic stress.

In our nearly three year experience with warm preservation, all of the surgeons in our group are satisfieded with its approach and have deemed it the best method for myocardial preservation. In fact, it is advantageous to the slow surgeon who takes a considerably longer period of time to perform his complete operation. There are no deleterious effects noted associated with longer cardioplegic arrest times of 2 to 3 hours, whereas with cold preservation, such prolonged arrest would routinely necessitate intra-aortic balloon pumping and a large volume of inotropes.

ACKNOWLEDGMENTS

Supported by NIH Grant #HL 22559.

REFERENCES

1. Melrose DG, Dryer B, Bentall HH, Baker JBE: Elective cardiac arrest. Lancet 1955; 2:21.

2. Helmsworth JA, Kaplan S, Clark L Jr, McAdams AJ, Mathews EC, Edwards FK: Myocardial injury associated with asystole induced with potassium citrate. Ann Surg 1959; 149:200.

3. Tyers GFO, Todd GH, Niebauer IM, et al: The mechanism of myocardial damage following potassium citrate (Melrose) cardioplegia. Surgery 1975; 78:45.

4. Hirose T, Bailey CP: Coronary arterial perfusion during aortic valve surgery. J Thorac Cardiovasc Surg 1969; 57:164–70.

5. McGoon DC, Pestona C, Moffitt EA: Decreased risk of aortic valve surgery. Arch Surg 1965; 91:779.

6. Hayward RH, Korompai FL: A new coronary perfusion cannula. Ann Thorac Surg 1978; 25:258.

7. Reed GE, Spencer FC, Boyd AD, Engelman RM, Glassman E: Late complications of intraoperative coronary artery perfusion. Circulation (Suppl III) 1973; 48:80–85.

8. Buckberg GD, Brazier JR, Nelson RL, Goldstein SM, McConnell DH, Cooper N: Studies of the effects of hypothermia on regional myocardial blood flow and metabolism during cardiopulmonary bypass. I. The adequately perfused beating, fibrillating, and arrested heart. J Thorac Cardiovasc Surg 1977; 73:87–94.

9. Karp RD, Lell W: Evaluating techniques of myocardial preservation for aortic valve replacement: Operative risk. J Thorac Cardiovasc Surg 1976; 72:206–8.

10. Cooley DA, Reul GJ, Wukasch DC: Ischemic contracture of the heart: 'stone heart'. Am J Cardiol 1972; 29:595–7.

11. Shumway NE, Lower RR: Topical cardiac hypothermia for extended periods of anoxic arrest. Surg Forum 1960; 10:563–6.

12. Kirsch U, Rodewald G, Kalmar P: Induced ischemic arrest. Clinical experience with cardioplegia in open heart surgery. J Thorac Cardiovasc Surg 1972; 63:121–30.

13. Kalmar P, Bleese N, Döring V, Gercken G, Kirsch U, Lierse W, Pokar H, Polonius M-J, Rodewald G: Induced ischemic cardiac arrest. Clinical and experimental results with magnesium aspartate procaine solution (Cardioplegin®). J Cardiovasc Surg 1975; 16:470–5.

14. Bretschneider HJ: Überlebenszeit and Wiederbelebungszeit des Herzens bei Normo- und Hypothermie. Vehr Dtsch Ges Kreislaufforschg 1964; 30:11–34.

15. Gay WA Jr, Ebert PA: Functional, metabolic and morphologic effects of potassium-induced cardioplegia. Surgery 1973; 74:284–90.

16. Jynge MI, Hearse DJ, de Leiris J, Feuvray D, Braimbridge MV: Protection of the ischemic myocardium. Ultrastructural, enzymatic, and functional assessment of the efficacy of various cardioplegic infusates. J Thorac Cardiovasc Surg 1978; 76:2–15.

17. Buckberg GD: Progress in myocardial protection during cardiac operations. Cardiovasc Clin 1981; 12:9–30.

18. Salerno TA, Houck JP, Barrozo CAM, et al: Retrograde continuous warm blood cardioplegia: a new concept in myocardial protection. Ann Thorac Surg 1991; 51:245–7.

19. Lazenby WD, Ko W, Weksler BB, Weiner M, Zelano JA, Lynch C, Isom OW, Krieger KH: Platelet function and hemostasis after cardiopulmonary bypass: a comparison of hypothermic and normothermic cardiopulmonary bypass. Surg Forum 1990; 41:307–9.

20. Butler BD, Kurusz M: Gaseous microemboli: a review. Perfusion 1990; 5:81–99.

21. Rousou JA, Engelman RM, Flack JE III, Deaton DW, Liu X, Das DK: Comparison of normothermic vs hypothermic cardioplegia in patients undergoing coronary artery bypass grafting. Surg Forum 1991; 42:239.

22. Flack JE III, Hafer J, Engelman RM, Rousou JA, Deaton DW, Pekow P: Effect of normothermnic blood cardioplegia on postoperative conduction abnormalities and supraventricular arrhythmias. Circulation 1992; 43(Suppl II):385–392.

23. Engelman RM, Rousou JA, Flack JE III, Deaton DW, Liu X, Das DK: A prospective randomized analysis of cold crystalloid, cold blood, and warm blood cardioplegia for coronary revascularization. In: Engelman RM, S Levitsky, (Eds.) A Textbook of Cardioplegia for Difficult Clinical Problems. Futura Publishing Co., Mt. Kisco 1992:159–71.

24. Rousou JA, Parker T, Engelman RM, Breyer RH: Phrenic nerve paresis associated with the use of iced slush and the cooling jacket for topical hypothermia. J Thorac Cardiovasc Surg 1985; 89:921–5.

25. Pratt FH: The nutrition of the heart through vessels of thebesius and the coronary veins. Am J Physiol 1898; 1:86–9.

26. Blanco G, Adam A, Fernandez A, Raffucci F: A direct experimental approach to the aortic valve. II. Acute retroperfusion of the coronary sinus. J Thorac Surg 1956; 32:171–5.

27. Gott VL, Gonzalez JL, Zuhdi MN, Varco RL, Lillehei CW: Retrograde perfusion of the coronary sinus for direct vision aortic surgery. Surg Gynecol Obstet 1957; 104:319.

28. Gates RN, Laks H, Drinkwater DC, Pearl JM, Zatagoze AM, Lewis W, Sorensen T, Kaczer E, Chang PA: Gross and microvascular distribution of retrograde cardioplegia in explanted human hearts. Ann Thorac Surg (In Press).

29. Okamoto F, Allen BS, Buckberg GD, Young H, Bugyi H, Leaf J: Studies of controlled reperfusion after ischemia. XI. Reperfusate composition: Interaction of marked hyperglycemia and marked hyperosmolarity in allowing immediate contractile recovery after four hours of regional ischemia. J Thorac Cardiovasc Surg 1986; 92:583–93.

30. Flack JE III, Kimura Y, Engelman RM, Rousou JA, Iyengar J, Jones R, Das DK: Preconditioning the heart by repeated stunning improves myocardial salvage. Circulation 1991; (Suppl III) 84:369–74.

PHARMACOLOGIC MANIPULATION TO MINIMIZE BLOOD LOSS IN CARDIAC SURGERY

Aurel C. Cernaianu, M.D. and Anthony J. DelRossi, M.D.

University of Medicine and Dentistry of New Jersey
Robert Wood Johnson Medical School
Cooper Hospital/University Medical Center
Camden, New Jersey

Despite the widespread clinical success of open heart surgery, bleeding and related complications are persistent cause for concern. The hemorrhagic tendency accompanying cardiopulmonary bypass is a complex reflection of multiple hemostatic defects including thrombocytopenia[1], qualitative defects in platelet function[2], mainly attributed to partial activation of platelets with release of platelets constituents[3], reduced number of platelets fibrinogen receptors and alpha-adrenergic agonist receptors and perhaps generation of platelet inhibiting factors, fibrinolysis[4,5], or the presence of unneutralized heparin or excessive protamine and maybe other factors. In essence, these bleeding problems may be caused by inadequate surgical technique or from an increased utilization or destruction of hemostatic factors. The result is usually excessive bleeding from an open vessel, or an excess of circulating fibrinogen split products, or fibrinolysis, or excessive heparin or protamine effect, or an intrinsic or extrinsic factor defect or any combination of the above findings.

Annually, more than 350,000 cardiac operations are performed throughout the United States alone. According to the National Center for Health Statistics, these cases consume over 25 percent of all blood used or 10 percent of the estimated 3.2 million annual recipients of blood[6]. More importantly, patients who receive blood are exposed to an increased risk of transmitted viral diseases and adverse reactions[7]. Most of the blood banks are presently facing severe shortages and an imbalance between the blood supply and demand[8–10].

Cardiopulmonary bypass has deleterious effects on blood and its constituents. Contact between blood and synthetic surfaces activate platelets, induces the release of their granular contents[2], stimulates thromboxane generation[3,11], disrupts the subcellular architecture, and reduces their sensitivity to acting agents[12]. Cardiopulmonary bypass may induce platelets aggregation on foreign surfaces[13] and in the microcirculation resulting

Cardiac Surgery: Current Issues 2, Edited by A. C. Cernaianu and A. J. DelRossi,
Plenum Press, New York, 1994

in a decreased platelet number and thus, contributing to an increased blood loss after cardiac operations. Cardiopulmonary bypass also activates the alternate pathway of the complement. {14}

Complement-mediated stimulation of leukocytes and the release of anaphylatoxines C3a and C5a may also contribute to increased postoperative capillary permeability and transient postoperative multiorgan coagulation dysfunction{15}. Cardiopulmonary bypass produces a dilutional effect of the coagulation factors. {16} Due to centrifugal forces, erythrocyte membranes are destroyed, thereby decreasing red cell survival, which in turn may contribute to an increased requirement for postoperative transfusion{17}.

Intraoperative measures which may conserve blood in cardiac surgery consist of general surgical principles of avoiding and controlling blood loss by performing careful hemostasis, hemodilution{19–21}, platelets sequestration{22}, intraoperative autotransfusion{23}, the use of artificial oxygen carriers{24} and their alternatives or pharmacologic manipulation of the coagulation cascade. All these techniques have been advocated to reduce the loss of blood post cardiac surgery and the need for blood transfusion.

In recent years, research has focused on several drugs which can minimize blood loss and eliminate the need for blood transfusion. This communication will focus only on those drugs where more clinical experience has been accumulated. Some old drugs like epsilon-amino caproic acid (EACA){25,26} and tranexamic acid{27} which are synthetic antifibrinolytic amino acids have been re-evaluated for their role in inhibiting the coagulation defects seen with cardiopulmonary bypass surgery. Other drugs like desmopressin{28} or aprotinin{29} have been recently promoted as useful therapeutic agents in reducing blood loss associated with cardiac surgery.

Hemorrhagic diathesis after cardiopulmonary bypass has been ascribed in part to hyperfibrinolysis{30} due to increased plasminogen activator activity{31}. This appears after sternotomy, and reaches a maximal intensity during and immediately upon termination of cardiopulmonary bypass. EACA inhibits the proteolytic activity of plasmin and the conversion of plasminogen to plasmin by plasminogen activator. EACA is a synthetic monoamine carboxylic acid which has a structure related to lysine, which appears to interact with fibrin protecting it against proteolysis. Plasmin exerts it's proteolytic effect on several plasma proteins including the coagulation components, for example fibrinogen, Factor V, and Factor VIII. EACA prolongs partial thromboplastin time and one stage prothrombin time. It has direct anti-plasmin activity which inhibits it's release. Investigators have found that EACA may decrease lysosomal release from cells which is a reflection of changes in membrane permeability and a diminishing process of cellular disruption{32}.

Data from DelRossi et al. {33} on 350 patients undergoing cardiac surgery with cardiopulmonary bypass, and random prophylactic treatment with EACA has shown that EACA-treated patients have statistically significant less bleeding, required statistically significant less homologous blood, and presented no case of re-operation for bleeding.

Desmopressin acetate, also known as DDAVP, is a synthetic vasopressin analogue which lacks vasoconstrictor activity{28}. It has been employed to improve hemostasis in patients with mild hemophilia or von Willebrand's disease in whom it shortens the bleeding time apparently by inducing the release of Factor VIII{34}. The exact biological mechanism behind all these effects of desmopressin on the coagulation remains obscure. It has been emphasized that the likely mechanism relays on the optimization of platelet-endothelial interaction{34}. It is important to emphasize that desmopressin remains a drug with an effect of major clinical importance that has not yet been fully explained{35}. In addition, its role in blood conservation is still controversial. {36,37} Side–effects of desmopressin include facial flushing, transient headache, increase in heart rate and slight increases in blood pressure. Tachyphylaxis has been reported with repeated doses over a short time period. {38} Moreover, a decrease in systemic vascular resistance and increased cardiac output associated with administration of desmopressin has been reported. {38} DDAVP may have prothrombotic potential secondary to the increases in circulated procoagulant factors, however this is a purely theoretical concern, because there are no reports of thrombotic complications associated with desmopressin administration.

Another agent which has been shown to have therapeutic potential in reducing blood loss after cardiopulmonary bypass operations particularly in Europe and has been recently approved by the FDA in the United States, is aprotinin which is a naturally occurring inhibitor of proteolytic enzymes. {29} Aprotinin acts as an inhibitor of human trypsin, plasmin, plasma kallikrein, and tissue kallikreins by forming reversible enzyme-inhibitor complexes. {39} These enzymes play a major role in the kallikrein-kininogen-kinin system, the complement system, the coagulation system, and the fibrinolytic system where plasmin and plasma kallikrein hold key positions.

Trials including cardiac surgical patients have shown that aprotinin reduces blood loss by 45 - 80 percent and the transfusion need by up to 75 percent when compared to control groups. {40–42}

Bidstrup and co-workers{43,44} studied the amount of chest drainage after return to ICU for all primary patients having bypass grafting and /or the subgroup of patients who had autologous blood retransfused. Blood losses were significantly reduced in the patients receiving aprotinin. The authors have demonstrated that the aprotinin treated group had a reduced hemoglobin level into the chest drains. The use of autologous blood did not alter the differences.

van Oeveren and colleagues{40} have shown that platelet's adherence is maintained when aprotinin is given to patients treated with aspirin before coronary bypass surgery. In their randomized study of 80 patients, bleeding time was 30 percent lower and blood loss was reduced significantly.

The evaluation of functional integrity of platelets in patients treated with aprotinin during cardiopulmonary bypass has been studied in 20 patients by Lavee et al. {45} who demonstrated that all 10 patients treated with aprotinin revealed normal unchanged platelet aggregation whereas all placebo treated patients showed severely disturbed aggregation. The total 24 hour postoperative bleeding and blood requirement was significantly lower in the aprotinin group compared with the placebo group. This study demonstrates that improved postoperative hemostasis is directly related to the complete preservation of platelet function achieved by the protective properties of aprotinin. Similar conclusions have been reached by Sunamori et al. {46}

Recent data published by Hovel and co-workers{47} showed that the addition of aprotinin to cultured human umbilical and endothelial cells produces an increasing concentration of thromboxane B_2 which has a major role in platelet aggregation and vasoconstriction as well as an increase in the eicosanoids 6-keto-prostaglandin F_1 alpha which usually mediates vasodilation and inhibition of platelet aggregation. It appears that one mechanism of the clinically observed effectiveness of aprotinin lies in the altered ratio of 6-keto-prostaglandin F_1 alpha to thromboxane B_2 in endothelial cells which leads to enhanced aggregation and improved vessel sealing. This can explain the decreased bleeding tendency after operations when aprotinin is used. On the other hand, the authors raised the issue that the use of aprotinin may potentially result in thrombotic vessel occlusion and a note of caution has been inserted in their discussions as to further clinical studies may be necessary related to the use of aprotinin and specifically to look into the question if there is any higher rate of early graft closure, especially for coronary bypass operations.

Unfortunately, aprotinin therapy is not without side effects and potential risks. The drug must be given intravenously in large amounts and frequently may cause severe hypotension. The drug is eliminated via the kidney and has a tendency to accumulate in the proximal renal tubes where it may produce acute tubular necrosis. [48,49] However, these concerns remain controversial. [50]

In conclusion, pharmacologic manipulation of blood loss after cardiac operations should be part of the therapeutic arsenal available for cardiac surgical patients and should be used in conjunction with other preoperative, intraoperative and postoperative measures for blood conservation. Blood conservation with pharmacologic manipulation remains controversial. Some investigators have raised the issue of using certain drugs only if a specific coagulation defect has been positively identified. [51] As we know, this issue is very complex due to the multifactorial nature of the coagulation defect seen after cardiopulmonary bypass. Also, it remains to validate the fact that blood conservation with the pharmacologic manipulation is cost effective.

REFERENCES

1. Holloway DS, Summaria L, Sandesara J, Vagher JP, Alexander JC, Caprini JA: Decreased platelet number and function and increased fibrinolysis contribute to postoperative bleeding in cardiopulmonary bypass patients. Thromb Haemost 1988; 59:62–7.

2. Edmunds LH, Ellison N, Colman RW, et al: Platelet function during cardiac operation: comparison of membrane and bubble oxygenators. J. Thorac Cardiovasc Surg 1982; 83:805.

3. Davies GC, Salzman EW, Sobel M: Elevated plasma fibrinopeptide A and thromboxane A_2 levels during cardiopulmonary bypass. Circulation 1980; 51:808.

4. Mori F, Nakahara Y, Kurata S, Furukawa S, Esato KF, Mohri M: Late changes in hemostatic parameters following open heart surgery. J Cardiovasc Surg 1982; 23:458–62.

5. Porter JM, Silver D, Durham NC: Alterations in fibrinolysis and coagulation associated with cardiopulmonary bypass. J Thorac Cardiovasc Surg 1968; 56:869–78.

6. Lawrence L: Detailed diagnoses and procedures for patients discharged from short stay hospitals, United States. 1984 Hyattsville, MD: National Center for health Statistics, 1986:169. Vital and health statistics. Series 13: Data from the National Health Survey; no. 86 (DHHS publication No. (PHS)86–1747).

7. Cohen ND, Munoz A, Reitz BA, et al: Transmission of retroviruses by transfusion of screened blood in patients undergoing cardiac surgery. N Engl J Med 1989; 320:1172–6.

8. Cosgrove DM, Thurer RL, Lytle BW: Blood conservation during myocardial revascularization. Ann Thorac Surg 1979; 28:184–9.

9. Breyer RH, Engelman RM, Rousou JA, Lemeshow S: Blood conservation for myocardial revascularization. J Thorac Cardiovasc Surg 1987; 93:512–22.

10. Goodnough LT, Shuck JM: Review of risks, options, and informed consent for blood transfusion in elective surgery. Am J Surg 1990; 159:602–9.

11. Addonizio VP Jr, Smith JB, Strauss JF III, et al: Thromboxane synthesis and platelet secretion during cardiopulmonary bypass with a bubble oxygenator. J Thorac Cardiovasc Surg 1980; 79:91.

12. Harker LA, Malpass TW, Bronson HE, et al: Mechanism of abnormal bleeding in patients undergoing cardiopulmonary bypass: acquired transient platelet dysfunction associated with selective granule release. Blood 1980; 56:824.

13. Dutton RC, Edmunds LH Jr, Hutchinson JC, Roe BB: Platelet aggregate emboli produced in patients during cardiopulmonary bypass with membrane and bubble oxygenators and blood filters. J Thorac Cardiovasc Surg 1974; 67:158.

14. Kirklin JK, Westaby S, Blackstone EH, et al: Complement and the damaging effects of cardiopulmonary bypass. J Thorac Cardiovasc Surg 1983; 86:845.

15. Hammerschmidt DE, Stroncek DF, Bowers TK, et al: Complement activation and neutropenia occurring during cardiopulmonary bypass. J Cardiovasc Surg 1981; 81:307.

16. McKenna R, Bachman F, Whitaker B, et al: The hemostatic mechanism after open-heart surgery. J Thorac Cardiovasc Surg 1975; 70:298.

17. Tabak C, Eugene J, Stemmer EA: Erythrocyte survival following extracorporeal circulation: a question of membrane versus bubble oxygenator. J Thorac Cardiovasc Surg 1981; 81:30.

18. Baron JF, Samama ChM: Hémodilution, auto-transfusion, hémostase. Anesthésie et Réanimation d'aujourd'hui, ed. Arnette, 1989.

19. Robertie PG, Gravlee GP: Safe limits of isovolemic hemodilution and recommendations for erythrocyte transfusion. International Anesthesiology Clinics 1990; 28:197–204.

20. Trouwborts A, Van Woerkens ECSM, Van Daele M, et al: Acute hypervolaemic haemodilution to avoid blood transfusion during major surgery. Lancet 1990; 336:1295–1297.

21. DelRossi AJ, Cernaianu AC, Vertrees RA, et al: Platelet-rich plasma reduces postoperative blood loss after cardiopulmonary bypass. J Thorac Cardiovasc Surg 1990; 100:281–286.

22. Chambers LA, Kruskall MS: Preoperative autologous blood donation. Transf Med Rev 1990; 4:35–46.

23. Toy PT, Stehling LC, Strauss RG, et al: Underutilizatin of autologous blood donation among eligible elective surgical patients. Am J Surg 1986; 152:483–486.

24. Cernaianu AC, Spence RK, Vassilidze T, et al: Improvement in circulatory and oxygenation status with perflubron (Oxygent-HT) in a canine model of surgical hemodilution. Biomat Art Cell Immob Biotech, 1994; 22(4): (in press).

25. Kaplan AP, Austen KF: The fibrinolytic pathway of human plasma: isolation and characterization of the plasminogen proactivator. J Exp Med 1972; 136:1378–93.

26. Soter NA, Austen KF, Gigli I: Inhibition by E-aminocaproic acid of the activation of the first component of the complement system. J Immunol 1975; 114:928–32.

27. Plötz FB, van Oeveren W, Aloe LS, et al: Prophylactic administration of tranexamic acid preserves platelet numbers during extracorporeal circulation in rabbits. ASAIO J 1992; 38(2):M416–417.

28. Soslau G, Schwartz AB, Putatunda B, et al: Desmopressin-induced improvement in bleeding times in chronic renal failure patients correlates with platelet serotonin uptake and ATP release. Am J Med Sci 1990; 300(6):372–379.

29. van Oeveren W, Jansen NJ, Bidstrup BP, et al: Effects of aprotinin on hemostatic mechanism during cardiopulmonary bypass. Ann Thorac Surg 1987; 44:640–645.

30. Gibbon JA Jr, Camishion R: Problems in hemostasis with extracorporeal bypass. Ann NY Acad Sci 1964; 115:195.

31. Bachmann F, McKenna R, Cole ER, Najafi H: The hemostatic mechanism after open-heart surgery: I. Studies on plasma coagulation factors and fibrinolysis in 512 patients after extracorporeal circulation. J Thorac Cardiovasc Surg 1975; 70:76–85.

32. Ambrus JL, Ambrus CM, Stutzman L, et al: Treatment of fibrinolytic hemorrhage with proteinase inhibitors: a preliminary report. Ann NY Acad Sci 1988; 146:625–41.

33. DelRossi AJ, Cernaianu AC, Botros S, Lemole GM, Moore R: Prophylactic treatment of postperfusion bleeding using EACA*. Chest 1989; 96:27–30.

34. Mannuci PM: Desmopressin (DDAVP) for treatment of disorders of hemostasis. Progress in Hemostasis and Thrombosis, ed. Grune & Stratton, 1986:19–45.

35. Salzman EW, Weinstein MJ, Wientraub RM, et al: Treatment with desmopressin acetate to reduce blood loss after cardiac surgery: a double blind randomized trial. N Engl J Med 1986; 314:1402–1406.

36. Rocha E, Llorens R, Paramo JA, et al: Does desmopressin acetate reduce blood loss after surgery in patients on cardiopulmonary bypass? Circulation 1988; 77:1319–1323.

37. Hackman T, Gascoyne RD, Naiman SC, et al: A trial of desmopressin (1–desamino–8–D–arginine vasopressin) to reduce blood loss in uncomplicated cardiac surgery. N Engl J Med 1989; 321:1437–1443.

38. Stimate™ (desmopressin acetate) injection and control of bleeding following cardiac surgery. Transcript of a panel discussion held at the Sixty-Seventh Annual Meeting of The American Association for Thoracic Surgery, Chicago, April 1987.

39. D'Ambra MN, Risk SC: Aprotinin, erythropoietin, and blood substitutes. Int Anesthesiol Clin 1990; 28:237–240.

40. van Oeveren W, Harder MP, Roosendaal KJ, Eijsman L, Wildevuur CR: Aprotinin protects platelets against the initial effect of cardiopulmonary bypass. J Thorac Cardiovasc Surg 1990; 99(5):788–96.

41. de Smet AA, Joen MC, van Oeveren W, et al: Increased anticoagulation during cardiopulmonary bypass by aprotinin. J Thorac Cardiovasc Surg 1990; 100(4):520–7.

42. Harder MP, Eijsman L, Roozendaal KJ, van Oeveren W, Wildevuur CRH: Aprotinin reduces intraoperative and postoperative blood loss in membrane oxygenator cardiopulmonary bypass. Ann Thorac Surg 1991; 51:936–41.

43. Bidstrup BP, Royston D, Sapsford RN, Taylor KM: Reduction in blood loss and blood use after cardiopulmonary bypass with high dose aprotinin (Trasylol). J Thorac Cardiovasc Surg 1989; 97:364–72.

44. Bidstrup BP, Royston D, Taylor KM, Sapsford RN: Effect of aprotinin on need for blood transfusion in patients with septic endocarditis having open heart surgery. Lancet 1988; 1:366–7.

45. Lavee J, Savion N, Smolinsky A, Goor DA, Mohr R: Platelet protection by aprotinin in cardiopulmonary bypass: electron microscopic study. Ann Thorac Surg 1992; 53(3):477–81.

46. Sunamori M, Sultan I, Suzuki A: Effect of aprotinin to improve myocardial viability in myocardial preservation followed by reperfusion. Ann Thorac Surg 1991; 52:971–8.

47. Havel M, TeufelsbauerH, Knöbl P, et al: Effect of intraoperative aprotinin administration on postoperative bleeding in patients undergoing cardiopulmonary bypass operation. J Thorac Cardiovasc Surg 1991; 101(6):

48. Dudziak R, Kirchhoff PG, Reuter HD, Schumann F: Proteolyse und Proteaseninhibition in der Herz- und Gefässchirurgie. Stuttgart:FK Schattauer, 1985.

49. Verstraete M: Clinical application of inhibitors of fibrinolysis. Drugs 1985; 29:236–61.

50. Blauhut B, Gross C, Necek S, et al: Effects of high-dose aprotinin on blood loss, platelet function, fibrinolysis, complement, and renal function after cardiopulmonary bypass. J Thorac Cardiovasc Surg 1991; 101:958–67.

51. Jones RE, Cohn LH: Prophylaxis for post-perfusion CABG bleeding. Chest 1990; 98(2):516–18.

SUTURELESS INTRALUMINAL RING GRAFTS FOR AORTIC REPLACEMENT

Gerald M. Lemole, M.D.

The Medical Center of Delaware
Wilmington, Delaware

This chapter presents our experience of over 15 years with a sutureless intraluminal ring graft (Figure 1) for replacement of the descending aorta, aortic arch and abdominal aorta. During this time, we have used this prosthesis in almost 150 cases and have learned the advantages and pitfalls of this technique.

Abbe first used a vitrilline hourglass tube to repair femoral vessels in 1894, followed by Alex Carrel, in 1912, who attempted intubation of the aorta with metallic tubes. More recently, Blakemore and Hufnagle, in the fourth and fifth decades of the 20th century used rigid fixation of prosthesis in the thoracic aorta. We developed the intraluminal prosthesis in the laboratory at Temple University in 1974 (Figure 2) and since 1980 have been using a commercially available prosthesis manufactured by Bard and Company.

The most important principle in the use of this type of prosthesis is a rapid repair of aortic pathology with minimal interruption of blood flow to the tissues. In the case of an aortic dissection, it excludes the tear of the false lumen from the blood flow. The rapidity of insertion helps prevent distal ischemia which still represents one of the serious complications related to this type of surgery. Spinal cord ischemia associated with extended aortic cross clamp time may result in spinal cord paralysis. Renal or hepatic failure, and gastrointestinal ischemia and/or necrosis may also occur. Moreover, this technique has the advantage of decreasing post-operative bleeding and pseudoaneurysm formation because sutures are not required to hold the friable tissues of the dissected aorta.

Repair of the ascending aorta and arch has been associated with an overall mortality rate of 10 percent. A 38 percent mortality for arch replacement and an 18 percent mortality for dissecting aneurysms have been reported. Our results for resection of the arteriosclerotic aneurysm of the aorta has a mortality rate of approximately 4 percent which compares favorably with the results in the literature. Complications such as pseudoaneurysm formation, thrombosis or graft migration were not encountered in our series, nor in our follow-up. Moreover, bleeding necessitating

Cardiac Surgery: Current Issues 2, Edited by A. C. Cernaianu and A. J. DelRossi,
Plenum Press, New York, 1994

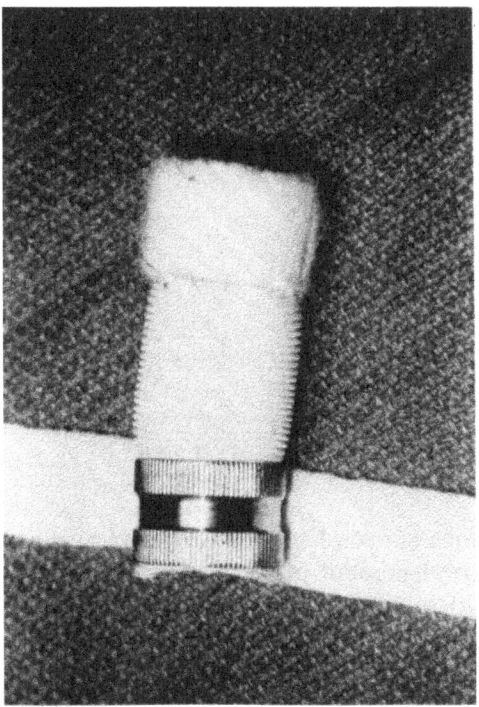

Figure 1. Appearance of the prototype sutureless prosthesis originally used in study. One spool has already been completed; the other is being prepared. (Reprinted with permission from J Vasc Surg 1990; 11:331–8.)

reported in 11 percent of the patients in past studies, was not a serious problem in our patients.

Several technical developments have helped us obtain these results. We use a woven Dacron graft which has a preclotted minimized blood loss. During the early phases of the operation, a unit of the patient's blood is withdrawn and centrifuged to separate the plasma in which the graft is then bathed and autoclaved for three minutes to effectively preclot the Dacron.

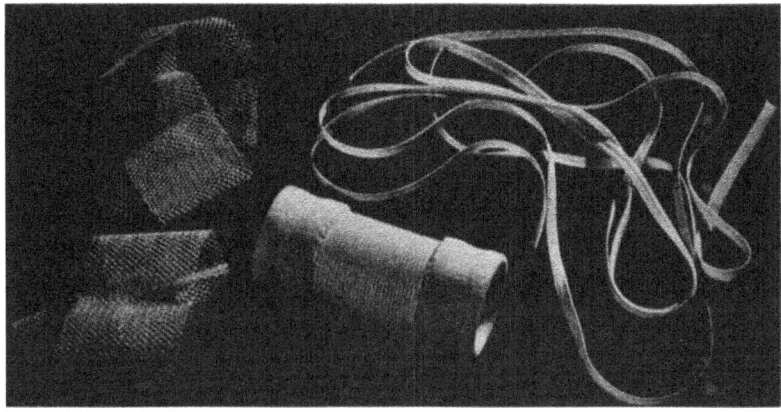

Figure 2. Bard prosthesis with nylon tapes and mesh. (Reprinted with permission from Ann Thorac Surg 1989; 39:47–52.)

Additionally, the outer surface of the spools is lined with Dacron cloth which induces sufficient scarring to hold the prosthesis in place. Moreover, the broad design of the spool and the vascular nature of the aortic wall make erosion unlikely after tying of the spools. We never encountered spool erosion in our series.

DESCENDING AORTA

The overall mortality for aortic replacement is approximately 10 percent, 8 percent for aortic atherosclerotic descending aortic aneurysms, and 14 percent for dissecting aneurysms, including thoraco-abdominal aneurysms. The five-year actuarial survival for this group is 56 percent. Myocardial infarction and pulmonary insufficiency are the primary cause of death in this group. In comparison, the five-year survival of patients undergoing repair of the ascending aorta and arch aneurysms is approximately 64 percent. Death is usually caused by arrhythmia and myocardial infarction. In the abdominal aorta, the sutureless ring graft has limited use when the aortic lesion involves the bifurcation. However, if the lesion is not located at the bifurcation, a ring graft can be used in a normal fashion. The early mortality in our series with ring grafts used for repair of the abdominal aorta including ruptured aorta was 6 percent with a five-year actuarial survival rate of 79 percent. We encountered no incidence of renal failure or other ischemic complications when this technique was employed.

Problems related to the use of the sutureless intraluminal graft often occur when the device is used by unexperienced surgeons who may choose an inappropriate size (too wide or too long) graft for the involved segment of the aorta. Reduction of the aortic lumen by up to 70 percent has not been shown to increase intravascular hemolysis but the choice of a smaller size graft diameter is generally preferable. The size of the ascending aortic lumen should be assessed with valve obturators and the graft diameter that fits comfortably within the diseased vessel should be chosen. In our experience, a 24 mm graft is used most often; infrequently, we use 22 and 26 mm diameter prostheses. The use of a longer than 7 to 8 cm graft may result in kinking and serious hemodynamic complications. The Dacron graft stretches approximately 30 percent after intraaortic insertion; therefore, a graft length that is shorter than the diseased aortic segment should be selected. Again, a shorter graft is better than a longer one. If a composite PTFE graft device is used (Figure 3), the PTFE can be fixed to the ring after insertion, when a more precise determination of the optimal graft length has been made.

Incorrect placement of fixation ligatures on the spools is a common problem encountered during the learning process. We routinely place two ties on the spools and sometimes apply a third tie on the graft material itself between the spools to prevent blood leakage through the graft-spool interface. When stabilizing the spool, care must be taken to ensure that the posterior surface of the spool is in contact with the tie before tension is applied on the ligature. This avoids dislodgement of the device and prevents inadvertent injury to the aortic wall by the shearing force of the ligatures pulling the aortic back wall over the spool.

Although the sutureless intraluminal devices are especially useful in aortic dissections, we are now using these grafts routinely in aortic aneu-

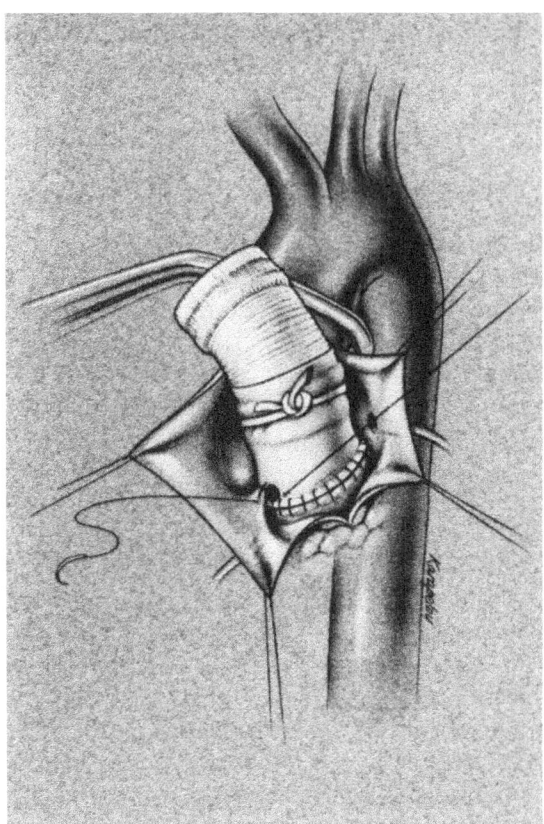

Figure 3. Alternatively, a prosthetic valve attached to polytetrafluoroethylene material is inserted and the proximal spool of a sutureless device is secured within the free end of the polytetrafluoroethylene graft with a Dacron tie. (Reprinted with permission from Ann Thorac Surg 1990; 50:74–9.)

rysms and also infected aortitis. The advantages over sutured anastomoses are not as great. However, the reduction in operative time warrants the use of a sutureless graft in these situations, especially if the patient is hemodynamically unstable. This graft is especially useful in fabricating composite connections between long portions of the aorta. There is a recent trend towards total replacement of the thoracic aorta in certain conditions such as Marfan's syndrome because of the potential for long-term multiple redissections during follow-up. Most people advocate simultaneous operations for replacing the ascending aorta and arch, followed by the replacement of the descending aorta through a left thoracotomy. Moreover, the use of the intraluminal rigid prosthesis is especially useful in replacing the entire thoracic aorta from the annulus to the diaphragm (Figure 4).

During arch replacement, the use of the intraluminal graft may decrease the sewing time for the distal and proximal anastomosis of the cerebral vessels and greatly decreases the ischemic time to the central nervous system. A thoraco-abdominal aneurysm can be more rapidly sewn, requiring only approximately 25 to 30 minutes of ischemic time, with a resultant lower incidence of intraoperative ischemia to distal organs. This in turn may result in a great reduction of the complication rate for this procedure. However, it must be remembered that the outcome of patients undergoing aortic repair with this technique, like anything else in our surgical armamentarium, is

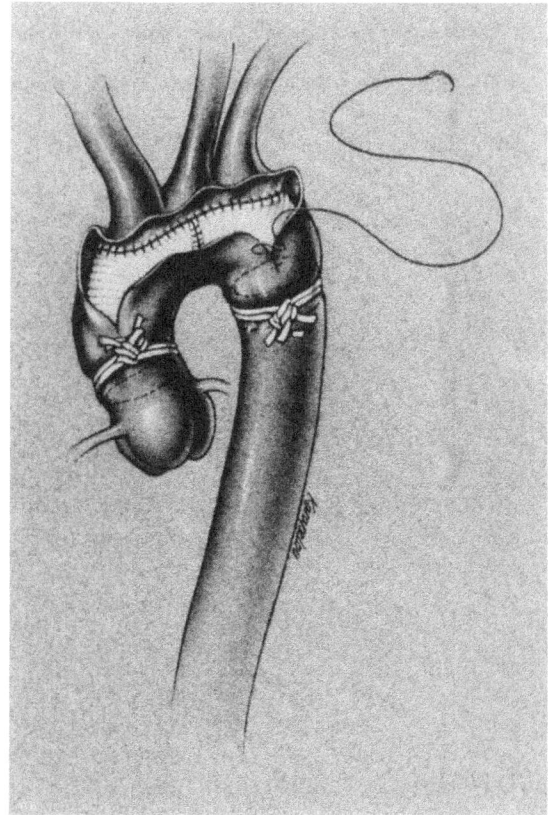

Figure 4. Two sutureless devices are joined together by removing adjoining rings and suturing the free ends together, thus leaving intact rings on either side. An island of tissue incorporating the arch vessels is anastomosed to the spools within the ascending and descending aorta. (Reprinted with permission from Ann Thorac Surg 1990; 50:74–9.)

dependent not only upon the pathological findings but, also on the experience and judgment of the operating surgeon.

References

Crawford ES, Crawford JL: Diseases of the aorta: including an atlas of angiographic pathology and surgical technique. Williams & Wilkins Baltimore, 1984; 14:134–66.

Crawford ES, Crawford JL, Safi JH, et al: Thoracoabdominal aortic aneurysms: preoperative and intraoperative factors determining immediate and long-term results of operations in 605 patients. J Vasc Surg 1986; 3:389–404.

Goddard MB, Lucas AR, Curletti L, Cohn MS, Sdaighi PJ: Sutureless intraluminal graft for repair of abdominal aortic aneurysm. Arch Surg 1984; 120:791–3.

Kouchoukos NT, Marshall WG Jr, Wedige-Stecher TA: Eleven-year experience with composite graft replacement of the ascending aorta and aortic valve. J Thorac Cardiovasc Surg 1986; 92:691–705.

Lemole GM: Aortic replacement with intraluminal grafts. Tex Heart Inst J 1990; 17:302–309.

Lemole GM, Strong MD, Spagna PM, Karmilowicz NP: Improved results for dissecting aneurysms: intraluminal sutureless prosthesis. J Thorac Cardiovasc Surg 1979; 83:249.

Lemole GM, Spagna PM, Strong MD: Sutureless graft replacement of descending thoracic aortic aneurysms. In: Cohn LH, (ed) Cardiac and Thoracic Surgery. Futura, New York, 1983:52:2–9.

Matsumae M, Oz MC, Lemole GM: A flexible sutureless intraluminal graft that becomes rigid after placement in the aorta. J Thorac Cardiovasc Surg 1990; 100:787–92.

Oz MC, Ashton RC Jr, McNicholas KW, Lemole GM: Sutureless ring graft replacement of ascending aorta and aortic arch. Ann Thorac Surg 1990; 50:74–9.

Oz MC, Ashton RC Jr, Oz M, et al: Replacement of the abdominal aorta with a sutureless intraluminal ringed prosthesis. Am J Surg 1989; 158:121–6.

IMMUNOLOGIC CONSEQUENCES OF TRANSFUSION

Paul I. Tartter, M.D.

Mount Sinai Medical Center
New York, New York

THE EFFECTS OF SURGERY AND BLOOD TRANSFUSIONS ON IMMUNE FUNCTION

The effect of blood transfusion on immune function in normal man is unknown-transfusions have never been given to normal volunteers followed by measurement of immune function. One must study patients who receive transfusions, measure the changes observed in immune cells and their function within the context of whatever disease they are being transfused for, and extrapolate this information to the effect of transfusing blood in the absence of disease. In observing similar changes in immune cells following transfusion for a variety of diseases, one can assume that these changes usually follow transfusion. Neither patients nor volunteers will ever be randomized to be transfused or untransfused. Patients scheduled for elective surgery can be randomized to participate in an autologous donation program or to receive blood prepared in some unique manner by filtering and/or washing. The changes in immune function following transfusion with their own blood or washed/filtered blood can be compared to patients who are receiving routinely prepared whole blood or packed cells. In this instance, the blood is given within the context of a surgical procedure as a consequence of operative blood loss which is due to trauma and trauma itself is associated with changes in immune cells and their function.

In Vitro Lymphocyte Response

Generally, a profound depression in *in vitro* lymphocyte responsiveness is noted within hours of surgery which recovers over the next several days. [1-4] Some of this inhibition is due to plasma factors since lymphocyte responsiveness can be partially restored by testing in plasma from normal blood donors. Blood transfusion seems to add to the depressed state of the lymphocytes, at least initially, but may cause stimulation in unoperated patients. [5] Testing of lymphocytes *in vitro* with ConA, PHA and PWM or homologous lymphocytes does not yield consistent results and there is no real-life counterpart *in vivo*. One is not exposed to mitogen during the natural course of life so the significance of these tests for the whole organism is unknown. There has been no evolutionary pressure for lymphocytes to be more or less responsive to mitogen or homologous lymphocytes. For these and other reasons, *in vivo* testing of lymphocytes has been developed in the form of delayed cutaneous hypersensitivity to antigens.

Delayed Hypersensitivity Skin Testing

Delayed hypersensitivity skin testing has been used to predict sepsis and mortality. {6} Anergic patients have significantly higher rates of sepsis and mortality than normal responders but careful study of the temporal relationship between skin reactions and clinical events in individual patients suggest that these differences are not of value in clinical practice. Abnormal reactions usually follow obvious complications such as sepsis or secondary hemorrhage rather than predict them. {7}

The effect of perioperative blood transfusion on delayed hypersensitivity skin test response has been studied by Nielson et al. {8} in 24 transfused and 26 untransfused patients, 16 in each group with colorectal cancer. They were skin tested with tetanus and diphtheria toxoid, streptococcus, tuberculin, Proteus, candida and trichophyton antigens 24 hours before surgery, immediately before surgery, and one and three days after surgery. Mean postoperative skin test response area decreased 57 percent in transfused patients compared to a 38 percent decrease in untransfused patients.

Since transfused and untransfused patients differed significantly in duration of surgery, preoperative blood hemoglobin and serum albumin, the authors reanalyzed their data with 64 pairs of patients matched for these variables with the same results.

Lymphocyte Subsets

Fernandez et al. {9} studied lymphocyte subsets following vascular surgery in 17 transfused patients and 21 untransfused patients. Lymphocytes, B cells, T cells, helper cells and suppressor cells had all dropped significantly five days after surgery and the decline was twice as great in the transfused patients compared to the untransfused. The helper cell number declined sufficiently in transfused patients to cause the helper/suppressor ratio to decrease significantly despite a significant decline in suppressor cell number. These changes in cell numbers had recovered somewhat by ten days so the difference between transfused and untransfused patients was no longer statistically significant although cell numbers in transfused patients were still lower than those in untransfused patients. Lymphocyte responses to ConA and PHA declined significantly in both groups and remained below preoperative levels even one year following surgery.

Despite differences among studies of lymphocyte subsets following surgery, generally surgery is followed by significant decreases in peripheral blood lymphocyte numbers affecting all lymphocyte subsets to some degree. In several studies a disproportionate decline in helper cell numbers was associated with a significant decrease in the helper/suppressor ratio.

Transfused patients exhibited greater declines in lymphocytes but it is not clear if this decline is due to the transfusion or due to the operative trauma or pre–existing anemia which caused physicians to transfuse blood.

Natural Killer Cytotoxicity

Natural killer cells have been shown in experimental animals to play a role in the prevention of spontaneously arising tumors and in controlling metastatic spread of implanted tumors. For this reason, we and others have examined natural killer cytotoxicity in patients undergoing surgery for malignancies and in relation to receiving blood. Preoperative suppressor cells and natural killer cells were significantly increased in colorectal patients who subsequently recurred. Despite increased numbers of natural killer cells, natural killer cytotoxicity was significantly depressed in the 18 patients who recurred. Using multivariate analysis, Dukes' stage, peripheral lymphocyte count, number of suppressor cells, number of natural killer cells and natural killer cytotoxicity were statistically significant prognostic factors. In addition, it was noted that 14 of 115 colorectal cancer patients had received blood for unrelated problems an average of 19 years previously. Helper T cells were significantly lower in number in patients previously transfused and natural killer cytotoxicity was significantly inhibited despite higher total numbers of natural killer cells in transfused patients.

In a prospective study[12] of colorectcal cancer patients randomized to receive whole blood or filtered whole blood, natural killer cytotoxicity declined significantly in patients receiving whole blood and remained significantly depressed 30 days following surgery. Natural killer cytotoxicity in untransfused patients and patients receiving filtered blood declined significantly with surgery (p < 0.001) but had fully recovered by 30 days (p < 0.001). Since natural killer cytotoxicity is of proven prognostic significance, filtered blood may improve the outcome for patients with malignancies.

Collectively, these studies indicate that surgery depresses immune function because both anesthetic agents and physical trauma cause circulating levels of all lymphocyte subsets to decline after surgery with general anesthesia causing a panlymphoyctopenia. In addition to declines in lymphocyte number, lymphocyte function, independent of cell number, is inhibited whether measured *in vitro* by lymphocyte responses to mitogen, antigens or homologous lymphocytes or measured *in vitro* by loss of response to skin testing. Lymphocyte functional inhibition may be related to disproportionate declines in T cell subsets-helper cell number decreases following surgery are much greater than declines in suppressor cell numbers—or related to the appearance of immunosuppressive serum factors which inhibit lymphocytes. Transfusion seems to potentiate whatever mechanism is responsible for lymphocyte inhibition; surgery accompanied by transfusion is followed by more profound decreases in lymphocyte numbers and in lymphocyte functional activity than surgery without transfusion. The prospective study by Jensen et al. suggests that use of leukocyte-free blood will prevent transfusion-associated adverse clinical phenomena, but this study needs to be replicated. The data certainly favors avoiding the use of homologous blood whenever possible.

CLINICAL CONSEQUENCES OF BLOOD TRANSFUSION INDUCED IMMUNE SUPPRESSION

Blood transfusion is the earliest form of organ transplant but until recently the immunologic effects of blood transfusion were not appreciated.

Transfusion is associated with immune suppression in dialysis patients and prolongation of survival of subsequently transplanted renal allografts; numerous multivariate studies have linked transfusion to recurrence of a variety of malignancies following potentially curative surgery; some women suffering from recurrent abortion can be induced to carry to term by transfusion with spouse leukocytes; and transfusion may play a role in the clinical course of autoimmune disease such as Crohn's. However, the area in which transfusion most convincingly plays a role is in increasing susceptibility to infection, particularly postoperative infections. Blood transfusions are commonly received by patients admitted for both elective and emergency surgery and the most common complications following surgery are infections. Infectious complications not only cause morbidity, but contribute to postoperative mortality and significantly increase hospital costs by prolonging hospital stays.

Clinical Studies Linking Blood Transfusion and Infection

The hypothesis that transfusion causes immune suppression leading to infections is confounded by the observation that the magnitude of the injury, whether accidental or intentional, as with elective surgery, directly correlates with the degree of immune suppression. Trauma indices have been developed to account for bone, soft tissue and visceral injuries, quantifying tissue destruction and degree of bacterial contamination, but these indices are no more than estimates of the number of cells damaged or eliminated by the insult. Nevertheless, these potential confounders must be considered in any study of infections following surgery: confounders in one clinical situation are not significant or non-existent in another. For example, re-operation is reproducibly associated with infection in patients undergoing cardiothoracic surgical procedures, whereas in abdominal surgery where re-operation is much less common, it is not a significant variable or risk factor for infection. On the other hand, creation of an ostomy is a very significant risk factor for infection in patients undergoing abdominal surgery, but cardiothoracic patients do not need ostomies. Each field of surgery has its own risk factors for infection which must be controlled. These factors are often associated with transfusion as well as with infection.

The contribution of transfusion to the risk of infection independent of the risk from variables reflecting tissue destruction and bacterial contamination can be calculated statistically using stepwise logistic regression. [13] This analysis is a highly complicated chi square which examines the relationship between each independent variable, such as re-operation or ostomy or transfusion and the dependent variable, in this case infection. An equation is created relating the most significant independent variable to infection and the significance of the remaining independent variables is recalculated. Independent variables are added to the equation, one at a time in order of significance, recalculating the significance of the remaining variables at each step. Variables are added at a preset p value, usually < 0.05, and may be removed if the significance deteriorates. The analysis can also be run backwards: first creating an equation relating infection to all the potential independent variables and removing the least significant in a stepwise fashion. Finally, by creating such an equation leaving out one variable like transfusion, for example, one can evaluate the significance of a single independent factor after the contributions to infection of all the other variables are considered.

This type of analysis is commonly used, or misused, in medical studies, ignoring the basic precept that the independent variables must be truly independent. In fact, most of the independent variables are not independent: the magnitude of the procedure, the duration of surgery, the blood loss and the tissue damage are all related to one another and all are related to the number of units of blood given as well as to the risk of infection. However, the analysis is still useful as long as one is aware that all conclusions drawn are subject to limitations. I have gathered the multivariate studies linking transfusion to risk of infections and listed them by disease.

"Rank" refers to the step in which transfusion enters the stepwise logistic regression equation referred to above. For example, in my own study of colorectal cancer patients, 42 (12 percent) of the 343 patients developed infections after surgery, 25 percent of the 134 transfused patients compared to only 4 percent of the 208 untransfused patients. The mean number of blood transfusions among patients with infectious complications was 2.3 units compared to 0.74 units among patients without complications. Transfusion was associated with low admission hematocrit, high operative blood loss, tumor stage of B2 or greater, poor tumor differentiation and length of specimen. None of these variables was significantly related to infection. Resection of the left colon, sigmoid or rectum was associated with increased

Table 1. Multivariate Studies Linking Transfusion with Infection

Author	Number	Disease	Transfusion's Rank	p
Ottino[14]	2579	Open Heart	5	0.03
Miholic[15]	246	Open Heart	1	0.006
Murphy[16]	238	Coronary Bypass	1	0.017
Nichols[17]	145	Abdominal Trauma	4	0.0519
Dellinger[18]	338	Abdominal trauma	1	0.0001
Dawes[19]	137	Colonic injury	1	0.0004
Tartter[20]	169	Crohn's	1	0.0007
Tartter[21]	343	Colon Cancer	1	<0.0001
Pinto[22]	196	Gastric Cancer	2	0.015
Maetani[23]	565	Major Abdominal Surgery	1	<0.001
Wobbes[24]	548	Abdominal Surgery	3	0.003
NORGAS[25]	1537	Abdominal Surgery	1	<0.001
Jensen[26]	311	Colon Cancer	1	<0.001
Jensen[12]	197	Colon Cancer	1	<0.01
Fernandez[27]	376	Spinal, Hip, Knee	1	0.0001
Dellinger[28]	240	Open fractures	2	0.003
Triulzi[29]	102	Spinal fusion	1	0.016
Murphy[30]	100	Hip Replacement	1	0.0029
Graves[31]	594	Burns	3	<0.05
Agarwal[32]	5366	Trauma	1	<0.001
Mezrow[33]	100	Miscellaneous	1	0.05

risk of infection but this could not be related to the creation of a stoma. Prolonged surgery was also associated with increased infection risk. Multivariate analysis identified transfusion ($p < 0.001$) and hematocrit ($p = 0.024$) as significant independent risk factors for infection. However, the statistical significance of hematocrit was not due to increased infection in patients with low hematocrit as some would predict: the highest risk of infection (33 percent) was seen in transfused patients admitted with normal hematocrit! The multivariate analysis was utilized to investigate the significance of blood transfusion after consideration of all the other variables. After forcing in age, sex, blood loss, procedure, tumor differentiation, stage, admission hematocrit, duration of surgery, length of specimen and tumor size, the association of blood transfusion with infectious complications was highly significant ($p \leq 0.0001$). This study illustrates the value of narrowly defining the population under study in order to eliminate potential confounding variables and isolate the effect of blood transfusion. It also demonstrates the value of computerized multivariate analysis for evaluating the significance of a risk factor within the context of all the other risk factors. As noted previously, all data must be available on all patients.

This type of analysis has been applied to 21 populations of patients undergoing procedures ranging from bone marrow harvesting to coronary artery bypass graft. In all 21 studies, transfusion was a statistically significant risk factor for infection and in 15 of the 21, it was the most significant determinant of infectious complications in stepwise logistic regression. Fourteen studies calculated a p value for the relationship between transfusion and infection of 0.001 or less. All of these studies are excellent and well worth reading.

However, retrospective studies in medicine cannot prove a cause and effect relationship between transfusion and infection because they are susceptible to observer bias in collecting data. The causative factor for infections may be associated with transfusion causing transfusion to be associated with infection, yet may still not be identified in all these studies or transfusion may simply reflect the sum of weak associations of various variables with infection causing transfusion to be more significant than any other single variable. To prove a cause and effect relationship between transfusion and infection, one must randomize patients to receive nor not receive blood or some substitute for blood presumably not associated with increased susceptibility to infections. Patients have not been randomized in the United States but several studies have attempted matching recipients of autologous blood to recipients of homologous blood.

A study of hip replacement surgery at the University of Rochester compared homologous and autologous blood recipients. [30] There were 16 infections in the 50 homologous recipients (32 percent) and only one infection among 34 autologous recipients (3 percent). Eleven of the 17 infections were not wound related. Homologous recipients averaged more days of antibiotics and significantly longer hospital stays. The only significant risk factor for infection in this study was transfusion with homologous blood.

In a second study from the University of Rochester, the association between transfusion and infection in spinal surgery was prospectively studied in 102 consecutive patients undergoing spinal fusion by Triulzi et al. Seventy-one patients donated blood for subsequent autologous blood transfusion and 60 were transfused exclusively with autologous blood, 24 patients received homologous blood, and 25 were not transfused. Since the infection rate in untransfused patients was 4 percent and in patients receiving exclusively autologous blood it was 3.6 percent, these were combined and compared to patients who received any homologous blood. Patients who received homologous blood had five times more infections (21 vs 4 percent), increasing their hospital stays (12 vs 10 days), days of fever (4 vs 3 days), days of antibiotics (4 vs 2 days), length of surgery (308 vs 230 minutes), and blood loss (1343 vs 870 mL). Using multivariate analysis only homologous blood transfusion was a significant predicator of infection (p = 0.016), length of stay and days of antibiotics. All of these relationships were dose-response. The authors noted that patients who had received blood in the distant past for elective surgery or obstetrical bleeding (mean 14 years previously) had more infectious complications than other transfused patients making *previous homologous transfusion* the most significant factor in logistic regression affecting risk of infection (p = 0.004).

In Europe, colorectal cancer patients have been randomized to receive autologous or homologous blood. In Munich, (34) the incidence of infection amongst 58 recipients of homologous blood was double the incidence among 62 autologous recipients, while in Holland, the incidence of infection was the same in both autologous and homologous recipients.

In Denmark, Jensen et al. conducted a prospective randomized trial comparing the infection rates among colorectal cancer patients receiving filtered and unfiltered blood. (12) Blood was filtered by passage through a Pall-filter (MEDA, Copenhagen, Denmark) which reduced the leukocyte and platelet count by 99.98 percent leaving approximately 10(6) white cells. Ninety-three patients were not transfused, 56 received whole blood and 48 received filtered whole blood. There were 17 infectious complications among the recipients of whole blood including 13 wound infections and 3 intraabdominal abscesses. There was only one infectious complication, a wound infection, among the 48 recipients of filtered blood!

These clinical studies are very convincing: homologous blood transfusion was associated with increased risk of infection in every clinical situation examined. In virtually all multivariate analyses, transfusion was a significant predictor of infection after consideration of all other variables measured and in the majority of those studies transfusion was the single most significant factor. In studies where patients received both autologous and homologous blood, patients receiving homologous blood exhibited an incidence of infectious complications that was approximately four times higher than patients receiving autologous blood. The association of transfusion with infection was found among patients undergoing surgery for cardiac, orthopedic and gastrointestinal disorders and for trauma as well as among unoperated patients transfused for burns and gastrointestinal bleeding. No clinician can read these studies and continue to give homologous blood to patients without symptomatic anemia.

The observation that nosocomial infections were increased in these studies argues strongly that the association of transfusion with infection is not simply a reflection that transfusion is a marker of tissue destruction and contamination. Infections that develop in transfused patients away from the site of trauma, whether accidental or intentional, or in the absence of trauma, cannot be attributed to the quantity of tissue destroyed or to the degree of bacterial contamination.

Finally, the very promising work of Jensen et al. using filtered blood to remove leukocytes and prevent postoperative infections is the clearest evidence of a cause and effect relationship between transfusion and infection. If filtering blood can significantly reduce the incidence of infection among transfused patients, all transfused blood will be passing through one of these filters in the very near future.

Experimental Studies Relating Blood Transfusion to Increased Risk of Infection

Patients are extremely heterogeneous and even in prospective randomized trials, factors which influence patients' participation may affect the outcome despite double-blinding and randomization. The hospital course of patients is full of countless unmeasured variables which cannot possibly be controlled in a free society. Clinicians make anecdotal associations from their patients, support or refute the observation with retrospective and eventually prospective randomized studies, and finally develop an animal model to "prove" the observation. Only in animal studies using syngeneic strains with identical housing, lighting, access to food and water, control over the extent of injury, use of antibiotics and exposure to other variables can the influence of a single variable such as blood transfusion be measured. Unfortunately, and perhaps surprisingly, there is no animal model for infections which is analogous to the human clinical experience. Rats and mice are notoriously resistant to bacterial pathogens. Enormous quantities of bacteria must be injected into the peritoneal cavity in order to simulate peritonitis, quantities which would be invariably fatal in man are associated with survival in rodents. Attempting to create wound infections in rats, I once injected 10^9 E-coli subcutaneously with no observable infections after one week. Frustrated, I implanted stool pellets in the subcutaneous tissue. Imagine my surprise when not only did the animals survive, but I could find no evidence of intervention.

Rodents seem to require a double insult to produce measurable infections. For example, ligating the cecum in rats, comparable to appendicitis in humans, causes virtually no untoward sequelae. However, puncturing the ligated cecum, comparable to perforated appendicitis and usually fatal in man, results in less than 20 percent mortality. We used this model to study the effect of allogeneic and syngeneic transfusion on the cell mediated immune function of Lewis rats and their survival following cecal ligation and puncture. [36] One week following transfusion, lymphocyte response to concanavalin A was significantly reduced in recipients of allogeneic blood compared to recipients of syngeneic blood. All animals were subjected to cecal ligation and puncture and survival in the recipients of syngeneic blood was 82 percent compared to 48 percent in recipients of allogeneic blood.

Surprisingly similar survival rates were observed by Waymack et al. [37] in a completely different experimental model using the same strains for donor and recipient. Lewis rats were subjected to full-thickness 30 percent body surface area burn by immersion in 95°C water for 20 seconds. On post burn days 1, 4 and 7 the animals were transfused with 1 mL allogeneic ACI blood or 1 mL saline. Burn wounds were then contaminated with 10^8 pseudomonas 1244 organisms on post-burn days one or two. If contaminated on day one transfused animals had 47 percent mortality compared to 19 percent in saline recipients. Contamination on day two mortality was 26 percent with blood and 8 percent with saline.

Dr. Waymack's group followed up this study with a series intended to identify variables which interact with transfusion in affecting survival following septic challenge in animal models. {38} Using the pseudomonas contaminated burn model described above they gave transfusions of allogeneic blood ranging from 0.1 mL to three transfusions of 1 mL and found significantly increased mortality in comparison to animals receiving comparable amounts of Ringer's lactate. The effect of transfusion was not dose-related: survival of animals receiving 0.1 mL was the same as those receiving 3 mL. This group also demonstrated with this model that transfusion within 2 hours of pseudomonas challenge did not affect survival, suggesting that a time dependent interaction of the recipient and the transfused blood takes place resulting in increased susceptibility to bacteria challenge. {39} The interaction between anesthesia and transfusion was demonstrated in subsequent stud-ies using intravenous injection of 10^8 E-coli as a model of sepsis and a second model created by injecting 10^7 E-coli directly into the peritoneal cavity. {26}

Neither anesthesia (methoxyflurane) nor transfusion significantly affected survival of animals given intravenous injections in comparison to untransfused, unanesthetized animals given the same intravenous dose of E coli. However, both allogeneic transfusion and anesthesia caused significantly increased mortality compared to controls when 10^7 E-coli were injected into the peritoneal cavity. Survival in animals receiving allogeneic blood one week prior to intraperitoneal challenge was 21 percent compared to 73 percent for control animals transfused with saline (p = 0.029). This interaction was further explored with intraperitoneal injections of 10^7 or 10^8 E-coli the same day or four days following anesthesia with metaphane or transfusion with saline, syngeneic blood or allogeneic blood. {40} There was no significant difference in survival between the groups given 10^8 organisms on the same day as the anesthesia or transfusion. Same day injection of 10^7 organisms yielded 21 percent survival in allogeneic blood recipients compared to 0 percent in saline recipients (p = 0.029), 46 percent in syngeneic blood recipients, and 38 percent in animals anesthetized. Challenge with 10^8 organisms four days following treatment resulted in significantly decreased survival when followed at four days with 10^7 E-coli: allogeneic 33 percent, syngeneic 51 percent, anesthesia 42 percent and saline 63 percent survival. This series of studies indicates that the timing of transfusion relative to septic challenge and the severity of the septic challenge interact in determining the significance of allogeneic blood for increasing susceptibility to infectious agents.

Waymack's group investigated potential mechanisms of the transfusion effect both on local factors such as neutrophil chemotaxis and macrophage function and on systemic factors such as endotoxin and tumor necrosis factor. {41} Macrophage migration into the peritoneal cavity is significantly reduced in animals previously transfused with allogeneic blood. Macrophages from animals previously transfused with allogeneic blood also exhibit impaired ability to phagocytose and kill bacteria in culture. Waymack and co-workers{43} showed that immunosuppressive thromboxane and pro-staglandin E and F1α production by macrophages is significantly increased following allogeneic transfusion. Macrophage and macrophage supernatant from transfused rats whether allogeneic or syngeneic recipients, suppress lymphocyte responses for PHA. {43} Recently, Waymack's group {44} has become interested in the systemic immunosuppressive effects of blood trans-fusion. In the contaminated burn model they demonstrated that significant elevations of serum corticosterone accompanies declines in leukocyte counts in animals transfused with allogeneic blood in comparison to syngeneic recipients.

These experimental studies reproducibly demonstrate that allogeneic blood transfusion causes inhibition of cellular antibacterial mechanisms which cause increased susceptibility to bacterial pathogens. Certainly, none of these models accurately reproduces human infections. The cecum of rodents is disproportionately larger than the appendix in man so although the survival rates following cecal ligation and puncture in the rat may approximate that of untreated appendicitis in man, the septic insult of the experimental model is much great and the rodents' survival is probably due to their greater resistance to bacterial pathogens. Similar comments can be made concerning the contaminated burn wound or burn injury with gastric lavage. Certainly 30 percent full thickness burn followed by swabbing the burn with pseudomonas or acute peritonitis induced by injecting bacteria directly into the peritoneal cavity would be uniformly fatal in man if left untreated. Nevertheless, these models are all that is available to us and offer the best possible control over confounding variables which are unmanageable in human studies. All of the models support the hypothesis that transfusion-induce immune suppression leads to enhanced susceptibility to bacterial pathogens in the recipient. The mechanism may be inhibition of lymphocytes due to prostaglandin E production by macrophage or increased secretion of corticosterone, but whatever the mechanism, generally the receipt of blood must precede the infecting insult by 24 hours or more and it must be accompanied by some form of trauma, burn injury, operative intervention, general anesthesia, etc.

BLOOD TRANSFUSION AND RECURRENCE OF MALIGNANCY

The most controversial area in which transfusion may play a role is in the outcome for patients undergoing surgery for malignancy. Many of the same variables which confound studies relating transfusion to infection also confound the relationship between transfusion and malignancies. Duration of surgery, blood loss, magnitude of the procedure and stage of disease are all related to each other and to the administration of blood. Stepwise logistic regression is also capable here of ranking the "independent" variables in order of significance but stage of disease is invariably more important than trans-fusion. In addition, patients with cancers are commonly lost to follow-up or die of unrelated causes, only contributing to statistical error in calculations of relative significance of the various variables for outcome. Large numbers of patients are required to detect differences in recurrence in the order of 25 percent possibly due to transfusion with a good probability of detecting true differences—if they exist! Finally, patients with malignancies do not often respond to the presence of their tumors as patients with infections respond to bacteria. Factors which alter immune function in cancer patients potentially can affect the outcome only in the small proportion of patients whose immune cells have identified the malignant cells and are responding to it.

Colorectal Cancers

The most highly studied malignancy is colorectal cancer (Table 2). The majority of retrospective studies observed a significant relationship between transfusion and adverse outcome and in the majority of multivariate studies transfusion ranked second to stage in level of significance. Only two retrospective studies observed that transfusion was associated with improved outcome and neither study was statistically significant. Few clinicians will be swayed by retrospective studies.

My own contribution to this field is a prospective study begun in 1983{69} comparing packed cell recipients to patients not receiving blood. Three hundred thirty-nine patients were accrued between 1983 and 1986 and followed up to 1991. Six patients were lost to follow-up. The five year disease-free survival of the 40 percent of the patients transfused was 57 percent compared to 77 percent for untransfused patients (p < 0.001). Forty percent of transfused patients have recurred compared to 22 percent of untransfused patients (p < 0.001). Numerous other potential prognostic variables were examined for their relationship to transfusion. Using Cox proportional hazards model only stage (p < 0.001) and transfusion (p < 0.001) were significant and independently related to outcome. The Cox analysis was also used to calculate the prognostic significance of blood transfusion after consideration for all the other variables. After consideration for age, sex, blood loss, procedure, tumor differentiation, stage, admission and discharge hematocrit, duration of surgery, length of specimen and tumor size, the association of blood transfusion with disease-free survival was statistically significant (p = 0.0196). Blood transfusion were associated with recurrence when given pre-, intra- or postoperatively. The risk of recurrence did not increase with the number of units of blood given, one unit of packed cells had the same impact in disease-free survival as few or more units.

Two groups have addressed the influence of transfusion on the growth of colorectal cancers by studying recurrence after resection of colorectal liver metastases. Stephenson et al. {70} from the National Cancer Institute found that the amount of blood transfused was a significant prognostic factor (p = 0.0015) when applying the Cox proportional hazards model to 59 patients. Rosen et al. {71} recently presented data from 270 liver resections for metastatic colorectal carcinomas which supports the findings above. Eighty-one patients who were not transfused had 60 percent survival at three years and 32 percent at five years compared to 40 percent and 21 percent for transfused patients.

Numerous other malignancies have been studied in a retrospective manner and these are included for completeness' sake but actually do not contribute to our understanding of this phenomenon beyond showing that it is not limited to colorectal cancer (Table 3).

The preliminary results of a randomized prospective study of colorectal cancer patients was recently presented at the American Society of Clinical

Table 2. Colorectal Cancer Studies Multivariate Studies

Author	Number of Patients	Percent Transfused	% Difference in Survival or DFS between Transfused and untransfused Patients	Rank
Significant Multivariate Studies				
van Lawick van Pabst(45)	164	71	12	2
Tartter(69)	339	32	20	2
Blumberg(48)	197	65	32	1
Foster(49)	146	45	17	4
Arnoux(53)	198	94	50	3
Corman(50)	281	84	21	2
Liewald(61)	439	69	16	2
Voogt(56)	113	76	16	2
Wobbes(58)	270	68	20	5
Beynon(59)	519	55	20	2
Creasy(47)	68	49	25	2
Significant Univariate Studies				
Burrows(46)	295	60	14	
Waymack(60)	155	65	40	
Parrott(59)	517	72	23	
Mecklin(65)	520	68	15	
Francis & Judson(54)	87	61	10	
Insignificant Multivariate Studies				
Cheslyn-Curtis(67)	961	61	4	
Weiden(66)	171	60	−13	
Nathanson(63)	366	54	14	
Bentzen(62)	468	67	Not given	
Hermanek(51)	598	87	38	
Marsh(52)	224	47	Not given	
Insignificant Univariate Studies				
Ross(57)	159	60	13	
Vente(63)	212	75	0	
Ota(68)	207	78	5	

Oncology meeting. {34} This study by Weiss et al., from Munich randomized 120 patients to receive either homologous or autologous blood if transfusion were needed. With median follow-up of only 21 months (9–48), the recurrence rate among homologous recipients is 29 percent compared to 17 percent among autologous recipients and was significant in both B ($p = 0.032$) and C ($p = 0.006$) tumors. Multivariate regression identified receipt of homologous blood as an independent prognostic factor ($p = 0.008$). These results are very exciting. A second prospective trial of 500 colorectal cancer patients randomized between autologous and homologous blood is nearing completion in Holland. In this study, no difference in outcome can be attributed to receipt of homologous or autologous blood. {35} It is only through this type of

Table 3. Miscellaneous Retrospective Studies Linking Transfusion to Cancer Recurrence

Attributed to Disease	Number	Survival Difference Transfusion in Transfusion	Rank of p for Stepwise Analysis	Transfusion
Colorectal/Liver Metastases				
Stephenson (70)	59	19		0.0015
Rosen(71)	270	–		
Gastric Cancer				
Kaneda(72)	231	–		0.002
Sugegawa(73)	298	13		0.05
Kampschoer(74)	1000	24		0.28
Gynecologic Cancer				
Dalrymple(75)	142	15		<0.05
Blumberg(76)	130	–	3	0.05
Eisenkop(77)	126	10		0.025
Breast Cancer				
Nowak(78)	81	8		0.29
Foster(79)	226	1		<0.07
Tartter(80)		14		0.02
Voogt(56)	383	4		0.74
Eichoff(81)	1599	1		0.90
Crowe(82)	823	–		0.02
Salsali(83)	901	–		0.01
Saromas				
Rosenberg(84)	156	22	2	0.006
Chesi(85)	155	19	1	0.05
Lung				
Tartter(86)	165	14	2	0.08
Moores(87)	330	17	2	0.039
Hyman(88)	105	17	2	0.02
Little(89)	117	38	1	0.0278
Keller(90)	252	2		0.23
Pastorino(91)	282	0		NS
Prostate				
Heal(92)	262	23		0.2135
McClinton(93)	246		4	10^{-5}
Davies(94)	71	51	21	0.001
Ness(95)	309	2		0.748
Head And Neck Cancers				
Johnson(96)	179			0.0042
Jackson(97)		50		0.001
Bock(98)	174	7		0.053
Jones(99)	94	43	2	0.045
Renal				
Moffat(100)	126	20		NS
Mayonda(101)	80			0.04

prospective randomized study that the significance of transfusion for cancer patients will be determined.

These studies will no doubt convince many that a cause and effect relationship exists between homologous blood transfusion and recurrence of malignancy. Certainly this association has been subjected to greater statistical scrutiny than almost any other observation in medicine. Physicians have already dramatically cut their use of blood in cancer surgery for fear of transmitting AIDS and the immunosuppressive consequences of blood transfusion only reinforce this behavior. However, many academicians will never be convinced by retrospective studies that transfusion is anything other than a marker of stage disease and extent of surgery. In answer, I can only point to the prospective randomized trial comparing autologous to homologous recipients undergoing colorectal cancer surgery in Munich. {34} Significant differences in recurrence and survival are already apparent despite short follow-up and small numbers of patients.

Numerous variables affect the outcome of cancer surgery and prospective clinical studies of the prognostic significance of a singe variable such as transfusion are difficult to design. The ideal study would be of surgery for malignancy which required transfusion in the majority of instances, where the number of surgical procedures is very limited, and the malignancy would have to be sufficiently common that the necessary number of patients could be accrued in a short period of time. Randomizing patients between autologous and homologous units as has been done in Rotterdam and Munich would be ideal although hardly ethical in the Untied States since autologous blood is already proven to be superior to homologous blood with respect to risk of postoperative infection. Jensen et al in Denmark have randomized patients with colorectal cancer to receive either whole blood or filtered whole blood. Filtering removes 99.98 percent of the leukocytes and platelets. In their study, recipients of whole blood exhibited significant inhibition of natural killer cytotoxicity three days following surgery which remained suppressed even 30 days postoperative. This exciting study is continuing to follow these patients for recurrence. Hopefully, filtering will reduce recurrence and improve survival.

Until the results of this study and others like it become available, it is prudent to avoid the use of homologous blood. This includes maximum utilization of autologous pre–donation programs and maximum use of intraoperative and postoperative blood salvage techniques. Physicians have been found legally liable for transmission of disease by inappropriate transfusions and they will most certainly be held liable for failure to use autologous blood and/or blood salvage when failure to use these techniques results in disease transmission.

Experimental Studies of Blood Transfusion and Tumor Growth

The relationship of blood transfusion to the growth of tumors seems like an ideal clinical observation for experimental modelling. The major problems with clinical studies of the prognostic value of blood transfusion are due to transfusion's association with numerous other factors which may be prognostic and may account for the observed association between transfusion and outcome. Retrospective clinical studies, despite multivariate analysis,

Table 4. Studies in Which Transfusion Enhances Experimental Tumor Growth

Donor	Recipient	Tumor	Reference
Mice Studies			
CBA	C57B1/61	B16 Melanoma	110
ATL	C57B1/61	B16 Melanoma	110
ATH	C57B1/61	B16 Melanoma	110
BALB/c (NK deficient)	C57bg	B16 Melanoma	108
BALB/c	C57BL/61	B16 Melanoma	108
BDF1	C3h	MHh134	107
AKR	(C57BL/6X BDA/2)F1	LLC	107
AKR	C3H	MH134	107
C57/BL6	C3H	Neuroblastoma UV2237 Fibrosarcoma	105
B10BR	C3H	Neuroblastoma UV2237 Fibrosarcoma	105
BALB/c	C3H	Neuroblastoma UV2237 Fibrosarcoma	105
BALB/b	C3H	Neuroblastoma UV2237 Fibrosarcoma	105
DBA/2	C3H	Neuroblastoma UV2237 Fibrosarcoma	105
BALB/c	C57B1/61	Methylcholanthrene Induced Fibrosarcoma	105
C57/BL6	A/J	Neuroblastoma C1300	110
Rat Studies			
Fischer (344)	Fischer 344	Methylcholanthrene induced saromas	108
PVC	WAG	MC7 Sarcoma	104

Experimental Studies Which Did Not Observe Tumor Growth following Allogeneic Transfusion

Donor	Recipient	Tumor	Reference
Rat (BN)	WAG	Basal Cell Carcinoma1618	112
Rat (BN)	WAG		112
Rat (SD)	B09		111
Rat (SD)			109
Mice (C57BL10)			111
Mice (BALB/c)			112
Rat (Katsukabe)			102
Rat (Donryu)			102
Rat (Donryu)			103
Rat (Kyoto)			103
Rat (Tokyo)			103
Rat (Fischer)			103
Rat (ACI)			103
Mice (R)	C57b1		106
Mice	(C B A)	C3H	106
Mice	(NZW)	C3H	105
Mice (B10.D2)	C3H		105

begin with two separate patient populations, the transfused and untransfused, and the initial differences in these patients which leads to transfusion can never be controlled. In prospective studies, one may be aware of the causes for transfusion yet the two populations, transfused and untransfused, differed in those cases. The advantage of randomizing between autologous and homologous blood is that at least at entry into the study, the patients should be comparable. However, even with randomized prospective trials, it is unknown if the observed outcome is due to homologous blood or due to preparation for the patients who receive autologous blood. Experimental models of blood transfusion and tumor growth offer the opportunity for controlling the numerous potential prognostic factors which sabotage clinical studies. Animals are transfused whether it is needed or not, tumor burden can be measured by counting the number of malignant cells used, no one is lost to follow-up and non-cancer deaths are not a problem. Statistical error due to lost patients and non-cancer deaths is eliminated, reducing the number of animals required to demonstrate significant differences between groups. However, one must be aware that experimental studies are not otherwise completely analogous to clinical studies. The tumor has been present for some interval, usually years, in patients with malignancies and some immunologic interaction between the host and the tumor has preceded the effect of surgery and blood transfusion; whereas, in experimental studies tumor growth is measured in an immunologic milieu made receptive to tumor antigens by prior transfusion. Implanting tumor cells and measuring their growth in an animal model is not really analogous to removing spontaneously arising tumor in man, and measuring the rate of recurrence.

These studies collectively indicate that transfusion of allogeneic blood prior to tumor inoculation promotes tumor growth in most animal models. Immune function is suppressed following allogeneic transfusion as measured by lymphocyte response to ConA and PHA and by natural killer cytotoxicity, although Francis and Purcell[108] clearly show that natural killer cell activity is not necessary for a transfusion effect. Allogeneic transfusion promoted growth of both antigenic chemically induced tumors and syngeneic spontaneously arising tumors. By choosing the appropriate tumor and timing the transfusion relative to tumor inoculation, one can observe tumor growth promotion, inhibition, or no effect. Surgical trauma, blood loss and allogeneic transfusion independently promoted tumor growth and their effects on tumor growth seem to be additive. Promotion of tumor growth by allogeneic blood transfusion is by no means a universal finding.

Miscellaneous Phenomena Associated with Blood Transfusion

Recurrent Abortion. One of the most exciting, intriguing and controversial areas in which transfusion may affect the outcome and have a therapeutic role is in the treatment of recurrent abortion. That immune factors play a role in allowing the antigenic fetus to reach term without rejection cannot be argued. During pregnancy, lymphocyte function as measured by responses to antigens, mitogen and homologous lymphocytes (MLR), is suppressed just as it is following homologous blood transfusion. A large part of this inhibition of lymphocyte function is due to serum factors since sera from pregnant women will cause the same type of inhibition when added to lymphocytes from women who are not pregnant. Serum of some women experiencing recurrent spontaneous abortion is similar to that of non-pregnant women: they do not develop the factors which suppress cell mediated immunity present during normal pregnancy. Normal pregnant women's sera will block mixed lymphocyte reactions whereas male sera, sera from nulliparous women and sera from women suffering from recurrent spontaneous abortion will not.

In 1981, Taylor and Faulk{113} attempted to induce suppressive sera in women suffering from recurrent spontaneous abortion and sharing HLA antigens with their spouse by transfusing the women with leukocyte–enriched plasma from multiple donors. Three of four women had normal pregnancies and deliveries at term. These results have been replicated and expanded by several groups (Table 5).

These studies clearly show that during normal pregnancy antibodies appear in the maternal serum which block cell mediated immunity. Absence of these antibodies is associated with early fetal loss and with sharing of HLA antigens with the spouse. Transfusing these women causes the production of blocking antibodies allowing the blastocyte to implant and preventing it from being rejected and the pregnancy to reach term. Although only a small number of women can potentially benefit from this type of therapy, this clearly illustrates that immune suppression induced by blood transfusion can be used to advantage.

Crohn's Disease

Crohn's disease is an inflammatory condition of the gastrointestinal tract which presents clinically with diarrhea and crampy abdominal pain. Any section from mouth to anus can be affected but typically it is the small and large bowel which develop skip areas of chronic inflammation of unknown etiology. The disease often progresses to complete obstruction or intestinal perforation, complications which require surgical intervention. Recurrence of disease following surgery is not uncommon—nearly half of the patients will develop symptoms of recurrence within ten years of surgical resection of all diseased bowel. Immune function is abnormal in patients with Crohn's disease and patients have significantly decreased total lymphocyte and t cell counts compared to controls. {118} Following surgery when patients are clinically well, lymphocyte and t cell counts of transfused patients remain significantly depressed compared to normal levels in untransfused patients and controls. Increasing numbers of units of blood received are associated with progressively lower numbers of lymphocytes at follow-up.

Table 5. Studies of Transfusions for Spontaneous Recurrent Abortion

Authors	Number	Deliveries	%
Taylor and Faulk{113}	4	3	75
McIntyre{114}	26	20	77
Takakuwa{115}	10	5	50
Unander and Linholm{116}	37	25	65
Mueller-Eckhardt{117}	14	11	79

Several groups have studied the effect of blood transfusion on the outcome Crohn's disease, hypothesizing that the immunosuppressive effects of transfusion might benefit patients in the same way steroids effect the course to the disease (Table 6).

These studies are suggestive that transfusion may influence the course of diseases which are thought to have an immune or autoimmune basis and clinically respond to steroids. For Crohn's disease, one would expect patients with more severe disease, those with lower hemoglobin and serum albumins, undergoing resection of more bowel, to have higher recurrence rate. Yet, these patients when transfused, have recurrence rates comparable to untransfused patients with higher hemoglobin and albumins and less bowel resected. The work of Tartter et al. showing that lymphocyte counts remain depressed in transfused patients is strong evidence that homologous blood should have some effect. It will be interesting to follow Crohn's disease patients who receive autologous transfusions and compare them to patients receiving homologous blood.

Wound Healing

Recently it has been recognized that lymphocytes contribute to wound healing which is primarily mediated by macrophages. Activated lymphocytes secrete lymphokines which enhance fibroblast replication, migration and collagen synthesis. *In vivo* depletion of lymphocytes impairs skin wound healing. Since transfusions inhibit lymphocyte function it seems logical that transfusion-induced inhibition of lymphocyte function would lead to impaired wound healing.

Tadros et al. {123} studied the effects of allogeneic and syngeneic transfusions on healing of experimental intestinal anastomoses. Anastomotic abscesses were common in the transfused animals. Bursting pressure was significantly lower following transfusion with either syngeneic or allogeneic blood in comparison to saline. At day seven the site of rupture in saline recipients shifted away from anastomosis—more of the bowel segments ruptured within the segment of attached normal bowel before anastomosis breakdown. In contrast, two of seven syngeneic recipients and seven of ten allogeneic recipients ruptured at the anastomosis (p = 0.004). The study was repeated with inverted anastomoses rather than everted and the results were comparable with respect to origin of transfusion. The authors also measured hydroxyproline content of the ileal and colonic anastomoses and found that transfusion with either syngeneic or allogeneic blood reduced the hydroxyproline content of colonic anastomoses on day three but ileal anasto-

Table 6. Studies of Transfusion and Recurrence of Crohn's Disease

Authors	Number	Recurrence Rate	
		Transfused	**Untransfused**
Peters{8}	79	22%	44%
Williams & Hughess{9}	60	16%	59%
Steup{10}	104	38%	44%
Scott{11}	97	37%	37%

moses and colonic anastomosis on day seven were not affected. This study clearly implicates blood transfusion in impaired wound healing.

Diabetes

Insulin dependent diabetes mellitus is associated with decreases in both the number and functional activity of suppressor T lymphocytes in man. In the Bio-Breeding rat, diabetes develops spontaneously when the animals develop pancreatic insulitis, suggesting a cell-mediated immune pathogenesis. Diabetes can be prevented in these animals by treating them with immunosuppressive agents such as anti-lymphocyte serum, steroids, cyclosporin, irradiation, or neonatal thymectomy. Rossini et al. [124] investigated the influence of blood transfusions on the development of diabetes in a colony of inbred Bio-Breeding/Worcester rats (BB/W). Blood was obtained from a line of BB/W animals resistant to the disease and given to BB/W animals from diabetes-prone lines. Lymphocyte or splenocyte transfusions completely prevented the development of diabetes.

All recipients of white cells were free of insulitis. This phenomenon may not be due to transfusion-induced immunosuppression. Transfused animals had higher total lymphocytes and helper T cells than untransfused animals and their lymphocyte response to ConA was enhanced. In this experimental situation, it appears that diabetes-prone BB/W rat lines have a deficit in immunity which is restored by transfusing lymphocytes. This study may not have analogy for human insulin dependent diabetes mellitus.

SUMMARY

These studies at the very least indicate that homologous blood transfusion is capable of affecting the outcome of clinical diseases in both beneficial and adverse ways. These experimental situations are not suitable for randomized clinical trials—it is unlikely that transfusions will be given to prevent the onset of diabetes or that wound strength will be measured in man following receipt of homologous and autologous blood. However, these experimental observations suggest that the outcomes of numerous clinical diseases which have not been studied may be manipulated by the use of homologous blood or that transfusion should be avoided. Several studies suggest that some changes in immune function following transfusion are permanent. The field of clinical phenomena associated with immune suppression and attributable to blood transfusion is fertile, waiting for interested investigators.

REFERENCES

1. Riddle PR: Disturbed immune reactions following surgery. Brit J Surg 1967; 54:882–886.

2. Park SK, Brody JL, Wallace HA, Blakemore WS: Immunosuppressive effect of surgery. Lancet 1971; i:5455.

3. Jubert AV, Lee ET, Hersh EM, McBride CM: Effects of surgery, anesthesia and intraoperative blood loss on immunocompetence. J Surg Res 1973; 15:399–403.

4. Roth JA, Golub SH, Grimm EA, Eilber FR, Morton DL: Effects of operation on immune response in cancer patients: Sequential Evaluation of *in vitro* lymphocyte function. Surgery 1976; 79(1):46–57

5. Hunt PS, Trotter S: Lymphocyte response after surgery and blood transfusion. J Surg Res 1976; 21:57–61.

6. Meakins JL, Pietsch JB, Bubenick O, Kelly R, Rode H, Gordon J, MacLean LD: Delayed hypersensitivity: indicator of acquired failure of host defenses in sepsis and trauma. Ann Surg 1977; 186(3):241–250.

7. Brown R, Bancewicz J, Hamid J, Tillotson G, Ward C, Irving M: Delayed hypersensitivity skin testing does not influence the management of surgical patients. Ann Surg 1982; 196(6):672–676.

8. Nielsen HJ, Hammer JH, Moesgaard F, Kehlet H: Ranitidine prevents postoperative transfusion-induced depression of delayed hyper-sensitivity. Surgery 1989; 105(6):711–719.

9. Fernandez LA, MacSween JM, You CK, Gorelick M: Immunologic changes after blood transfusion in patients undergoing vascular surgery. Am J Surg 1992; 1613:263-270.

10. Tartter PI, Steinberg B, Barron DM, Martinelli G: The prognostic significance of natural killer cytotoxicity in patients with colorectal cancer. Arch Surg 1987; 122:1264–1268.

11. Tartter PI, Steinberg B, Barron DM, Martinelli G: Transfusion history, T cell subsets and natural killer cytotoxicity in patients with colorectal cancer. Vox Sang 1989; 56:80–84.

12. Jensen LS, Andersen AJ, Christiansen PM, Hokland P, Juhl CO, Madsen G, Morgensten J, Moller-Nielsen C, Hanberg-Sorensen F, Hokland M:Postoperative infection and natural killer cell function following blood transfusion in patients undergoing elective colorectal surgery. Br J Surg 1992; 79:513–516.

13. Cox DR: Analysis of binary data, Methuen: London, 1970.

14. Ottino G, De Paulis R, Pansini S, Rocca G, et al: Major sternal wound infection after open-heart surgery: A multivariate analysis of risk factors in 2,279 consecutive operative procedures. Ann Thoracic Surg 1987; 44:173–179.

15. Miholic J, Hudec M, Domanig E, Hiertz H, Klepetko W, Lackner F, Wolner E: Risk factors for severe bacterial infections after valve replacement and aortocoronary bypass operations: Analysis of 246 cases by logistic regression. Ann Thoracic Surg 1985; 40:224–228.

16. Murphy PJ, Connery C, Hicks GL Jr., Blumberg N: Homologous blood transfusion as a risk factor for postoperative infection after coronary artery bypass graft surgery. J Thoracic Cardiovasc Surg 1992; 104:1092–1099.

17. Nichols RL, Smith JW, Klein DB, Trunkey DD, Cooper RH, Adinolfi MF, Mills J: Risk of infection after penetrating abdominal trauma. New Engl J Med 1984; 311(17):1065–1070.

18. Dellinger PE, Millder SD, Wertz, MJ, Grypma M, Droppert B, Anderson PA: Risk of infection after open fracture of the arm or leg. Arch Surgery 1988; 123(11):1320–1327.

19. Dawes LG, Aprahamian C, Condon RE, Malongi MA: The risk of infection after colon injury. Surgery 1986; 100:796–803.

20. Tartter PI, Dreifuss RM, Malon AM, Heimann TM, Aufses AH Jr: Relationship of postoperative septic complications and blood transfusions in patients with Crohn's disease. Am J Surg 1988; 155:43–48.

21. Tartter PI: Blood transfusion and infectious complications following colorectal cancer surgery. Br J Surg 1988; 75:789–792.

22. Pinto V, Baldonedo R, Nicholas C, Barez A, Perez A, Aza J: Relationship of transfusion and infectious complications after gastric carcinoma operations. Transfusion 1991; 31:114–118.

23. Maetani S, Nichikawa T, Tobe T: Role of transfusion in organ system failure following major abdominal surgery. Ann Surg 1986; 203(3):276-281.

24. Wobbes T, Bemelmans BLH, Kuypers JHC, Beerthuizen IGJM, Theeuwes GM: Risk of postoperative septic complications after abdominal surgical treatment in relation to perioperative blood transfusion. Surg Gyneco Obstet 1990; 171:59–62.

25. The Norwegian Gastro-Intestinal Group (NORGAS). Infectious problems after elective surgery of the alimentary tract: the influence of perio-operative factors. Curr Med Res Opin 1988; 11:179–195.

26. Jensen LS, Andersen A, Fristrup SC, Holme JB, Hvid HM, Kraglund K, Rasmussen PC, Toftgaard: Comparison of one dose versus three doses of prophylactic antibiotics, and the influence of blood transfusion on infectious complications in acute and elective colorectal surgery. Br J Surg 1990; 77:513-418.

27. Fernandez MC, Gottlieb M, Menitove JE: Blood transfusion and postoperative infection in orthopedic patients. Transfusion 1992; 32:318–322.

28. Dellinger EP, Miller SD, Wertz MJ, Grypha M, Droppert B, Anderson PA: Risk of infection after open fracture of the arm or leg. Arch Surg 1988; 123:1320–1325.

29. Truilzi DJ, Vanek K, Ryan DH and Blumberg N: A clinical and immunologic study of blood transfusion and postoperative bacterial infection in spinal surgery. Transfusion 1992; 32:517–524.

30. Murphy P, Heal JM, Blumberg N: Infection or suspected infection after hip replacement surgery with autologous or homologous blood transfusions. Transfusion 1991; 31:212–217.

31. Graves TA, Cioffi WG, Mason AD, McManus WF, Pruitt BA: Relationship of transfusion and infection in a burn population. J Trauma 1989; 29(7):948–953.

32. Agarwal N, Murphy JG, Cayten CG, Stahl WM: Blood transfusion increases risk of infection in trauma. Presented to the Surgical Infection Society, Los Angeles, April 1992.

33. Mezrow, Bergstein NB, Tartter, PI: Postoperative infections following autologous and homologous blood transfusions. Transfusion 1992; 32:27-20.

34. Weiss MM, Jauch KW, Delanoff CL, Memple W, Schildberg FW: Blood transfusion modulated tumor recurrence—a randomized study of autologous versus homologous blood transfusion in colorectal cancer. Proc ASCO 1992; 11:172.

35. Marquet RL, van Papendcecht H, Busch ORC, Jeekel J: The Immunologic consequences of blood donation. in Transfusions medizin 92/93, pp. 179–185, Kretschmea, Stangel and Reckstein, eds., Karger: Basel, 1993.

36. Tartter PI, Maidman DC: Allogeneic blood transfusions suppress immunity and increase mortality in a septic rat model. Surg Res Comm 1989; 5:30.

37. Waymack JP, Robb E, Alexander JW: Effect of transfusion on immune function in a traumatized animal model. Arch Surg 1987; 122:935–939.

38. Waymack JP, Warden GD, Miskell P, Gonce S, Alexander JW: Effect of varying number and volume of transfusions on mortality rate following septic challenge in an animal model. World J Surg 1987; 11:387–391.

39. Waymack JP, Miskell P, Gonce S: Alterations in host defense associated with inhalation anesthesia and blood transfusion. Anesth Analg 1989; 69:163–168.

40. Waymack JP, Warden GD, Alexander JW, Miskell P, Gonce S: Effect of blood transfusion and anesthesia on resistance to bacterial peritonitis. J Surg Res 1987; 42:528–535.

41. Waymack JP, Yurt RW: The effect of blood transfusions on immune function. J Surg Res 1990; 48:147–153.

42. Waymack JP, McNeal N, Warden GD, Balakrishnan K, Gonce S, Alexander JW, Miskell P: Effect of blood transfusions on macrophage-lymphocyte interaction in an animal model. Ann Surg 1986; 204(6):681–685.

43. Waymack JP, Moldawer LL, Lowry SF, Guzman RF, Okerberg CV, Mason AD, Pruitt BA: Effect of prostaglandin E in multiple experimental models. J Surg Res 1990; 49:328–332.

44. Waymack JP, Fernandez G, Cappelli PJ, Burleson DG, Guzman RF, Mason AD Jr, Pruitt BA Jr: Alterations in host defense associated with anesthesia and blood transfusions. Arch Surg 1991; 126:59-62.

45. van Lawick van Pabst WP, Langenhorst BL, Mulder PG, Marquet RL, Jeekel J: Effect of perioperative blood loss and perioperative blood transfusions on colorectal cancer survival. Eur J Cancer Clinical Oncology 1988; 24(4):741-747.

46. Burrows L, Tartter P, Aufses AH Jr: Increased recurrence rates in perioperatively transfused colorectal malignancy patients. Cancer Detect Prev 1987; 10:361.

47. Creasy TS, Veitch PS, Bell PR: A relationship between perioperative transfusion and recurrence of carcinoma of the sigmoid colon following potentialy curative surgery. Ann Roy Soc Surg Eng 1987; 69:100.

48. Blumberg N, Agarwal MM, Chuang C: Relation between recurrence of cancer of the colon and blood transfusion. Br Med J 1985; 390:1037.

49. Foster RS Jr, Costanza MC, Foster JC, Wanner Mc, Foster CB: Adverse relationship between blood transfusions and survival after colectomy. Cancer 1985; 55:1195.

50. Corman J, Arnoux R, Peloquin A, St.-Louis G, Smeesters C. Giroux L: Blood transfusions and survival after colectomy for colorectal cancer. Can J Surg 1986; 29:325.

51. Hermanek P, Guggenmoos-Holzmann I, Schricker KTH, et al: Der [Influence of blood and hemoderivatives on the prognosis of colorectal carcinomas.] Langenbecks Arch Chir 1989; 374:118.

52. Marsh J, Konnan PT, Hamer-Hodges DW: Association between transfusion with plasma and the recurrence of colorectal carcinoma. Br J Surg 1990; 77:623.

53. Arnoux R, Corman J, Peloquin A, Smeesters C, St-Louis G: Adverse effect of blood transfusions on patient survival after resection of rectal cancer. Can J Surg 1988; 131:121.

54. Francis D, Judson R: Relation between recurrence of cancer of the colon and blood transfusion. Br Med J 1985; 291:544.

55. Parrot NR, Lennard T. WJ, Taylor RMR, Proud G, Shenton BK, Johnston IDA: Effect of perioperative blood transfusion on recurrence of colorectal cancer. Br J Surg 1986; 73:970.

56. Voogt PJ, van de Velde C. JH, Brand A, et al: Perioperative blood transfusion and cancer prognosis. Different effects of blood transfusion on prognosis of colon and breast cancer patients. Cancer 1987; 59:836.

57. Ross WB: Blood transfusion and colorectal cancer. J Roy Col Surg Edin 1987; 32:197.

58. Wobbes T, Joosen KHG, Kuypers HHC, et al: The effect of packed cells and whole blood transfusions on survival after curative resection for colorectal carcinoma. Dis Colon Rectum 1989; 32:743.

59. Beynon J, Davies PW, Biol M, et al: Perioperative blood transfusion increases the risk of recurrence in colorectal cancer. Dis Colon Rectum 1989; 29:975.

60. Waymack JP, Moomaw CJ, Popp MB: The effect of perioperative blood transfusions on long-term survival of colon cancer patients. Milit Med 1989; 154:515.

61. Liewald F, Wirshing RP, Zulke C, Demmel N, Hempel W: Influence of blood transfusions on tumor recurrence and survival rate in colorectal carcinoma. Eur J Cancer 1990; 26:327.

62. Bentzen SM, Balslev I, Pedersen M, et al: Blood transfusion and prognosis in Dukes' B and C colorectal cancer. Eur J Cancer 1990; 26:457.

63. Nathanson SD, Tilley BC, Schultz L, Smith RF: Perioperative allogeneic blood transfusions and survival in patients with resected carcinomas of the colon and rectum. Arch Surg 1985; 120:734.

64. Mecklin JP, Jarvinen HJ, Ovaska JT: Blood transfusion and prognosis in colorectal carcinoma. Scand J Gastroenterol 1989; 24:33.

65. Vente JP, Wiggers TH, Weidema WF, Jeekel J, Obertrop H: Peri-operative blood transfusions in colorectal cancer. Eur J Surg Oncol 1989; 15:371.

66. Weiden PL, Bean MA, Schultz P. Perioperative blood transfusions in colorectal cancer recurrence. Cancer 1987; 60:870.

67. Cheslyn-Curtis S, Fielding LP, Hittinger R, Fry JS, Phillips RKS: Large bowel cancer: the effect of perioperative blood transfusion on outcome. Ann Roy Col Surg Eng 1990; 172:53.

68. Ota D, Alvarez L, Lichtiger B, Giacco G and Guinee V: Perioperative blood transfusions in patients with colon carcinoma. Transfusion 1985; 25:392.

69. Tartter PI: The association of perioperative blood transfusion with colorectal cancer recurrence. Ann Surg 1992; 216:633–638.

70. Stephenson KR, Steinberg SM, Hughes KS, et al: Perioperative blood transfusions are associated with decreased time to recurrence and decreased survival after resection of colorectal liver metastases. Ann Surg 1988; 208:679.

71. Rosen CB, Nagorny DM, Taswell ML, van Heerden JA: Perioperative blood transfusion and determinants of survival after tumor resection for metastatic colorectal carcinoma. Presented to the American Surgical Association, May 1992.

72. Kaneda M, Horimi T, Ninomiya M, Mukai K, Chono S, Orita K. The effect of perioperative blood transfusion on patients' survival rate after gastric cancer surgery. Transfusion 1987; 27:373.

73. Sugezawa A, Kaibara N, Sumi K, Ohgta M, Osamu K, Nichodoi H, Koga S: Blood transfusions and the prognosis of patients with gastric cancer. J Surg Oncol 1989; 42:113.

74. Kampschoer GHM, Maruyama K, Sasako M, Kinoshita T, van de Velde CJH: The effects of blood transfusion on the prognosis of patients with gastric cancer. World J Surg 1989; 13:637.

75. Dalrymple JC, Monaghan JM. Recurrent carcinoma of the vulva: relationship with operative blood transfusion. J Obstet & Gyn 1986; 7:65.

76. Blumberg N, Agarwal M, Chuang C. A possible association between survival time and transfusion in patients with cervical cancer. Transfusion (in press).

77. Eisenkop SM, Spirtos NM, Montag TW, Moossazedeh J, Warren P, Hendrickson M: The clinical significance of blood transfusion at the time of radical hysterectomy. Obset & Gynecol 1990; 76(1):110–113.

78. Nowak MN, Ponsky JL: Blood transfusion and disease-free survival in carcinoma of the breast. J Surg Oncol 1984; 27:124.

79. Foster RS Jr., Constanza MC: Blood transfusion and survival after surgery for breast cancer. Arch Surg 1984; 119:1138.

80. Tartter PI, Burrows L, Papatestas AE, Lesnick G, Aufses AH Jr: Perioperative blood transfusion has prognostic significance for breast cancer. Surgery 1985; 97:225.

81. Eickhoff JH, Andersen PM, Norgard H: Effect of perioperative blood transfusion on recurrence and death after mastectomy for breast cancer. Acta Chir Scand 1988; 154425.

82. Crowe JP, Gordon NH, Gry DE, Shuck JM, Hubay CA: Breast cancer survival and perioperative blood transfusion. Surgery 1989; 106:836.

83. Salsali M, Bufalino R, Morabito A: Combined effect of transfusion and blood groups on the survival of patients with breast cancer. A clinical study of 901 patients. Vasc Surg 1988; 22(6):402–412.

84. Rosenberg SA, Seipp CA, White DE Wesley, R: Perioperative blood transfusions are associated with increased rates of recurrence and decreased survival in patients with high-grade soft-tissue sarcomas of the extremities. J Clin Oncol 1985; 3:698.

85. Chesi R, Cazzola A, Bacci G, et al: Effect of perioperative transfusions on survival in osteosarcoma treated by multimodaltherapy. Cancer 1989; 64:1727.

86. Tartter PI, Burrows L, Kirschner P: Perioperative blood transfusion adversely affects prognosis after resection of Stage I (subset N0) non-oat cell lung cancer. J Thorac Cardiovasc Surg 1984; 88:659.

87. Moores DWO, Plantadosi S, McKneally MF: Effect of perioperative blood transfusion on outcome in patients with surgically resected lung cancer. Ann Thorac Surg 1989; 47:346.

88. Hyman NH, Foster RS Jr, DeMeules JE, Costanza MC: Blood transfusions and survival after lung cancer resection. Am J Surg 1985; 149:502.

89. Little AG, Wu HS, Ferguson MK, et al: Perioperative blood transfusion adversely affects prognosis of patients with Stage I non-small-cell lung cancer. Am J Surg 1990; 160:630.

90. Keller SM, Groshen S, Martini N, Kaiser L. Blood transfusion and lung cancer recurrence. Cancer 1988; 62:606.

91. Pastorino L, Valente M, Cataldo I, Lequaglie C, Ravasi G: Perioperative blood transfusion and prognosis of resected stage Ia lung cancer. Eur J Clin Oncol 1986; 22:1375.

92. Heal JM, Chuang C, Blumberg N: Perioperative blood transfusion and prostate cancer recurrence and survival. Am J Surg 1988; 156:374.

93. McClinton S, Moffat LEF, Scott S, Urbaniaq SJ, Kerridge DF: Blood transfusion and survival following surgery for prostatic carcinoma. Br J Surg 1990; 77:140.

94. Davies AM, Ramarakha P, Cranston D, Clarke JP: Effect of blood transfusion on survival after radiotherapy as treatment for carcinoma of the prostate. Ann Roy Soc Surg Eng 1991; 73:116.

95. Ness PM, Walsh, PC, Zahurak M, Baldwin ML, Piantadosi S: Prostate cancer recurrence in radical surgery patients receiving autologous or homologous blood. Transfusion 1992; 37(1):31–36.

96. Johnson JT, Taylor FM, Therle PB: Blood transfusion and outcome in Stage III head and neck carcinoma. Arch Otolaryngol Head Neck Surg 173.

97. Jackson RM, Rice DH: Blood transfusion and recurrence in head and neck cancer. Ann Otol Laryngol 1989; 90:171–173.

98. Bock M, Grevers G, Koblitz M, Heim MU, Mempel W: Influence of blood transfusion on recurrence, survival and postoperative infections of laryngeal cancer. Acta Otolaryngol (Stockh) 1990; 110:115.

99. Jones KR, Weissler MC: Blood transfusion and other risk factors of cancer of the head and neck. Arch Otolaryngol Head Neck Surg 1990; 116:304–309.

100. Moffat LEF, Sunderland Gt, Lamont D: Blood transfusion and survival nephrectomy for carcinoma of kidney. Brit J Urol 1987; 60:316–319.

101. Manyonda IT, Shaw DE, Froulkes A, Osborn DE: Renal cell carcinoma: blood transfusion and survival. Br Med J 1986; 293:537–538.

102. Tsukada Y: An experimental study on the effect of blood or blood component transfusion to the transplanted tumor cell. GANN 1979; 61:105–120.

103. Oikawa T, Hosokawa M, Imamura M, Sendo F, Nakayama M, Gotohda E, Kodama T, Kobayashi H: Anti-tumor immunity by normal allogeneic blood transfusion in rat. Clin Exp Immunol 1977; 27:549–554.

104. Francis DMA, Shenton BK, Proud JG, Taylor RMR: Tumor growth and blood transfusion. J Exp Clin Cancer Res 1982; 1:1210–1216.

105. Clarke PJ, Wood KJ and Morris PJ. Increased tumor growth after blood transfusion. Transplantation Proceedings 1989; 21(1):584–585.

106. Judson RT, Robb L, A'Apice AJF. Blood transfusion and tumor growth: An experimental study. Surgical Research 1985; 55:503–506.

107. Horimi T, Kagawa S, Ninomiya M, Yoshida E, Hiramatsu S, Orita K: Possible induction by blood transfusion of immunological tolerance against growth of transplanted tumors in mice. Acat Med Okayama 1983; 37:259–263.

108. Francis DMA, Purcell L: Enhancement of tumor growth in natural killer cell-deficient mice by allogeneic transfusion. Am J Surg 1991; 161:411-412.

109. Younes RN, Rogatka A, Vydelingum NA, Brennan MF: Effects of hypovolemia and transfusion on tumor growth in MCA-tumor-bearing rats. Surgery 1991; 109:307–310.

110. Francis DMA, Burren CP, Clunie GJA: Acceleration of B16 melanoma growth in mice after blood transfusion. Surgery 11987; 2(3):485–492.

111. Rossler W, Kreikorn K, Lenhard V, Zeller W, Scholler P: Effect of allogenic blood transfusion on the growth of two different tumors in the rat. Urol Int 1985; 40:217–219.

112. Jeekel J, Eggermont A, Heystek G, Marquet RL: Inhibition of tumor growth by blood transfusion in the rat. Europ Surg Res 1982:113.

113. Taylor C, Faulk WP: Prevention of recurrent abortion with leucocyte transfusions. Lancet 1981; ii:68–69.

114. McIntyre JA, Faulke WP, Nichols-Johnson VR, Taylor CG: Immunologic testing and immunotherapy in recurrent spontaneous abortion. Obstet & Gynecol 1986; 67(2):169–175.

115. Takakuwa K, Kanazawa K, Takeuchi S: Production of blocking antibodies in vaccination with husband's lymphocytes in unexplained recurrent aborters: The role in successful pregnancy. AJRIM 1986; 10:1–9.

116. Unander AM, Lindholm A: Transfusions of leukocyte-rich erythrocyte concentrates: A successful treatment in selected cases of habitual abortion. Am J Obstet Gynecol 154(3).

117. Mueller-Eckhardt G, Neppert J, Kunzel W, Muller-Eckhardt C: Prevention of recurrent spontaneous abortion by intravenous immunoglobulin. Vox Sang 1989; 56:151–154.

118. Tartter PI, Heimann TM, Aufses AH Jr: Blood transfusion, skin test reactivity, and lymphocytes in inflammatory bowel disease. Am J Surg 1986; 151:358–361.

119. Peters WR, Fry RD, Fleshman JW, Kodner IJ: Multiple blood transfusions reduce the recurrence rate of Crohn's disease. Dis Col Rect 1989; 32(9):749–753.

120. Williams JG, Hughes LE: Effect of perioperative blood transfusion on recurrence of Crohn's disease. Lancet 1989; i:131–132.

121. Steup WH, Brand A, Weterman IT, Zwinderman KH, Lamers CBHW, Gooszen: The effect of perioperative blood transfusion on recurrence after primary operation for Crohn's disease. Scand J Gastroenterol 1991; 26:81–86.

122. Scott ADN, Ritchie JK, Phillips RKS: Blood transfusion and recurrent Crohn's disease. Br J Surg 1991; 78:455–4587.

123. Tadros Tamer, Wobbes T, Hendriks T: Blood transfusion impairs the healing of experimental intestinal anastomoses. Ann Surg 1992; 215(3):276–281.

124. Rossini AA, Faustman D, Woda BA, Like AA, Szymanski I, Mordes JP. Lymphocyte transfusions prevent diabetes in the bio-breeding/Worcester rat. J Clin Invest 1984; 74:39–46.

TRAUMATIC RUPTURE OF THE THORACIC AORTA

Rudolph C. Camishion, M.D. and James B. Alexander, M.D.

University of Medicine and Dentistry of New Jersey
Robert Wood Johnson Medical School
Cooper Hospital/University Medical Center
Camden, New Jersey

Thoracic injuries cause approximately one out of every four trauma deaths. Fifteen percent of all traffic fatalities are due to injuries of the great vessels of the aortic arch. Eighty percent of the people who have sustained this type of injury will die at the scene of the accident and never make it to the hospital. [1,2] Consequently, clinical series only report a very small proportion of those patients who sustain this type of injury. Of the 20 percent that arrive in the hospital, 50 percent will die within 24 hours if they are not operated upon. Ninety percent will die within four months, if left untreated. [3] Only 2 percent will survive with a chronic pseudoaneurysm. Conversely, early diagnosis and repair of major thoracic injuries results in survival in up to 86 percent of patients.

The mechanism of the aortic injury is a shearing effect at the sites of fixation of the aorta to the chest. Consequently, the sites of rupture are at the distal aortic arch where it is tethered between the left subclavian artery and the ligamentum arteriosum (in approximately 95 percent of the cases), the ascending aorta at the aortic valve where there is a fixation by the pericardium, or the descending aorta at the diaphragm as it passes through the aortic hiatus.

The patient with rupture of the thoracic aorta has typically sustained substantial blunt injury. This is usually the result of a motor vehicle accident or a vertical fall. Although, for obvious reasons, they may be in profound shock on presentation, most patients who survive to be seen at the hospital are relatively hemodynamically stable. They may complain of chest pain, difficulty breathing, hemoptysis (from associated pulmonary injury), hoarseness (from stretching of the recurrent laryngeal nerve as it passes around the aortic arch), or they may have no symptoms related to their aortic injury. [4] Not surprisingly, it is rare to have an isolated thoracic injury. The most common associated injuries are the orthopedic which occur in about 50 percent of the cases. Concomitant abdominal injuries occur in 30 percent and 40 percent have a neurologic deficit.

Cardiac Surgery: Current Issues 2, Edited by A. C. Cernaianu and A. J. DelRossi,
Plenum Press, New York, 1994

Disruption of the thoracic aorta should be seriously considered in all patients with evidence of severe blunt chest injury. The initial study most helpful in evaluating a patient with blunt chest injury in an erect chest x-ray. Any patient sustaining a significant blunt injury should have an erect chest x-ray if at all possible. [5] Findings on the erect chest film that may suggest aortic injury include mediastinal width greater than 8 cm, mediastinal/thoracic ratio greater than 0.25, obscuration of the aortic knob, widening of the right peritracheal stripe, deviation of the trachea to the left, elevation of the left mainstem bronchus, widening of the paravertebral stripe, deviation of a nasogastric tube to the right, and apical pleural cap. [6] If there is a widened mediastinum or other radiologic signs suggestive of this problem, contrast angiography is the most valuable study. Experience is still being accumulated with MRI, transesophageal echocardiography and, CT scanning, but aortogram is the current "gold standard". [3]

Although exclusion of the diagnosis of traumatic aortic disruption by angiography is the standard of care, contrast aortography is not perfect. There are a small number of patients who have multiple aortic tears that are not appreciated on the aortogram. If the additional aortic injuries are proximal to the left subclavian artery, into the transverse arch, then proximal aortic control and cardiopulmonary bypass may be necessary. [7] If there is any question of a thoracic aortic disruption, an aortogram should be performed to exclude the diagnosis. Admittedly, this may, result in a considerable number of negative aortograms. However, the risks of a negative aortogram are far less than the risks of a missed traumatic aortic disruption. [8]

There are causes of mediastinal widening that are not due to hemorrhage. For example, a supine film is almost impossible to interpret. The x-ray machine must be far from the patient and the film must be close or magnification will result. The heart or the aorta may be enlarged from atherosclerosis or hypertension, or the patient may actually have a pre–existing aortic aneurysm. The causes of actual mediastinal bleeding, on the other hand, include rupture of the thoracic aorta or brachiocephalic arteries but, also include venous bleeding and bleeding from fracture of the sternum, ribs, or vertebrae. Many of these do not require immediate repair, or even an eventual operation.

Some authors have suggested that if there is a fracture of the first or second rib, there's been sufficient force that there is very likely to be injury of the heart, aorta or great vessels. [9] However, there has been no greater incidence of traumatic rupture of the aorta with that injury than with any other injury of the ribs. [10–12]

The authors have had experience with 36 patients who were admitted to Cooper Hospital/University Medical Center over a period from 1985 through 1992. There were 30 males and 6 females. Of this group, 23 were transported to us directly from the site, 13 were transferred from other hospitals as long as 36 hours after injury. The mechanism of the injury, in most instances, was a motor vehicle accident, except two patients who had a fall. Most of the injuries occurred from a deceleration mechanism which is usually a head-on collision. Most patients arrived at the hospital hemodynamically stable. Patients surviving long enough to reach the hospital typically have a contained rupture. However, 5 patients in our series presented in profound shock. The most common symptom was chest pain.

On radiologic examination, 29 (80 percent) of our patients showed a widened mediastinum, 17 (47 percent) showed hemothorax, 14 (39 percent) lost the aortic knob and 8 (22 percent) pleural capping. In 8 (22 percent) there was no chest x-ray. In these last eight, suspicion of an aneurysm was raised on other studies such as CT scan. All patients had associated injuries, the most common being orthopedic. There were also a large number of central nervous system and abdominal injuries.

When the diagnosis is made, operation is indicated. However, many patients have associated injuries and it is important to decide which injuries should be treated first. In the seven patients in our series who had only thoracic trauma, only a thoracotomy was required. Of this group 5 were in profound shock and thoracotomy was performed in the emergency room. Three of the 5 survived.

Sixteen patients had associated orthopedic injuries. They were all operated on for aneurysm first and had the orthopedic repair later. Three patients had a thoracotomy followed by immediate laparotomy. One of these was a patient whose thoracotomy was initiated in the emergency room. The thoracic aorta was cross-clamped and the patient was resuscitated and brought to the operating room. He had resection of his aorta but exsanguinated from massive injuries of his liver and spleen. Seven patients had laparotomy first, followed by repair of the thoracic aorta.

The operative technique involves a posterolateral thoracotomy. Proximal control is obtained by clamping the aorta, usually, between the left carotid and left subclavian arteries. Distal control is usually obtained just beyond the point of rupture. In some instances, a Gott, heparinized shunt was used, however, most of these patients have large mediastinal hematomas which makes this technically difficult. All patients had interposition prostheses in this series.

We encountered 3 multiple tears in the aorta, proximal to the ligamentum. They require repair using cardiopulmonary bypass. The presence of these multiple aortic tears into the transverse arch was not predicted but pre-operative aortic angiography but was discovered intra-operatively.

We have evolved a philosophy that cardiopulmonary bypass may be required in any thoracic aortic injury and a perfusion team is on stand by. In most instances their intervention is not required but, if it is, they need to be immediately available.

Of 5 patients who underwent emergency room thoracotomy, 2 recovered. Three of the 5 patients presenting in shock died. Of the remaining 31 patients, in 25 a so-called "clamp and sew" technique was used. That is no surgical adjuncts were used to decrease afterload or augment the distal circulation. Of those 25, there were 3 deaths, four instances of spinal ischemia with paralysis including 1 patient who developed renal failure. In 5 additional patients we used a Gott shunt. In these 5 there were no deaths and no complications. Cardiopulmonary bypass was employed in only one patient, who survived without complications.

Analysis of the time of transport from the accident scene to our trauma center proved to be important. The average time for those patients who lived was 45 minutes as opposed to 75 minutes for those who did not survive. Additionally, the greater the Injury Severity Score, the greater the mortality.

This was statistically significant ($p < 0.05$). The multiplicity of injuries resulted in increased morbidity and mortality.

Overall, 30 of 36 patients survived, for a survival rate of 83 percent. We had an incidence of paraplegia of 9 percent in the survivors, which is consistent with current literature. {8} The average aortic cross-clamp time was 26 minutes. However, in those patients that developed spinal cord ischemia, the clamp time was prolonged as it was in 3 of the patients with multiple tears of the aorta. Of the 4 patients with spinal cord insult, 2 had permanent paraplegia and 2 had spasticity in the lower extremities. The one patient who had acute renal failure was also one of those who had paraplegia.

There were no complications when we used the Gott shunt. We found no complications in the one patient that underwent cardiopulmonary bypass. Prosthetic grafts were placed in all patients. No infections, late deaths, or reoperations have been observed. All the patients have been followed for over a year and all have done well.

Spinal cord ischemia continues to be a problem. {13,14} Despite reports of a variety of experimental modalities to provide protection, none of these have been proven consistently effective. {13,15} Important factors include the anatomic origin of the artery of Adamcawicz which is difficult to identify, and a speedy operation. We found that in those patients who had an expeditious procedure, resulting in a clamp time of approximately 26 minutes, there were few complications. When clamp time was prolonged, complications resulted. Similar findings have been reported in the literature. {8,15}

Thoracic aortic injury requires prompt diagnosis and surgical repair. The outcome is related to the time interval from injury to transport to the operating room. In the polytraumatized patient, even though signs and symptoms may be subtle, a high index of suspicion for this injury is necessary. At a minimum, an erect chest x-ray should be done. An aortogram should be performed if there is any suspicion whatsoever.

Important factors are the timing of the thoracotomy in relationship to the other injuries. There should be some attempt, if possible, to maintain circulation to the distal arteries, especially, if prolonged aortic cross-clamp time is anticipated. We believe the clamp and sew technique is safe. However, cardiopulmonary bypass may be required depending on operative findings and needs to be on hand for complicated aortic injuries. The operative technique has to be adjusted to the type of aortic injury found at exploration.

REFERENCES

1. Hartford JM, Fayer RL, Shaver TE: Transection of the thoracic aorta; assessment of a trauma system. Am J Surg 1986; 151:224–9.

2. Pate JW: Traumatic rupture of the aorta: Emergency operation. Ann Thorac Surg 1985; 39:531–7.

3. Avery JE, Hall DP, Adams JE, et al: Traumatic rupture of the thoracic aorta. South Med J 1979; 72:1238–40.

4. DelRossi AJ, Cernaianu AC, Madden LD, Cilley JH Jr, et al: Traumatic disruptions of the thoracic aorta: Treatment and outcome. Surgery 1990; 108(5):864–870.

5. Schwab CW, Lawson RB, Lind JF, et al: Aortic injury: Comparison of supine and upright portable chest films to evaluate the widened mediastinum. Ann Emerg Med 1984; 13:896–899.

6. Alexander JB and Camishion RC: Thoracic vascular trauma. Topics in Emerg Med 1990; 12:33–43.

7. DelRossi AJ, Cernaianu AC, Cilley JH, et al: Multiple traumatic disruptions of the thoracic aorta. Chest 1990; 97:1307–09.

8. DeBakey ME, McCollum CH, Graham JM: Surgical treatment of aneurysms of the descending thoracic aorta. Long-term results in 500 patients. J Cardiovasc Surg 1978; 19:571–6.

9. Richardson JD, McElvein RB, Trinkle JK: First rib fracture: a hallmark of severe trauma. Ann Surg 1975; 181:251–254.

10. Fisher RG, Wand RD, Ben-Menachem, et al: Arteriography and the fractured first rib: Too much or too little? AJR 1982; 138:1059.

11. Woodring JH, Fried AM, Hatfield DR, et el: Fracture of first and second ribs: predictive value for arterial and bronchial injury. AJR 1982; 138:211.

12. Fermanis GG, Deane SA, Fitzgerald PM: The significance of first and second rib fractures. Aust NZJ Surg 1985; 55:383–386.

13. Crawford ES, Feastermacher JM, Richardson W, et al: Reappraisal of adjuncts to avoid ischemia in the treatment of thoracic aneurysms. Surgery 1970; 67:182–96.

14. Marvasti MA, Meyer JA, Ford BE, Parker FB Jr: Spinal cord ischemia following operation for traumatic aortic transection. Ann Thoracic Surg 1986; 42:425–8.

15. Najafi H, Javid H, Hunter J, Serry C, et al: Descending aortic aneurysmectomy without adjuncts to avoid ischemia. Ann Thorac Surg 1980; 30:326–35.

CARDIOMYOPLASTY

Ray C.-J. Chiu, M.D., Ph.D.

McGill University
Montreal, Quebec, Canada

INTRODUCTION

Dynamic cardiomyoplasty is a relatively new and still evolving surgical procedure for patients suffering from heart failures. [1] This chapter attempts to address many clinical issues associated with this procedure, based primarily on the author's experience and bias. References[2] are provided for readers who wish to explore in depth some of the issues raised in this chapter.

CURRENT STATE

Although the concept of using skeletal muscle to assist circulation has been around for many decades, [3] dynamic cardiomyoplasty as we know now was developed in surgical research laboratories during the late 1970's to early 1980's. [4] A number of fundamental biological problems associated with the application of skeletal muscle for cardiac assist were addressed during this phase. The issue of skeletal muscle fatigue upon repetitive and prolonged stimulation was dealt with by skeletal muscle transformation induced by low frequency electrical stimulation. [5] In the meantime, a synchronizable burst stimulator was developed to recruit motor units of the skeletal muscle, in order to generate contractile duration and force analogous to those of the myocardium. [6] The early laboratory studies were rapidly applied to clinical patients in the mid 1980's, [7] which attracted interest for this operation in a number of cardiac centers around the world.

Since an electrical stimulator which can synchronize the skeletal muscle contraction with the cardiac cycle is required for the dynamic component of this procedure, the more than 200 patients operated on so far in many continents can be divided into three groups. The first group of patients, who were operated on in Europe, North America and most of South America, received a Medtronic SP1005(R) cardiomyostimulator. This is the largest group comprising almost 150 patients. Most of the scientific data available in the western countries come from these patients. The second group of 26 patients operated on in the republics of the old Soviet Union and in India, were implanted with the Russian made Stiminak stimulator and its successor devices. The third group of patients operated on in a few countries in South America, notably in Cuba, received the single pulse, double chamber (DDD) pacemakers. Rigorous scientific data from the latter two groups are scarce, and thus most of the discussions below will be based on patients who received the cardiomyostimulator SP1005(R). [8]

Medtronic Company, which manufactures the cardiomyostimulator SP1005(R), has been sponsoring an FDA approved program to test their device. The first phase, which ended in the spring of 1991, comprises of approximately 120 patients from centers in Europe, North and South America. [8] In North America, two centers, Allegheny General Hospital of Pittsburgh and the author's group at McGill University, Montreal, Canada, participated. The purpose of this phase was to evaluate the safety and function of the device as well as the feasibility of the procedure. In the last year, phase II study has been conducted with participation of four additional centers in the U. S. The data are now being collected according to protocol in a prospective manner, and case match controls are recruited. In entering phase III in the near future, in which a prospective randomized control study is expected, rapid but orderly expansion of participating centers is likely.

PATIENT SELECTION

The primary candidates for this procedure are patients who suffer from intractable heart failure. Although a few patients have been operated upon for right heart failure and as a reinforcement in Fontan procedure to overcome increased pulmonary vascular resistance, the great majority of patients were operated upon for left ventricular failures. [8] Most of them had either idiopathic dilated cardiomyopathy or ischemic cardiomyopathy. A few of them were operated on for cardiac tumors. One interesting group in South America is patients with Chagas disease, in whom cardiac transplantation is contraindicated as the new heart can be rapidly infected with the parasite. [9] Thus, the most common candidate for cardiomyoplasty is a patient with heart failure who is deteriorating in spite of maximum medical therapy. [1]

There are a number of obvious contra-indications, such as in one who had prior thoracotomy, resulting in transection of the latissimus dorsi muscle which is to be used for cardiomyoplasty. The experience in the phase I study has shown that terminal, New York Heart Association Functional Class IV patients, when operated upon, had early mortality exceeding 30 percent. By selecting patients in Class III, the operative mortality can be reduced to around 10 percent[8]. Thus, the candidates for cardiomyoplasty are not the same as those for heart transplantation, since the patients undergoing cardiomyoplasty have to survive with medical therapy alone for several weeks before benefit from surgery can be expected. In order to quantify the severity of heart failure for cardiomyoplasty, it had been suggested that only patients with left ventricular ejection fraction greater than 15 percent, and right ventricular ejection fraction greater than 35 percent should be chosen. [10] Although these guidelines have been developed in a few centers based on uni-variant analysis of a relatively small sample size, we have found these not to be reliable indicators of suitability for cardiomyoplasty. We have a number of patients with pre-operative left ventricular ejection fraction below

15 percent, and in a couple of them below 10 percent, who had excellent post-operative recovery following this procedure. Virtually all of our patients selected for this operation had a right ventricular ejection fraction below 35 percent. {11}

Another contra-indication is severe and poorly controlled arrhythmias. Sudden death due to ventricular tachyarrhythmia and fibrillation continues to be a threat intra-operatively and following operation. Due to the high incidence of serious arrhythmias in the target population, it is recommended that routine electrophysiological consultations be obtained prior to the selection of patients, and continued collaboration with cardiologists with expertise in electrophysiology, during both the peri- and post-operative periods. Certain intra- and post-operative precautions to prevent fatal arrhythmias will be discussed in the following section.

A number of factors would make surgery technically more difficult. One of them is the severe adhesion in the pleural space and pericardium, as extensive dissection may be required to allow the transposition of the latissimus dorsi muscle flap into the pleural cavity, and then wrapping it around the heart. Patients with severely restricted pulmonary function will be a poor candidate, in part because of the risk of hypoxia and arrhythmia associated with compression of the left lung by a bulky muscle mass, both intra-operatively and in the early post-operative period.

We do not consider controllable diabetes, hypertension and other systematic diseases, which are thought to be unfavorable factors in selecting patients for heart transplantation, to be necessarily contra-indications for cardiomyoplasty. We and others have operated on patients with a history of diseases such as diabetes, ulcerative colitis, {11} Chagas disease, {9} etc., provided these conditions are medically controlled.

We also entertain certain "temporary" contra-indications. {1} They are temporary because the cardiomyoplasty procedure is still in an experimental trial stage of development. Once fully established as a viable therapeutic modality, these factors will no longer be considered contra-indications. For example, if a relatively young patient who is an optimal candidate for heart transplantation is presented to us, we would prefer to offer cardiac transplantation as the procedure of choice, simply because transplantation is a more established operative procedure at this time than dynamic cardiomyoplasty. Likewise, patients with conditions which can benefit from conventional procedures, such as coronary artery bypass, ventricular aneurysmectomy and valve surgery, are temporarily excluded from our cardiomyoplasty program, as these concurrent procedures would become confounding factors in analyzing the outcome of patients, thus making the scientific evaluation of the efficacy of cardiomyoplasty more difficult. Again, once the clinical merit of cardiomyoplasty is established, concurrent surgery may be not only permissible, but also desirable for many of such patients.

PRE- AND INTRA-OPERATIVE MANAGEMENT

Pre-operatively, a detailed history and cardiology consultations are essential to verify that the patients are in deteriorating heart failure in spite of optimal medical therapy. Both indications and contra-indications discussed above are verified. Routine pre-op studies for open heart surgery are carried out, including cardiac catheterization, ultrasound studies, as well as other procedures which are mandated by the protocol. In view of the high incidence and seriousness of complications associated with tachyarrhythmia, we routinely obtain Holter monitoring of cardiac rhythms and electrophysiological consultation.

The detailed operative procedure will not be discussed here as it has been described elsewhere. {12,13} Some variations exist on the operative approach, depending on the centers. {14} The most commonly used method involves the use of the left latissimus dorsi, with a two-stage operation carried out in the same setting. {13} First the patient is placed in the right lateral position and the left latissimus dorsi muscle flap raised. The muscle stimulating electrodes are implanted, and both the muscle and the electrodes are then introduced into the left pleural cavity through the bed of a resected rib. Following closure of the wound, the patient is turned to the supine position and a sternal splitting incision carried out to expose the heart, implanting the sensing electrodes on the ventricle, and wrapping the latissimus dorsi muscle around the heart. Both clockwise and counter-clockwise wrap (as seen from the apex) have been carried out. We have used clockwise wrap to ensure adequate muscle mass over the left ventricle and, if the muscle length is not sufficient to achieve complete wrap, a pericardial flap is used to supplement the wrap, usually over the right ventricular outflow tract. Both the sensing and stimulating electrodes are connected to the cardiomyostimulator which is then implanted into a subcutaneous pocket in the upper abdomen.

The cardiopulmonary bypass machine has always been fully primed and on standby, but would be rarely needed in properly selected patients who are not undergoing concomitant cardiac surgery. We also prophylactically introduce a guide wire through a femoral artery to allow for rapid percutaneous access for insertion of an intra-aortic balloon pump if required. During the procedure, after the stimulating electrodes have been placed into the latissimus dorsi muscle near the thoracodorsal nerve, electrical stimulations are delivered to test both the threshold and the contractile pattern of the muscle to assure the proper positioning of the electrodes. It is important to remember that at this point, muscle relaxants either are not used, or are neutralized appropriately, since otherwise the muscle would not respond to electrical stimulation. Following the introduction of the muscle flap into the left pleural cavity, appropriate ventilatory control by the anesthesiologist needs to be assured in order to avoid hypoxia, as these hearts are sensitive to such insults. We routinely use a double lumen endotracheal tube so that the ventilation to the right lung, at least, can be fully controlled by the anesthesiologist. {15} During the early phase of muscle wrapping, when a portion of the muscle is to be slipped behind the heart and transfixed along the posterior AV groove, the heart may be irritated and develop arrhythmias as it needs to be elevated and manipulated. First, we start xylocaine drip prior to such maneuver to reduce ventricular irritability. Second, the procedure is planned in such a way that elevation and irritation of the heart is kept as brief as possible. In completing the wrap of the muscle around the heart, we approximate the muscle edges together over the heart snugly, but without undue tension. The earlier concern that lack of resting tension may reduce the efficacy of muscle contraction upon electrical stimulation in accordance with Frank-Starling's law appears to be irrelevant for this procedure. There are a number of experimental evidence indicating that, over time, the skeletal muscle can conform to its new geometric configuration and resting length by altering the number of sarcomeres, so that an optimal resting tension can be restored. {16} Experimentally as well as in anecdotal clinical cases where the muscle had been wrapped too tight around the heart, acute reduction in cardiac function was observed.

Recently, we have proposed that one of the reasons that patients, after cardiomyoplasty, demonstrated varying degrees of clinical and hemodynamic improvements may be in part related to the completeness of muscle wrap around the heart. {17} Thus, we attempt to introduce virtually all the latissimus dorsi muscle available into the chest cavity for wrapping purpose, and transfer the humerus tendon of this muscle to the periosteum of the resected rib, rather than to the rib above as we and others have done previously. {1}

POST-OPERATIVE CARE AND MUSCLE TRANSFORMATION

In the intensive care unit, medical management needs to be optimized to support the cardiac function and control rhythm disturbances. Appropriate inotropic and anti-arrhythmic drugs are used, and ventilator supports are continued until spontaneous breathing assures that hypoxia would not develop. Seroma in the back where the latissimus dorsi muscle was dissected out occurs frequently, which could usually be managed with a closed drainage system and occasional late tapping. Hemorrhagic complications are rare as patients are usually not heparinized and cardiopulmonary bypass not employed. Upon returning to the ward, we allow a period of one to two weeks for "vascular delay", under the assumption that the extensively dissected latissimus dorsi muscle flap needs time to recover from peripheral ischemia, as some of the collaterals from intercostal vessels have been divided. After the vascular delay period, skeletal muscle transformation is initiated by weekly programming of the cardiomyostimulator, starting with a single pulse delivered every second heart beat, to three or four impulses delivered to every heart beat or every second heart beat, generally within three to four weeks of the initiation of the transformation protocol. {18} Burst frequency of 20 to 30 Hz is commonly used. {19} Although both the vascular delay and transformation protocols are based on some experimental laboratory observations in animals, these have not so far been verified as the optimal choice in patients, and it is possible that this preparatory phase may be speeded up in future trials.

Upon the completion of muscle transformation when the fatigue resistance of the skeletal muscle wrap is assured, the electrical burst stimulation parameters need to be adjusted periodically, preferably under ultrasonic guidance. The first important parameter is the delay between the sensing of R-wave and the initiation of burst stimulation. This is particularly important in patients with intra-ventricular conduction defects, since burst stimulation may occur prior to the closure of the mitral valve. This may aggravate mitral regurgitation which is commonly associated with markedly dilated hearts in such patients. The initiation of burst can be adjusted to follow immediately after the closure of the mitral valve and opening of the aortic valve as judged by ultrasound. The second stimulation parameter that has to be adjusted is the burst duration. It is important to remember that the cessation of electric burst does not coincide with the complete relaxation of the muscle. {20} This interval between the end of electrical burst stimuli and complete relaxation of the skeletal muscle becomes progressively prolonged during transformation of the skeletal muscle, since the Type I fatigue resistant muscles are composed of slow twitch fibers, with a markedly reduced rate of muscle contraction and relaxation. Long burst stimulation could lead to maintenance of muscle flap tension around the heart, thus impair the diastolic filling of the ventricle. The observation by many investigators that their patients' cardiac function appeared to be better with 2:1 ratio stimulation may be a reflection of this phenomenon. A third stimulation parameter which needs to be adjusted is the voltage delivered to stimulate the latissimus dorsi muscle flap. Too low a voltage would produce inadequate muscle contraction, whereas excessively high voltage would waste the battery life. Unfortunately, at this time, there seems to be no quantitative way to optimize the voltage required, and most of us use the quality of contraction which can be palpated under the axilla. This contraction is produced by the extra-thoracic end of the latissimus dorsi muscle being stimulated. There have been suggestions that radio-opaque markers be placed on the muscle, and a fluoroscope be used to observe the displacement of these markers and use this as a guide to adjust the required voltage. More documentation of the efficacy of such measures needs to be carried out.

FOLLOW-UP AND EVALUATION

The post-operative follow-up is similar to any cardiac surgery patient, with periodic monitoring and adjustment of the stimulation parameters to optimize cardiac function, as judged by the patient's clinical response, ultrasonography and radionuclide scan. With improvement, the patient's medication may be re-adjusted, and appropriate exercise encouraged. We have not excluded patients with atrial fibrillation from our acceptance criteria, and in most cases, this has not been a problem provided that the ventricular response rate is properly controlled with medications. {11} It is important to remember that attempted electrical conversion of atrial fibrillation may deplete the battery of the cardiomyostimulator. Likewise, defibrillation for ventricular tachyarrhythmia may cause immediate or premature cessation of cardiomyostimulator function. Although the cardiomyostimulator so damaged needs to be replaced, experience showed that the deterioration in the patient's condition following the dysfunction of the cardiomyostimulator seems to appear gradually over days, unlike those of patients with complete heart block who are completely dependent on pacemakers. {9} On the other hand, prolonged absence of stimulation of the skeletal muscle may cause, not only the deterioration of the hemodynamic condition of the patient, but also the reversal of the skeletal muscle fiber type to a more fatigue prone Type II fibers. Thus, theoretically, a skeletal muscle which has not been subjected to electrical stimulation for more than a couple of weeks may require re-transformation when stimulation is resumed.

The clinical endpoints used for follow-up and evaluation of a patient's clinical outcome need to reflect the mechanism of dynamic cardiomyoplasty currently postulated. Originally, cardiomyoplasty was thought to be beneficial to the heart failure patients through its systolic assistance. In many patients, this is probably true, as increase in stroke volume, and ejection fraction were associated with clinical improvement. {9,11} In others, gradual improvement seen clinically was not matched by corresponding increase in systolic function. These patients may in fact benefit from what we call "myocardial sparing effect" due to reduced myocardial strain. {17} The mechanism of improvement in these latter patients may be somewhat similar to those observed following vasodilator and ACE inhibitor therapies. As the ejection fraction correlates with exercise capacity poorly, other laboratory endpoints need to be used to gauge the progress of these patients. It has also been suggested that cardiomyoplasty delays the continued dilation of the ventricle, resulting in ventricular remodelling and prolonged survival. To confirm this theory, a prospective controlled study envisioned in the phase III trial will be required.

FUTURE PERSPECTIVE AND THE CONCEPT OF "HEART FAILURE SURGERY GROUP"

Further clinical experience and rigorous scientific trials are required to conclusively establish both the usefulness of this procedure and the precise target population to whom this operation can be applied. Experience so far has demonstrated the desirability of having more advanced capabilities for the cardiomyostimulator, including the self-adjusting of burst duration depending on the heart rate, and eventual incorporation of defibrillation capability, in view of the high incidence of sudden death in these patients. The optimal programming parameters for the stimulator, as well as the possible change over time of these parameters, need to be elucidated. {20} Ultimately, we envision the establishment in large cardiac centers of "heart failure surgical group". Patients with intractable heart failure will be scrutinized for the most appropriate surgical therapy, which may include heart transplantation, cardiomyoplasty and mechanical assist devices. Some of such mechanical devices may be powered by transformed fatigue resistant muscle, rather than by compressed air or electric motors. Each modality has its advantages and disadvantages, and an integrated approach may facilitate the selection of individualized, cost effective mode of therapy for each patient.

REFERENCES

1. Chiu RCJ: Dynamic cardiomyoplasty: An overview. Pacing & Clin. Electrophysiol 1991; 14:557.

2. Chiu RCJ: Dynamic cardiomyoplasty. Ann Thorac Surg 1992; 54:592.

3. Walsh G, Chiu RCJ: Skeletal muscle for cardiac repair and assist: Historical overview, in Biomechanical Cardiac Assist: Cardiomyoplasty and Muscle Powered Devices, RCJ Chiu, ed., Futura Publishing Co. Inc., Mount Kisco, New York 1986:1–18.

4. Dewar ML, Drinkwater D, Wittnich C, Chiu RCJ: Synchronously stimulated skeletal muscle graft for myocardial repair. J Thorac Cardiovasc Surg 1984; 87:325.

5. Salmons S, Sreter FA: Significance of impulse activity in the transformation of skeletal muscle type. Nature 1967; 263:30.

6. Drinkwater DC, Chiu RCJ, Modry D, Wittnich C, Brown PR: Cardiac assist and myocardial repair with synchronously stimulated skeletal muscle. Surg Forum 1980; 31:271.

7. Carpentier A, Chachques JC: Myocardial substitution with a stimulated skeletal muscle: First successful clinical case. Lancet 1985; 8440:1267.

8. Grandjean PA, Austin L, Chan S, Terpstra B, Bourgeois IM: Dynamic cardiomyoplasty: Clinical follow-up results. J Card Surg 1991; 6:80.

9. Jatene A, et al: Left ventricular function changes after cardiomyoplasty in patients with dilated cardiomyopathy. J Thorac Cardiovasc Surg 1991; 102:132.

10. Magovern JA, Furnary AP, Christlieb IY, Kao RL, Park SB, Magovern GJ: Indications and risk analysis for clinical cardiomyoplasty. Semin Thorac Cardiovasc Surg 1991; 3:145.

11. Chiu RCJ, Odim JNK, Burgess JH: Responses to dynamic cardiomyoplasty for dilated cardiomyoplasty. American J. Cardiology 1993; 72:475.

12. Chachques JC, Grandjean PA, Carpentier A: Latissimus dorsi dynamic cardiomyoplasty. Ann Thorac Surg 1989; 47:600.

13. Chiu RCJ, Odim JNK, Blundell PE, Williams HB: Dynamic cardiomyoplasty. In: Atlas on Heart and Lung Transplantation, AS Kapoor et al, (eds.). McGraw Hill, New York (in press), 1993.

14. Magovern JA, Furnary AP, Christlieb IY, Kao RL, Magovern GJ: Right latissimus dorsi cardiomyoplasty for left ventricular failure. Ann Thorac Surg 1992; 53:1120.

15. Robinson RJS, Truong DT, Odim JNK, Chiu RCJ: Anesthesia for dynamic cardiomyoplasty. J Cardiovasc Anaesth 1992; 6:476.

16. Herring SW, Grimm AF, Grimm BR: Regulation of sarcomere number in skeletal muscle: A comparison of hypothesis. Muscle & Nerve 1984; 7:161.

17. Chiu RCJ: Dynamic cardiomyoplasty: Efficacy and mechanisms. Card Chron (in press), 1993.

18. Carpentier A, Chachques JC: The use of stimulated skeletal muscle to replace diseased human heart muscle. In Biomechanical Cardiac Assist: Cardiomyoplasty and Muscle Powered Devices RCJ Chiu, ed., Futura Publishing Co. Inc., Mount Kisco, New York 1986:85–102.

19. Chiu RCJ, Walsh GL, Dewar ML, DeSimon JH, Khallafalla AS, Ianuzzo D: Implantable extra-aortic balloon assist powered by transformed fatigue resistant skeletal muscle. J Thorac Cardiovasc Surg 1987; 94:694.

20. Pekarsky VV, Akhmedov ShD, Dubrovsky IA, et al: The choice of optimal regimes of electrical stimulation for latissimus dorsi muscle in different periods after the operation of cardiomyoplasty. J Card Surg 1993; 8:172.

CURRENT STATUS OF AUTOTRANSFUSION

Roger A. Vertrees, B.A., C.C.P. and
Aurel C. Cernaianu, M.D.*

University of Texas Medical Branch
Galveston, Texas

*University of Medicine and Dentistry of New Jersey
Robert Wood Johnson Medical School
Camden, New Jersey

Predeposit autologous blood programs to collect and store blood and/or blood components for later reinfusion have become popular and widely available particularly since more information has become available in regard to the potential of such transfusion for alloimmunization, transmission of viral or bacterial diseases. The main purpose of autologous blood transfusion is to decrease the demand for banked blood. This chapter will discuss the techniques of autotransfusion developed especially for blood conservation.

The maintenance of red cell mass is accomplished by either preventing blood loss or salvaging blood for reuse. According to LaVeen, [1] the optimal hematocrit (Hct) for normal oxygen delivery is about 30 percent. At a Hct of 20 to 50 percent, oxygen delivery varies only slightly. Aside from restoring red cell mass, autotransfusion may be beneficial in preservation of other blood components and maintaining normal coagulation profile, and osmotic pressure. However, according to Klimberg, [2] the primary role of autotranfusion is to avoid the use of homologous blood products and reduce the complications associated with transfusion therapy.

Red cell mass augmentation may be accomplished by homologous, or autologous transfusions and blood component therapy. The advantages of conserving ones own blood rather than administering homologous transfusions are primarily related to the fact that autologous blood therapy does not cause significant morbidity resulting from rare blood types or transfusion reactions. The use of homologous blood products has been associated with febrile, allergic and hemolytic reactions, alloimmunization, and the transmission of viral disease such as hepatitis and acquired immune deficiency syndrome (AIDS). The use of these techniques in the management of cancer patients may avoid the occurrence of transfusion-induced immuno-suppression. [3] Autotransfusions are better accepted by patients with religious objections to blood transfusions. In addition, the autologous blood may be more readily available and perhaps of better quality. {4} Autologous transfusion, may be applied in the preoperative, intraoperative, and the postoperative period. Each phase of autologous blood conservation will be discussed individually with its own advantages and disadvantages.

PRE-OPERATIVE BLOOD DONATION

Preoperative blood donation represents the intentional collection and storage of blood in preparation for reinfusion at the time of operation or in the postoperative period. Unfortunately, only approximately 5 percent of the performed surgical procedures are combined with this technique, although almost any patient qualifies for preoperative donation, except for emergent cases or patients with concurrent anemias. {5} Scott et al. {6} studied the impact of blood predonation in cardiac surgery and demonstrated a reduction of 72 percent in the use of homologous blood, having patients donating only an average of 2 units of blood starting approximately 18 days prior to the surgical procedure. The predonation resulted in a decrease of only 2.2 g/dL in the preoperative hemoglobin level which is for most people usually clinically insignificant. Autologous blood predonation is a relatively safe and easy procedure to perform, requiring only simple monitoring similar to that used during any other blood donation. When a patient's baseline hemoglobin level is in normal range, donation can be performed as often as 1 unit every 4 days. Oral iron supplementation prior to donation and during the procedure and volume support with isotonic solution may increase the chance of maintaining normal Hct with no hemodynamic consequences.

Autologous predeposit has its own set of drawbacks. There are different requirements for the blood bank concerning handling of the autologous blood. Since autologous and homologous blood banking have different life spans, homologous blood is generally fractionated. Most importantly, the autologous blood is intended for use in a specific individual, therefore, there is a need for perfect coordination between the blood bank and the surgical team. A good and reliable system of labeling and tracking the blood is necessary. This may result in additional paperwork and costs. Generally, the cost charged to the patient is slightly higher than for each unit of homologous red cells. The safety of autologous predonation has been studied by Mann et al. {7} who demonstrated that, indeed, almost every patient undergoing cardiac surgery qualified for blood predonation. Hemodynamic instability and concurrent anemias with progressing angina occurred in only 3 to 7 percent of the patients.

The American Association of Blood Banks has developed guidelines for autologous predeposit programs. {8} There is basically no age limit for patients who want to donate blood. The maximum amount of blood drawn at one time should not exceed 450 mL or 12 percent of the patient's calculated blood volume. Simultaneous isovolemic fluid replacement should accompany blood predonation. The patient's Hct should be greater than 34 percent at the time of donation. Finally, there should be no more than one unit of blood collected every three days, and the patient should receive supplemental ferrous sulfate (325 mg three times daily) prior to the first donation which should be continued for several months thereafter.

INTRAOPERATIVE TECHNIQUES

Attempts to conserve blood intraoperatively has lead to the development of many different techniques which may focus on either limiting the amount of blood lost or on reclaiming the blood that was shed. Currently, approximately 75 percent of all blood administered during hospitalization is given in the perioperative period. [9] Therefore, any attempt to reduce blood loss during this time period would have a major impact on the nation's blood resources. Presently, there are numerous conservation techniques such as intraoperative phlebotomy and sequestration, cell saver, hemoconcentration, shed blood collection, and a newly introduced process of autologous whole blood processing.

Intraoperative Phlebotomy

Intraoperative phlebotomy is the removal of whole blood in the operating room after the induction of anesthesia. In most cases, 15 to 20 percent of the patient's blood volume can be collected. [10] This technique requires the insertion of a large bore central catheter for blood withdrawal, and an anticoagulated collection chamber for short-term storage. The collected blood is maintained at room temperature, and is agitated very gently to prevent platelet aggregation and rouleaux formation. As in the case of the predeposit program, simultaneous isovolemic replacement therapy is necessary. The blood is usually stored in the operating room, readily available during the surgical procedure, or, it can be saved and reinfused upon completion of the procedure. For cardiac surgical patients, intraoperative phlebotomy provides fresh and well-preserved autologous platelets, plasma proteins, and coagulation factors which have not been subjected to either cold temperatures, or to the effects of cardiopulmonary bypass. [11] The removal of the blood prior to the surgical procedure may result in a reduction of the blood cell mass which may be lost due to hemorrhage during surgery. According to Sherman et al. [10], the use of the intraoperative phlebotomy may result in a 20 to 58 percent reduction of homologous blood usage. There are, however, disadvantages associated with the intraoperative phlebotomy technique. The procedure cannot be offered to anemic patients, or in those who are hemodynamically unstable. Those with borderline hemodynamic stability, extensive monitoring is necessary. The collection of blood may take as long as 30 minutes. It should be remembered that the collected whole blood is anticoagulated, and this may influence the coagulation profile when it is returned to the patient.

Whole Venous Blood Sequestration

Venous sequestration is an alternative to the above–described technique and is mostly used in cardiac surgery. This procedure may result in the collection of approximately 4 units of blood immediately prior to bypass. The blood collection occurs after heparinization and cannulation, and usually immediately upon initiation of bypass. The initial blood venous return has a high Hct and it is diverted into a collection bag rather than the extracorporeal circuit. This results in a substantial sequestration of red cell mass. When the collection of approximately 800 to 1000 mL of blood is accomplished, the usual perfusion techniques are employed. This technique has been employed successfully with measurable amounts of blood being protected from the deleterious effects of bypass. {12–15}

Platelet-Rich Plasma

Platelet-rich plasma (PRP) sequestration is another technique that can be performed intraoperatively. Like intraoperative phlebotomy, approximately 20 percent of the patient's blood volume is slowly collected from a central catheter. The blood is then separated through a process of differential centrifugation, (a process which separates whole blood into its components according to the relative density of the components) into red blood cell concentrate and plasma. The red blood cell portion can be reinfused immediately or retained until its use is required. PRP, containing a large number of fresh platelets, is usually returned to the patient after the neutralization of heparin with protamine sulfate. Approximately 600 to 1000 mL of PRP may be sequestered and deposited in bags containing citrate, phosphate, and dextrose (CPD). A large number of platelets are preserved by this method. Giordono et al., {14} Jones et al., {15} and DelRossi et al. {16} were able to use this technique successfully for blood conservation. The technique may yield 5.5 to 7.7×10 viable platelets {11} with a reduced amount of contaminating white and red cells. {16}

During PRP sequestration, attention should be paid to establishing the appropriate withdrawal site, and monitoring the patient's hemodynamics. Anticoagulation is used to prevent clotting during sequestration and deposit, consequently, some anticoagulant will be returned to the patient at the time of PRP reinfusion.

Cell Saver Technique

Historically, the cell saver has played a major role in the reduction of homologous blood usage. {17,18} The shed blood is salvaged from the operative field with a special aspiration device and then collected and stored in a filtered reservoir. This filtration process removes debris such as bone fragments, suture material, or other foreign particles greater than 120 microns in size. The blood collected in the reservoir is then relocated into a Latham™ bowl and centrifuged at approximately 5,000 revolutions per minute for separation of blood into the red cells and plasma components (differential centrifugation). {19} The red cells are then washed with saline, and can be reinfused later as needed. Unfortunately, the remaining plasma portion is discarded, although it contains most of the platelets, coagulation factors, and other serum proteins. Typically, the volume of blood saved by this method is approximately 250 mL and has a hematocrit over 40 percent. {20} The red cells contain a higher level of 2,3-DPG and have a higher pH than stored blood. {3,21} The process does not substantially effect red cell survival{22} and the final product of cell-saving contains minimal red cell debris, plasma-free hemoglobin or anticoagulant. {23}

The technique's disadvantage consists in the fact that plasma component is discarded. The red cell concentrate contains no platelets, antithrombin III, protein C, plasminogen or other serum coagulation factors. {24} There is also a proportionate loss of serum elements and an increased activity of serum citrate. [25] Bull et al. [26] has recently demonstrated that washed and reinfused cell saver blood contains elements resulting from the destruction and activation of leukocytes which may initiate inflammatory processes such as those seen in adult respiratory distress syndrome. [26]

Ultrafiltration

Ultrafiltration is the process of removing particles according to their size. It requires the use of a hemoconcentrator. Since the technique is extracorporeal, the blood should be anticoagulated to prevent clotting. Ultrafiltration results from the pressure differential developed between the inlet and outlet ports. [27] Due to the differential pressure, plasma passes through a porous system separating it from the other blood components. The blood product is then reinfused into the patient. The most important factor which determines the efficacy of the ultrafiltration process is the pressure differential. Moreover, the size of the pores determine the size of the particles that are retained. Most hemoconcentrators remove molecules smaller than 17,000 daltons. This allows separating of such elements as plasma-free hemoglobin, and cell stroma. According to Boldt et al., [28] antithrombin III remains in the blood. Moreover, the hemoconcentrator may cause a slight reduction (6 to 7 percent) in the number of platelets. The degree of hemodilution contributes significantly to the device efficiency, i.e., the greater the degree of hemodilution, the more plasma water will be effectively removed. The ultrafiltration process becomes inefficient at Hct lower than 32 percent. Other major problems related to this technique are related to the fact that the procedure requires anticoagulation and is dependent upon the velocity of blood flow. [29]

The Salvage of Shed Blood

The collection of shed blood is a very important part of a perioperative blood conservation program. The typical collection device is basically composed of a holding chamber or reservoir, and a reinfusion device. An integral filter effectively removes particles greater than 250 microns. Hartz et al. [30] described the red cell product as "red cells suspended in serum." The typical unit of shed blood contains 20,000 to 100,000 platelets/mL. [31] According to Faris et al., [32] the filtered shed blood collected from orthopedic surgeries contains different amounts of fibrinogen. This technique of blood salvage does not affect the amount of protein C, however, it significantly decreases levels of coagulation factors including factors X, IX, VIII, VII, V and II. Antithrombin III and complement C3 and C5 have been found to be unaffected by the use of this technique. [32] To date, however, there is little information in the literature related to changes in the red cell survival with the shed salvage system. [33]

Shed blood is unwashed and may contain cellular debris, plasma-free hemoglobin and lysed cells, as well as anticoagulant. The blood/collection device interaction may activate the coagulation cascade and the reinfusion of large quantities of salvaged shed blood might initiate disseminated intravascular coagulopathy (DIC). [34,35] Shed blood obtained from orthopedic surgery contains large amounts of lipids and manufacturers, presently, try to develop and improve ways of removing it from the reinfused blood. Activation of complement and lipid peroxidase cascades by the reinfusion of the shed blood has also been suggested. {36} However, the use of reinfused shed blood has proved to be safe and effective, provided that the reinfused volume does not exceed 10 percent of the patient's blood volume.

Continuous Blood Filtration

Continuous blood filtration or autologous blood processing is a new technique currently entering in the blood conservation or salvage arena. The device employed in this technique uses a plasma filter instead of a spinning Latham™ bowl. The remaining hardware is similar to the cell saver. The main filter of the device is composed of two hollow disc shaped zones with a hydrophilic micro-pore filtering membrane located at the upper and lower surfaces of the membrane. Blood passes through these membranes propelled by a disc rotor. The supernatant is discharged into the waste bag. The filtration process results in a concentration of cellular components which are larger than the filter pores. The concentrated blood passes through a washing zone where saline is used for dilution of the previously concentrated cells. Two additional membranes serve again to remove the supernatant resulting in a reconcentrated, washed blood suspension of approximately 50 percent red blood cells. {37}

Autologous blood processing can be used continuously as a hemoconcentrator or intermittently as a cell saver. The process avoids cell spillage during the wash cycle, and may result in up to 72 percent of viable platelets. {38} Moreover, since the technique uses no spinning bowl, the red blood cells are not subjected to the usual centrifugation forces seen during cell washing. Although the resultant blood product is anticoagulated, most of the anticoagulant can be eliminated during the wash cycle. Serum proteins and other activated coagulation factors are also discarded, and the final product is a concentration of red and white blood cells and platelets.

Autologous Hemodilutional Autotransfusion

Autologous hemodilutional autotransfusion is a variation of the reinfusion process of the hemodiluted contents of the cardiopulmonary bypass circuit after completion of bypass without any further processing. No hemoconcentrator or cell saver is used. The benefits of this technique rest in the fact that generally large volume, usually in excess of 2 liters may be processed. The final product is anticoagulated and contains most of the coagulation factors and serum proteins. On the other side, the reinfused product contains anticoagulant, plasma-free hemoglobin, and some cell stroma. {39}

CONCLUSION

Blood conservation and the reduction of homologous blood usage has seen investigated by Boldt et al. {40} who studied six different techniques or combination of techniques for blood salvage. Patients in whom the technique of blood saver was used, presented with the least efficient blood conservation. This study demonstrated that different techniques and their combination may result in different degrees of effectiveness. Jones et al. {41} demonstrated a significant decrease in blood utilization only after maximum applications of a blood conservation program and acceptance of a lower Hct post-bypass, i.e., 20 percent instead of 25 percent. Ovrum et al. (42) analyzed 100 patients undergoing cardiac surgical procedures utilizing a blood conservation program consisting of preoperative predeposit, retransfusion of all pump contents, and the collection and the reinfusion of shed mediastinal blood. No patient received homologous blood postoperatively and only 5 patients received 1 to 2 units of fresh frozen plasma. The median Hct at discharge was 36 percent.

It is readily apparent that efforts to reduce the homologous blood usage may be successful. This may result in a decreased risk of transfusion-related morbidity and a reduction in related costs. Breyer et al. (43) demonstrated that regardless of the combination of the techniques used, a savings of 2 units of autologous blood, results in a significant reduction in hospital charges. A minimal efficient blood conservation program for a cardiac surgery patient consists in the limitation of unnecessary blood usage, and either, the use of predeposit in the preoperative period or venous sequestration immediately upon the initiation of bypass. When crystalloid cardioplegia is used, ultrafiltration of the bypass pump contents may be necessary. However, if blood cardioplegia is used, then reinfusion of all pump contents without further ultrafiltration or cell saving could be the best alternative (exceptions would be patients with large blood volumes). Finally, the collection and retransfusion of all shed mediastinal blood may be applied as long as the reinfused blood represents less than 10 percent of the patients blood volume. Should a larger volume be recovered, cell washing should be employed prior to reinfusion.

For the non-cardiac patient, i.e., vascular or orthopaedic, a minimal blood conservation approach should consist of a predeposit program, intraoperative cell saver, and the collection and reinfusion of shed blood.

According to Stehling(44) "it is often appropriate to employ more than one method of autologous transfusion, pharmacological measures and surgical hemostasis and the acceptance of lower hemoglobin levels, advice from transfusion medicine experts for homologous component blood therapy. Finally, the risk of homologous blood transfusion should not overshadow the life saving benefits."

REFERENCES

1. LaVeen HH: Normovolemic hemodilution and autotransfusion in surgery. In Haver JM, Thurer RL, Dawson RB (eds): "Autotransfusion" Elsevier, New York 1981:71–82.

2. Klimberg IW: Autotransfusion and blood conservation. Semin Surg Oncol 1989; 5:286–292

3. Martin E, et al: Autotransfusion systems (ATS). Crit Care Nur 1989; 9(7):65–73.

4. Dzik WH, Sherburne B: Intraoperative Blood Salvage: Medical Controversies. Trans Med Rev 1990; 4(3):208–235.

5. Toy PTCY, Strauss RG, Stehling LC, et al: Predeposited autologous blood for elective surgery. N Engl J Med 1987; 316:517–520.

6. Scott WJ, Kessler R, Wernly JA, et al: Blood conservation in cardiac surgery. Ann Thorac Surg 1990; 50:843–851.

7. Mann M, Sacks HJ, Goldfinger D: Safety of autologous blood donation prior to elective surgery for a variety of potentially "high-risk" patients. Transfusion 1983; 23:229–32.

8. Autologous transfusion. In: Walker RH, ed. American Association of Blood Banks (AABB) technical manual. Arlington, VA: American Association of Blood Banks 1990:433–448.

9. Wood L: Autotransfusion in the postanesthesia care unit. J Post Anesth Nurs 1991; 6(2):98–101.

10. Sherman MM, Dobrik DB, Dennis RC, Burger RL: Prediction of hematocrit changes in open heart surgery without blood transfusion. J Cardiovasc Surg (Torino) 1984; 25:545–548.

11. Aguilar C, Santos A, Sarrion MV, Pozo J, Timoned FL: Scheduled autotransfusion in orthopedic surgery. Rev Esp Anestesiol Reanim 1992; 39:19-21.

12. Dodrill FD, Marshall N, Nyboer J, Hughes CH, Derbyshire AJ, Stearns AB: The use of the heart-lung apparatus in human cardiac surgery. J Thorac Surg 1957; 33:60–73.

13. Cosgrove DM, Loop ID: Blood conservation in cardiac surgery. Cardiovasc Clin 1981; 12:165–175.

14. Giordano GF, Rivers SL, Chung GKT, et al: Autologous platelet-rich plasma in cardiac surgery: effect on intraoperative and postoperative transfusion requirements. Ann Thorac Surg 1988; 46:416–419.

15. Jones JW, McCoy TA, et al: Effects of intraoperative plasmapheresis on blood loss in cardiac surgery. Soc Thorac Surg 1990; 49:585-90.

16. DelRossi AJ, Cernaianu AC, Vertrees RA, Wacker C, Fuller SJ, Cilley JH Jr, Baldino WA: Platelet-rich plasma reduces postoperative blood loss after cardiopulmonary bypass. J Thorac Surg 1990; 100 (2):281–286.

17. Wilson JD, Taswell HF: Autotransfusion: historical review and preliminary report in a new method. Mayo Clin Proc 1968; 43:26–35.

18. Vertrees RA, Engelman RM, Johnson JW III, Auvil J, Breyer RH, Rousou JA: Blood conservation during open-heart surgery: A literature review. JECT 1986; 18:200–210.

19. Thurer RL, Lytle BW, et al: Reduction of postoperative donor blood requirement by use of the cell separator. Scand J Thorac Cardiovasc Surg 1985; 19:165–171.

20. Williamson KR, Taswell HF: Intraoperative blood salvage: a review. Trans Med 1991:16–29.

21. McCarthy PM, Popovsky MA, Schaff HV, Orszulak TA, Williamson KR, Taswell HF, Ilstrup DM: Effect of blood conservation efforts in cardiac operations at the Mayo Clinic. Mayo Clin Proc 1988; 63:225–229.

22. Ray JM, Flynn JC, Bierman AH: Erythrocyte survival following intraoperative autotransfusion in spinal surgery: an in vivo comparative study and 5-year update. Spine 1986; 11(9):879–882.

23. Elawad AA, Ohlin AK, Berntorp E, Nilsson IM, Fredin H: Intraoperative autotransfusion in primary hip arthroplasty. A randomized comparison with homologous blood. Acta Orthop Scand 1991; 62(6):557–562.

24. McShane AJ, Power C, Jackson JF, Murphy DF, MacDonald A, Moriarty DC, Otridge BW: Autotransfusion quality of blood prepared with a red cell processing device. Br J Anaesth 1987; 59:1035–1039.

25. Deleuze P, Intrator L, Liou A, Contremoulins I, Cachera JP, Loisance DY: Complement activation and use of a cell saver in cardiopulmonary bypass. ASAIO 1990; J:36:M179–181.

26. Bull BS, Bull MH: The salvaged blood syndrome: a sequel to mechanochemical activation of platelets and leukocytes?. Blood Cells 1990; 16(1):5–20.

27. Boldt J, Zickman B, Czeke A, Herold C, Dapper F, Hempelmann G: Blood conservation techniques and platelet function in cardiac surgery. Anesthesiology 1991; 75:426-32.

28. Boldt J, Zickman B, Fedderson B, Harold C, Dapper F, Hemplemann G: Six different hemofiltration devices for blood conservation in cardiac surgery. Ann Thorac Surg 1991; 51:747-53.

29. Shimizu T, Kudo T, Yamaguchi H, Ishimaru S, Furukawa K: Haptoglobin administration for hemolysis with autotransfusion of blood ultrafiltered after cardiopulmonary bypass. Kyobu Geka 1991; 44:206–210.

30. Hartz RS, Smith JA, et al: Autotransfusion after cardiac operation. Assessment of hemostatic factors. J Thorac Cardiovasc Surg 1988; 96(1):178–82.

31. Kongsgaard UE, Tilfsrud S, Brosstad F, Ovrum E, Bjrnskau L: Autotransfusion after open-heart surgery: characteristics of shed mediastinal blood and its influence on the plasma proteases in circulating blood. Acta Anaesthesiol Scand 1991; 35(1):71–6.

32. Faris PM, et al: Unwashed filtered shed blood collected after knee and hip arthroplasties. J Bone Joint Surg 1991; 73-A:1169–78.

33. Thorley PJ, Shaw A, Kent P, Ashley S, Parkin A, Kester RC: Dual tracer technique to measure salvaged red cell survival following autotransfusion in aortic surgery. Nucl Med Commun 1990; 11(5):369–74.

34. Schaff HV, Hauer JM, Bell WR, Gardner TJ, et al: Autotransfusion of shed mediastinal blood after cardiac surgery: a prospective study. J Thorac Cardiovasc Surg 1978; 75(4):632–41.

35. Cohen ND, Munoz A, Reitz BA, Ness PK, et al: Transmission of retroviruses by transfusion of screened blood in patients undergoing cardiac surgery. Ann Thorac Surg 1989; 47(3):400–6.

36. Fuller JA, Buxton BF, Picken J, Harris RA, Davies MJ: Hematological effects of reinfused mediastinal blood after cardiac surgery. Med J Aust 1991; 154(11):737–740.

37. The Plateletsplus™ Autotransfusion system. Technical manual. Advanced Haemotechnologies, 1992.

38. Gordon L: Laboratory evaluation of a compact autologous blood recovery system utilizing plasma filtration with continuous processing capabilities. AmSECT Proceedings 1992.

39. Soga K, Takigawa A, Nishihama M, Hirose Y: The efficacy of blood conservation technique for coronary artery bypass graft surgery. Jap J Anesthes 1991; 41(3):363–368.

40. Boldt J, Zickmann B, Herold C, Scholz S, Dapper F, Hempelmann G: Heparin management during cardiac surgery with respect to various blood conservation techniques. Surg 1992; 111(3):260–265.

41. Jones JW, Rawitscher RE, et al: Benefit from combining blood conservation measures in cardiac operations. Ann Thorac Surg 1991; 51:541–6.

42. Ovrum E, Holen EA, Lindstein-Rigndal MA: Heart surgery without blood transfusion. Eur J Cardiothorac Surg 1990; 110(6):694–697.

43. Breyer RH, Engelman RM, Rousou JA, Lemeshow S: Blood conservation for myocardial revascularization. Is it cost effective? J Thorac Cardiovasc Surg 1987; 93(4):512–522.

44. Stehling L: Autologous transfusion. Int Anesthesiol Clin 1990; 28(4):190–6.

TRANSESOPHAGEAL ECHOCARDIOGRAPHY IN CARDIAC SURGERY

William H. O'Connor, M.D.

University of Medicine and Dentistry of New Jersey
Robert Wood Johnson Medical School
Camden, New Jersey

Transesophageal echocardiography (TEE) involves the passage of a specialized endoscope into the esophagus and stomach to obtain ultrasound images of the heart. The TEE endoscope is equipped with one or more ultrasound transducers at the distal tip of the probe. Each transducer generates a wedge-shaped sector of ultrasound, as shown in Figure 1. The sector of ultrasound illustrated in this diagram is the horizontal or transverse

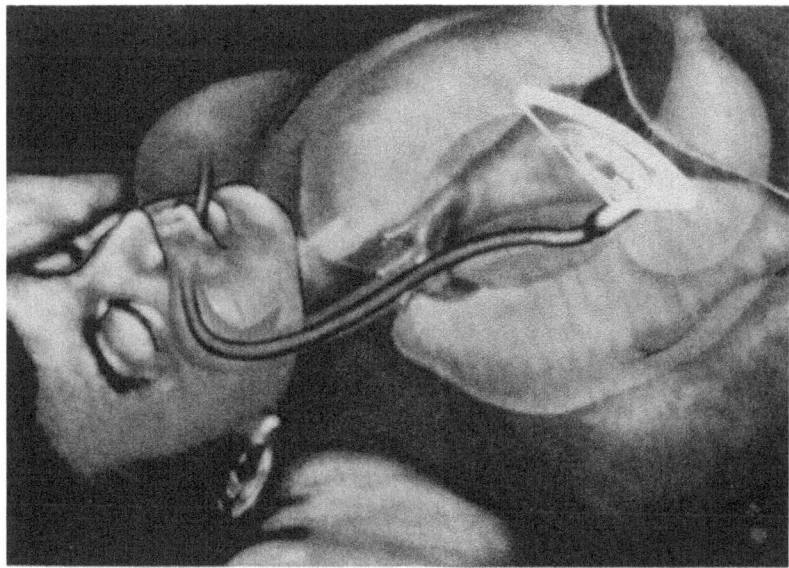

Figure 1. Diagram of a transesophageal echocardiography (TEE) probe in the esophagus with the horizontal imaging plane activated.

Cardiac Surgery: Current Issues 2, Edited by A. C. Cernaianu and A. J. DelRossi,
Plenum Press, New York, 1994

imaging plane, as will be described further below. The major advantage of the transesophageal window for ultrasound imaging is the proximity of the esophagus to the heart. This proximity allows the use of transducers of higher frequency, which have less depth of tissue penetration but are capable of producing images of significantly superior detail and resolution compared to standard transthoracic images. In addition, many of the obstacles to transmission of ultrasound encountered from the transthoracic window such as intervening bone, fresh surgical incisions, or air-filled lungs in patients on a respirator, do not affect imaging from the transesophageal window.

It should be noted that although esophageal intubation is quite easy well-tolerated, and safe in experienced hands, it does render the ultrasound examination "semi-invasive". Potential complications, which are similar to those of standard upper endoscopy, must always be weighed against the benefit of the information to be obtained in deciding which patients to perform this procedure on.

Table 1 lists some basic background information on TEE equipment and the type of information a TEE study is able to provide. There are three basic types of TEE probes currently available: 1. monoplane 2. biplane and 3. multiplane (also known as omniplane) probes. Also listed in this table are the ultrasound modalities available from the transesophageal window. Two-dimensional imaging only was available on the earliest generation of TEE probes. However all three Doppler blood flow modalities, i.e. color-flow, pulsed-wave and continuous-wave Doppler are also available on the newest generation of probes.

Although this discussion is not meant to be an exhaustive review of cardiac Doppler, the information on blood flow provided by the Doppler portion of the examination is a significant part of what makes TEE such a powerful tool in cardiac surgery patients. Examples of the use of each of these Doppler modalities will therefore be pointed out as appropriate throughout this discussion. Figure 2 illustrates the orthogonal planes of ultrasound that are generated by a biplane TEE probe. The horizontal plane is shown in the left half of the diagram, and is oriented perpendicular to the long axis of the probe shaft. This plane intersects the cardiac structures roughly in the transverse or horizontal plane of the body. The initial monoplane probes were designed to generate only this single transverse sector of ultrasound. In biplane probes, a second sector of ultrasound can be activated, which is parallel to the long-axis of the shaft of the TEE probe, as shown in the right half of Figure 2. This vertical plane is generated by a separate transducer

Table 1. Equipment and Type of Information Available

Probes	Monoplane
	Biplane
	Multiplane
Ultrasound Modalities Available	Imaging
	Doppler
	Color flow
	pulsed-wave
	continuous-wave

Figure 2. Diagram of biplane a TEE probe. Panel A
shows the horizontal ultrasound sector generated by
the distal transducer. Panel
B shows the vertical ultrasound sector generated by
the more proximal trans-
ducer. (From Dittrich HC
ed., "Clinical Transeso-
phageal Echocardiography,"
Mosby-Year Book, Inc., St.
Louis, 1992. Used by per-
mision.)

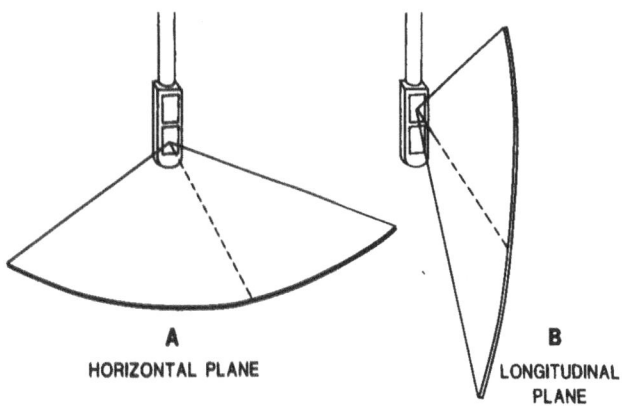

A
HORIZONTAL PLANE

B
LONGITUDINAL
PLANE

located about one centimeter more proximally on the probe shaft, and allows imaging in approximately the vertical or longitudinal plane of the body.

The ability to image structures alternately in these two perpendicular planes allows construction of a three–dimensional image of cardiac structures in the minds-eye. This multi-dimensional view often provides additional information on both cardiac structure and blood flow that is not obtainable with a single imaging plane. Figure 3 shows a photograph of the tips of several typical TEE probes.

Multiplane or omniplane probes represent the next step in the evolution of TEE technology. The capabilities and advantages of these probes will be discussed below under the topic of future directions in TEE.

The basic set-up for TEE imaging is shown in Figure 4. The operator controls the vertical position of the tip within the patient's esophagus by insertion or withdrawal of the probe shaft, performed by the operators left hand in this picture. The precise orientation of the probe tip, and therefore of the plane of ultrasound, is further controlled by rotation of the shaft of the probe.

There are also two control wheels mounted on the proximal end of the TEE probe which the operator is manipulating with the right hand in this case. These controls are similar to those used on a standard gastrointestinal endoscope, as shown in Figure 5. The larger wheel controls flexion and retroflexion of the tip of the probe. Clockwise rotation of this larger wheel can produce up to 90 degrees of forward flexion of the probe tip. Counterclockwise

Figure 3. Photograph of the distal tip of three representative TEE probes. 1. biplane probe showing
the distal horizontal or transverse (T) imaging
transducer and the more proximal vertical or longitudinal (L) imaging transducer. 2. monoplane probe
with a single horizontal or transverse (T) imaging
transducer. 3. pediatric monoplane transducer.
(From Bansal RC et al: J Am Soc Echocardiogr 1990;
3:348–366. Used by permission.)

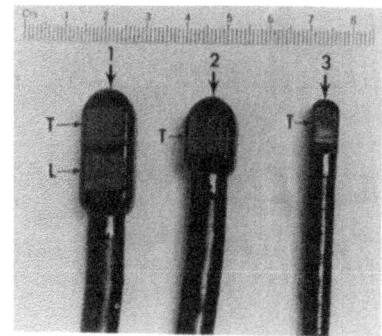

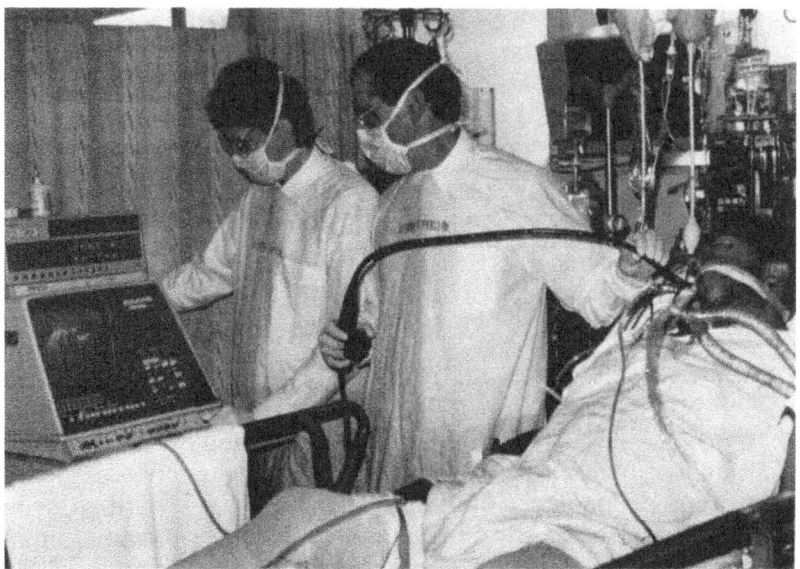

Figure 4. TEE probe in use in a patient on a respirator in the intensive care unit. The operator controls the depth of probe insertion and the rotational angle of the shaft of the probe with the left hand near the patient's mouth. The right hand is used to manipulate the control wheels at the proximal end of the shaft, which deflect the probe tip into the precise plane of imaging desired. The images are viewed in real-time on the monitor of the ultrasound machine seen at the left of this picture.

rotation of this larger wheel produces a similar deflection in the opposite direction (retroflexion). The smaller wheel controls deflection of the probe tip medially or laterally, also to a maximum angle of approximately 90 degrees. When combined with upward, downward and rotational motions of the shaft of the probe, the operator is able to image the heart and great vessels from a variety of different planes.

The images produced are viewed in real-time on the monitor screen of the ultrasound unit, which is seen at the far left in Figure 4. Despite the ability to manipulate the probe tip as outlined above, a full 90 degrees of deflection is often not feasible within the human esophagus. This limitation,

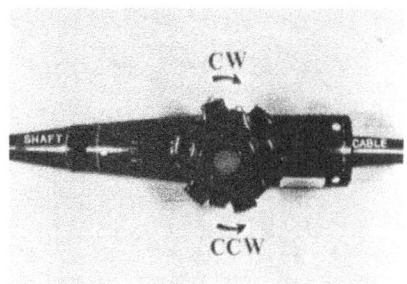

Figure 5. Close-up view of the typical TEE control wheels located on the proximal portion of the probe shaft. There is a large and a small control wheel, which are used to deflect the probe tip by rotation clockwise (CW), or counterclockwise (CCW)—see text for details. (Photograph courtesy of Marina N. Vernalis, M.D.)

Table 2. Overview of TEE in Cardiac Surgery

Pre-operative assessment
Intra-operative monitoring
Early post-operative management

and the presence of some intervening near-field obstacles such as the air-filled trachea, areas of intracardiac calcification or prosthetic heart valves, provided the impetus for development of biplane and multiplane TEE probes. In practice, the availability of two planes of imaging in biplane probes, and of multiple planes of imaging in multiplane probes, significantly expands the diagnostic power of transesophageal echocardiography.

The role of TEE in cardiac surgery can be organized into three general categories in cardiac surgery patients, as listed in Table 2: 1) pre-operative assessment; 2) intra-operative monitoring; and 3) early post-operative management.

For pre-operative assessment, TEE is most commonly used for the conditions listed in Table 3. One of the most important areas is evaluation of the mitral valve. As mentioned above, most currently-used TEE probes are capable of Doppler interrogation of blood flow, as well as two-dimensional imaging of cardiac structure. Using the color-flow Doppler modality, the severity of mitral regurgitation can be quantified as 1+ to 4+, similar to grading

Table 3. Pre-operative Assessment

Mitral Valve	Severity of MR/Structure (suitability for repair)
Vegetation/abscess	
Other Native Valves	
Prosthetic Valves	Stenosis
	Regurgitation
	Valvular
	Paravalvular
	Vegetations
	Abscess
Shunt Lesions	ASD
	Location
	Size
	Venous drainage
	VSD
	Location
	Size
	Associated Valvular lesions
Thoracic Aortic Disease	Dissection
	Aneurysm
	Traumatic Disruption
	Atherosclerosis
Miscellaneous	Cardiac Tumors
	IHSS

of regurgitation by left ventriculography. This assessment can be used with other clinical parameters to decide on the need for and timing of valve surgery. All three of the basic Doppler modalities (continuous-wave, pulsed wave and color-flow Doppler) are useful in the evaluation of mitral regurgitation, and of other regurgitant and stenotic lesions. Examples of the use of these Doppler modalities using the transesophageal window will be presented in the case studies below.

The structural information obtained pre-operatively by the two-dimensional imaging portion of the TEE examination of the mitral valve is also quite important. Since the esophagus lies directly behind the left atrium, the mitral valve is one of the first structures encountered by the beam of ultrasound. This proximity, as well as the lack of intervening obstacles to ultrasound, makes it possible to obtain extremely detailed, high-resolution images of the mitral valve apparatus. The level of detail is often equivalent to that provided by direct, close-up visual inspection. This allows precise pre-operative evaluation not only of the mitral leaflets themselves, but also the chordae tendineae, subchordal apparatus, papillary muscles and the mitral annulus. The precise abnormality responsible for mitral regurgitation can usually be ascertained, as well as the feasibility of mitral valve repair as an alternative to valve replacement.

The identification of mitral valvular vegetations, ring abscesses, fistula formation, and other complications of endocarditis is also much more reliably made from the TEE window.

Because of it's proximity to the TEE transducer, and the increasing utilization of mitral valve repair surgery, the mitral valve has received the most attention in evaluation by TEE. However, the other native valves (aortic, tricuspid and pulmonic) can also be well-visualized and evaluated by TEE, using both imaging and Doppler interrogation.

Another area of particular strength for TEE in pre-operative assessment is in suspected infection or malfunction of prosthetic heart valves. Attempts at imaging or Doppler of prosthetic valves using the standard chest wall windows is often severely limited by the prosthesis itself. Intense echo returns and reverberation artifacts from the stents, sewing ring, and mechanical leaflets often severely limit the information obtainable from transthoracic windows. The proximity, posterior location and higher frequency of the transesophageal probe overcomes many of these limitations, particularly for a prosthesis in the mitral position. TEE often permits precise pre-operative identification of the abnormality in a malfunctioning prosthetic valve. The severity of stenosis can be quantified by calculation of transvalvular gradient using continuous-wave Doppler. The severity of regurgitation can be quantified as 1+ to 4+ using color-flow Doppler. The site of regurgitation can also usually be identified as either trans-valvular or peri-valvular. Sewing ring dehiscence, even small degrees, can be identified and localized with much greater sensitivity and accuracy by TEE compared to transthoracic echocardiography. The presence or absence of valvular vegetations or prosthetic ring abscess, often impossible to identify by transthoracic imaging, can usually be identified by the TEE examination.

For shunt lesions, TEE is quite useful for both atrial and ventricular septal defects. The imaging portion of the study is useful in identifying the location and size of the defect. The presence of anomalous pulmonary venous drainage can be easily identified pre-operatively. Color-flow Doppler can be used to quantify the direction and magnitude of any shunt flow, and can be used to identify associated valvular lesions, such as aortic insufficiency associated with a membranous ventricular septal defect.

TEE is also extremely useful in the pre-operative assessment of diseases of the thoracic aorta. For suspected acute aortic dissection, TEE now stands on at least an equal footing with aortography, CAT scan and MRI imaging. In centers where TEE is available 24 hours a day on an emergency basis, it is often considered the procedure of first choice for possible acute aortic dissection. This is largely due to the portability of the equipment, the speed with which the images can be obtained, and the logistic difficulties often encountered when trying to place an acutely ill, intubated patient into a CAT scanner or MRI scanning equipment. TEE offers the additional advantage of providing immediate, real-time information on global and segmental left ventricular function, and the presence and severity of accompanying valvular heart disease, pericardial effusion or tamponade.

Other disorders of the thoracic aorta can also be readily identified and evaluated by TEE. Thoracic aortic aneurysm can be diagnosed and distinguished from acute aortic dissection. Traumatic aortic disruption can be quickly identified, even in patients too critically ill to be transported for emergency aortography. A case of such an aortic disruption identified by TEE is presented later in this discussion.

Finally, atherosclerosis throughout the course of the thoracic aorta can be recognized and localized by pre-operative TEE. Aortography primarily provides visualization of the lumen of the aorta, rather than the walls. TEE imaging allows visualization of the morphology of the walls of the aorta, including the thickness, shape and mobility of any atherosclerotic debris. Such detailed imaging not infrequently shows us quite frightening masses in the thoracic aorta, and may help us understand why some patients suffer embolic strokes following invasive vascular procedures or cardiopulmonary bypass. Attempts are being made to use this type of TEE imaging information to help guide the site of aortic cannulation or cross-clamping, with the hope of thereby reducing the incidence of embolic events.

Other miscellaneous conditions that can be assessed pre-operatively by TEE are cardiac tumors and idiopathic hypertrophic subaortic stenosis (IHSS). For the most common type of cardiac tumor, left atrial myxoma, the posterior position of the TEE probe provides very high resolution images of the size, extent and site of attachment of the tumor. In IHSS the severity and extent of septal hypertrophy can be assessed by the imaging portion of the study. The Doppler modalities can then be used to assess the severity of any outflow tract obstruction, and of the mitral regurgitation that nearly always accompanies IHSS.

Intra-operative monitoring is the next major use of TEE to be discussed. Table 4 lists a number of common intra-operative applications of TEE. The operating room is where TEE got its start in this country, much of it in the hands of anesthesiologists. TEE was initially used in the operating room as essentially a "high-tech" Swan-Ganz catheter, to monitor the volume status or filling of the left ventricle. In addition, the systolic function, global and segmental, of both the left ventricle and right ventricle can be assessed minute-to-minute by intra-operative TEE. A number of clinical research

Table 4. Intra-operative Monitoring

Volume Status (filling)	
Systolic Function	Global
	Segmental (ischemia)
New segmental wall motion abnormality	
Rapid assessment of sudden unexplained hypotension	
"De-airing" the heart	
Failure to wean from bypass	
Success of valve repair	
Prosthetic valve function	Sewing ring dehiscence
	Valve malfunction
	"IHSS"

IHSS = idiopathic hypertrophic subaortic stenosis.

studies have documented the fact that new segmental wall motion abnormalities identified by TEE provide the earliest indication of ischemia. Even before the Swan-Ganz catheter registers hemodynamic changes, and before ST segment deflections develop on the ECG, worsened segmental or global wall motion can be detected by intra-operative TEE monitoring. This allows the earliest possible intervention to correct the cause of the ischemia, in order to avoid prolonged ischemia or infarction. For this reason, we employ TEE monitoring in many of our peripheral vascular cases, since these patients often have concomitant coronary artery disease, to allow this early warning of the development of intra-operative ischemia. Although the initial intra-operative studies were done using monoplane TEE probes, the addition of biplane capability is likely to produce even more sensitivity in identifying intra-operative ischemia. The vertical imaging plane usually allows much better visualization of the apex of the left ventricle, and therefore of the territory served by the left anterior descending coronary artery.

Another important application of intra-operative TEE is for rapid assessment of sudden unexplained hypotension. TEE can obviously be used for this same indication both pre-operatively and post-operatively as well. In identifying the volume status of the left heart, the Swan-Ganz catheter has previously been the primary intra-operative monitoring device. Although the pulmonary artery wedge pressure does usually reflect the filling pressure of the left heart, it can be misleading, particularly in patients undergoing cardiac surgery. Specifically, in the presence of ischemia or other factors affecting cardiac compliance intra-operatively, an elevated wedge pressure may be recorded at a time when the heart is actually underfilled. Since the TEE image shows the size and volume of the heart chambers directly, it is able to provide accurate, minute-to-minute feedback on the volume status of the heart, and the need for volume replacement. In addition, the same minute-to-minute information is provided on overall left ventricular systolic function, to direct the use of inotropic agents to correct hypotension. Segmental or regional, rather than global areas of depressed systolic function can also be identified, to indicate when ischemia is the cause of the hypotension. This information can then be used to initiate intensified anti-ischemic therapy, or a search for technical problems indicating the need for revision of freshly-placed bypass grafts.

TEE is also used intra-operatively to help ensure adequate "de-airing" the heart. When coming off cardiopulmonary bypass, the passage of a small number of microbubbles of air is unavoidable. To minimize the chance of these microbubbles reaching the brain or other vulnerable organs in large numbers, attempts are made to remove as much air as possible from the heart. These microbubbles are easily seen by TEE and have a characteristic appearance, much like a swarm of bright white fireflies as they pass through the heart (Figure 15 below). Intra-operative monitoring for these microbubbles by TEE can be used to help assure adequate "de-airing" of the heart.

In failure to wean from bypass, TEE can be used to identify the cause of the problem. In this category are some of the same conditions mentioned above as causes of sudden unexplained hypotension, including hypovolemia, global or segmental abnormalities in systolic function, as well as technical or mechanical problems with newly repaired or replaced heart valves.

Intra-operative TEE is now used routinely in our center to evaluate the success of cardiac valve repair. One of the cases presented later in this discussion is a recent patient who underwent mitral valve repair. As you will see, TEE with color-flow Doppler allows accurate intra-operative assessment of the severity of mitral regurgitation prior to initiating cardiopulmonary bypass. The two-dimensional imaging portion of the study allows simultaneous assessment of the structural abnormality responsible for the regurgitation, and the possible suitability of the valve for repair rather than replacement. After open-heart surgery, but before the chest is closed, the success of the repair, and the presence of significant residual regurgitation or stenosis can be identified. If judged necessary, any such residual problems can be corrected at a second cardiopulmonary bypass run during the same operative procedure.

For prosthetic valve surgery, the same type of intra-operative assessment can be made immediately upon weaning from cardiopulmonary bypass, before the chest is closed. Mechanical or technical problems with a newly-implanted prosthesis can be identified, such as interference with proper leaflet opening or closure, unacceptable degrees of valvular or paravalvular regurgitation, or excessive sewing ring rocking or dehiscence. Occasionally, an IHSS type of physiology is identified by intraoperative TEE immediately upon weaning from cardiopulmonary bypass. This can occur, for example, after aortic valve replacement for aortic stenosis in a patient with left ventricular hypertrophy, particularly when the left ventricle is significantly underfilled or hypovolemic. The small left ventricular chamber size and narrowed left ventricular outflow tract with turbulent flow by Doppler can be readily identified by TEE as the cause of hypotension. This provides an immediate indication of the need for volume repletion to correct the problem. This is one of the situations where the pulmonary artery pressure may be elevated, making the diagnosis of underfilling difficult or impossible to make by modalities other than intra-operative TEE. In addition, if such a patient were hypotensive, the use of inotropic agents would be likely to aggravate the severity of dynamic outflow tract obstruction, worsening rather than improving any hypotension.

Outflow tract obstruction of this type may also occasionally occur during weaning from bypass in a patient with a relatively small left ventricle with a freshly-implanted bioprosthetic valve in the mitral position. Occasionally, the large stents of the mitral prosthesis protrude into and obstruct the outflow tract of the left ventricle, particularly in the presence of hypovolemia. Again, intra-operative TEE may be the only way to identify this problem so that appropriate measures can be taken to correct it.

TEE is not only useful for visualization of the heart chambers and valves intra-operatively. Because the aorta and great vessels are also well-visualized by TEE, it can be used to guide the placement of lines and catheters in the great vessels, as well as in the heart. TEE can be used to guide placement of Swan-Ganz catheters into the pulmonary artery, temporary or permanent pacemaker electrodes through the superior or inferior vena cavae into the right atrium or ventricle, retrograde cardioplegia catheters in the coronary sinus, or an intra-aortic balloon pump into the descending thoracic aorta. As part of the routine intra-operative evaluation, the entire thoracic aorta can be visualized to identify the rare occurrence of post-operative acute thoracic aortic dissection.

The uses of transesophageal echocardiography early post-operatively are listed in Table 5. Identification of the cause of sudden unexplained hypotension remains an important indication, just as it is intra-operatively. For years echocardiographers have brought their equipment urgently to the bedside of post-operative cardiac surgery patients in an attempt to help identify the cause of sudden hypotension. These bedside transthoracic studies, however, are almost always extremely technically limited by factors such as the inability to position the ventilated patient optimally, intervening lung tissue, the presence of chest tubes, and by early post-operative chest wall tenderness. Although TEE is somewhat more invasive than transthoracic echocardiography, it allows the echocardiographer to see the heart just as well the day after surgery as he could the day before. Hypovolemia and new segmental or global wall motion abnormalities can be readily identified as a cause of sudden hypotension, as well as post-operative pericardial or mediastinal tamponade, significant valvular regurgitation, or technical problems with newly-implanted prosthetic valves.

Source of embolism can be identified, both pulmonary and systemic. In patients with sudden post-operative hypotension due to pulmonary embolism, one may find evidence of acute right heart failure, with new dilatation and generalized hypokinesis of the right ventricle. Occasionally, in massive acute pulmonary embolism accompanied by hypotension, we have identified the embolic material in the proximal pulmonary artery branches, which are usually well-visualized by TEE.

Source of embolism also applies to patients who have suffered post-operative cerebrovascular events; either stroke or transient ischemic attacks.

Table 5. Early Post-operative Management

Rapid assessment of sudden unexplained hypotension
Pericardial/Mediastinal Tamponade
Source of embolism

Not infrequently, this occurs concomitantly with the development of post-operative atrial fibrillation. With the use of TEE, the left atrium and left ventricle can be thoroughly examined for the presence of clot. And the entire thoracic aorta can also be examined for potential source of atherosclerotic embolic material.

After that overview of what TEE has to offer in cardiac surgery patients, I would like to present five cases in which we have found TEE useful at our institution. In presenting these five cases, I will briefly review selected standard TEE imaging planes to help orient those who do not have the opportunity to view these images routinely. Since the purpose of this discussion is not to provide an exhaustive overview of TEE imaging planes, I have selected only a limited number of standard views. I will use only these few standard views to present the cases, and will try to describe the standard views using images taken from these same cases.

In all of the TEE sections that I will show, the image display format is that described in Table 6. The near field is at the top of the screen, at the apex or point of origin of the wedge-shaped sector of ultrasound. This apex or "point" of the sector always represents the location of the transducer, and is by convention displayed at the top of the monitor screen of the echocardiography machine. Since the TEE probe and transducer are located in the esophagus, and since the esophagus lies posterior to the heart, more posterior structures in the heart will always appear towards the top of the screen. This holds true for all TEE images, regardless of whether they are generated by a monoplane, biplane, or even a multiplane transducer.

In the horizontal imaging plane, leftward structures in the patient appear to the right of the screen. This left-to-right orientation should be familiar from other imaging modalities, such as standard chest x-ray, CAT scan and MRI images.

When the vertical TEE imaging transducer is activated, the standard convention is to display more superior structures to the right of the screen. One way to remember the orientation of the vertical plane images is to imagine that the patient is lying face down on a table. Imagine that you are an observer viewing this table from the patient's right side, and that the patient's head is towards your right. Now, with the TEE probe in the patient's esophagus, the images produced by the vertical ultrasound wedge will be displayed on the screen in precisely the same orientation as you are viewing the patient on the table. That is, structures closer to the head of the patient (i.e., more superior structures) will be displayed towards the right of the screen. And since the patient is envisioned lying face down with the probe in the esophagus (which is posterior to the heart) more posterior structures will be displayed towards the top of the screen, as is always the case in TEE images (unless the image is electronically inverted, which is not the practice in most laboratories).

Table 6. Image Display Format

Near field at top of screen	
Transverse plane	Leftward structures to the right of screen
Longitudinal plane	Superior structures to the right of screen

Once the basic left-right and superior-inferior orientation is understood, the next step in becoming oriented to TEE images is to begin to recognize a few of the generally-accepted standard TEE views of the heart. I will present only two of the standard horizontal plane views of the heart. The first is the short-axis or "doughnut" view of the heart, obtained with the TEE probe positioned in the stomach. This view is quite similar to the transthoracic short-axis view, except that it is displayed "upside down" compared to chest wall imaging (because the transducer is now on the opposite side of the heart). The second standard transverse TEE view to be presented is the four chamber view. Again this should be familiar from standard chest wall echocardiography, and again it appears inverted for the same reason. But in all of these images, whether transthoracic or transesophageal, leftward structures are displayed to the right of the screen, as is the standard convention used for x-ray, CAT scan and MRI images.

The five cases to be described are of patients with the following conditions: Case 1: acute myocardial infarction complicated by ventricular septal defect, left ventricular rupture, and hemorrhagic cardiac tamponade; Case 2: mitral valve repair for severe mitral regurgitation secondary to mitral valve prolapse with torn mitral chorda tendinea; Case 3: bioprosthetic aortic valve with suspected stenosis; Case 4: traumatic aortic disruption; and 5: cardiac tamponade related to chest wall trauma with right ventricular contusion.

Case 1 is a TEE study done emergently in the cardiac catheterization laboratory in an extremely ill patient with an inferior myocardial infarction which had been complicated by a ventricular septal defect, as well as cardiac tamponade from rupture of the inferior wall of the left ventricle. Figure 6 is the horizontal plane short- axis or "doughnut" view of the left ventricle in this patient, obtained with a biplane probe advanced from the esophagus into the stomach. The horizontal imaging plane is activated, and the left ventricle appears as a black annular (doughnut-shaped) structure towards the right side of the wedge of ultrasound. The endocardium and epicardium appear as white echogenic circles defining the margins of the left ventricular myocar-

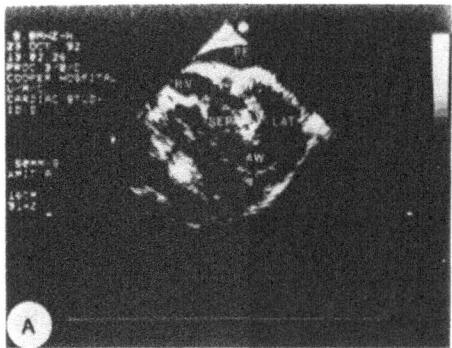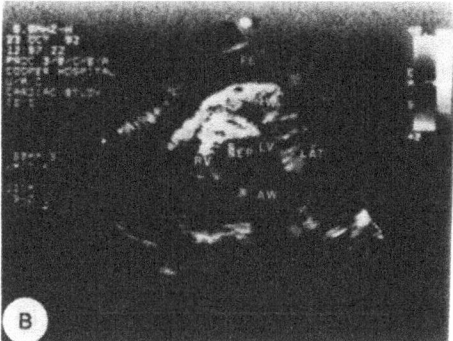

Figure 6. A. Short-axis or "doughnut" view of the left ventricle obtained from the transgastric TEE window in case 1. This patient has a large circumferential pericardial effusion (PE) which surrounds the left ventricle (LV) and right ventricle (RV). The walls of the left ventricle are labeled as follows: IW = inferior wall; AW = anterior wall; LAT = lateral wall and SEP = septum. B. The same view with color-flow Doppler activated. The bright turquoise color-flow signal indicates turbulent shunt flow from left to right through the defect in the ventricular septum.

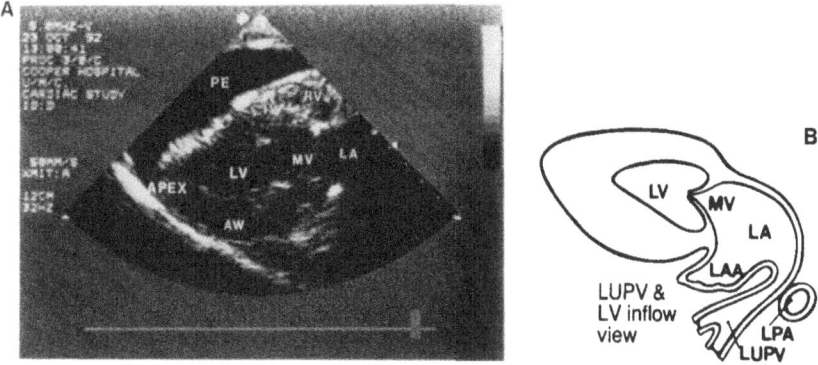

Figure 7. Vertical plane left ventricular (LV) inflow view A. TEE image in this view taken from case 1 with large pericardial effusion (PE). B. Illustration of the standard vertical plane LV inflow view. LA = left atrium; LAA = left atrial appendage; MV = mitral valve; LPA = left pulmonary artery; LUPV = left upper pulmonary vein; RV = right ventricle; APEX = LV apex; IW = inferior wall of LV; AW = anterior wall of LV.

dium. As the labels on the figure show, the inferior wall (IW) of the left ventricle is towards the top of the sector of ultrasound, since it is the wall of the left ventricle closest to the TEE probe. The anterior wall (AW) of the left ventricle appears toward the bottom of the screen, since it is further away from the TEE transducer located posterior to the heart. As noted above, structures on the patient's left are displayed to the right in the horizontal imaging plane, therefore the lateral wall (LAT) is on the right of the screen while the septum (SEP) is towards the left of the screen.

With these orienting features in mind, one can appreciate in Figure 6A that there is a break or gap in the epicardium, myocardium and endocardium of the left ventricle, between the inferior wall and the septum. This is the ventricular septal defect. This horizontal plane short-axis view of the left ventricle allows the echocardiographer to see myocardium supplied by all three of the major coronary arteries, and has therefore been most commonly employed for intra-operative monitoring for ischemia using TEE. Figure 6B shows the same TEE image with the color-flow Doppler function activated. Information on intracardiac blood flow is now displayed in color simultaneously with the imaging information. The bright turquoise color-flow signal indicates significant left-to-right shunt flow through the ventricular septal defect.

Figure 7A is a TEE vertical plane view from the same patient with acute inferior myocardial infarction complicated by ventricular septal defect. This view is obtained by activating the vertical imaging transducer of a biplane TEE probe.

Starting in the horizontal plane "doughnut" view of the left ventricle (Figure 6), a switch is flipped to activate the vertical imaging transducer from the same probe position. This produces the left ventricular (LV) inflow standard TEE view as illustrated in Figure 7B. In this view, the more superior left atrium appears on the right side of the screen, while the apex of the left ventricle, a more inferior structure, appears on the left. As in the previous

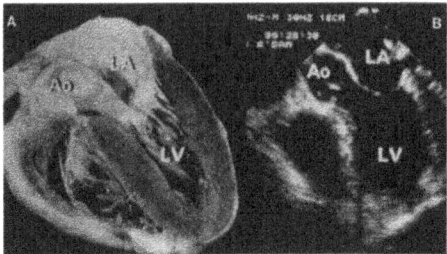

Figure 8. Horizontal plane four-chamber view. A. Anatomic section cut in this plane. B. TEE image in the four-chamber view. LA = left atrium; LV = left ventricle; Ao = aortic root.

images from this patient, all the cardiac chambers are shown outlined by a black echo-free space, which represents a large pericardial effusion (labelled PE). The mitral valve leaflets can also be seen (MV). The anterior wall (AW) of the left ventricle is displayed towards the bottom of the screen, with the inferior wall (IW) closer to the TEE probe, and therefore appearing near the top or origin of the ultrasound sector. This vertical or longitudinal view of the left ventricle provides a good look at the apex of the left ventricle. The true apex of the left ventricle is often difficult to visualize with the single horizontal plane, and this ability to image the apex is an example of one of the many advantages of biplane (and multiplane) TEE over monoplane imaging.

Figure 8 illustrates the horizontal plane standard four-chamber TEE view. The left panel (Figure 8A) shows an anatomic section cut in this plane. The right panel (Figure 8B) shows the corresponding ultrasound section. This standard TEE view is similar to the familiar transthoracic apical four-chamber view, except that it appears inverted top to bottom. This is again a result of the fact that the transducer is now located posterior to the heart, rather than on the anterior chest wall as it is in transthoracic echocardiography.

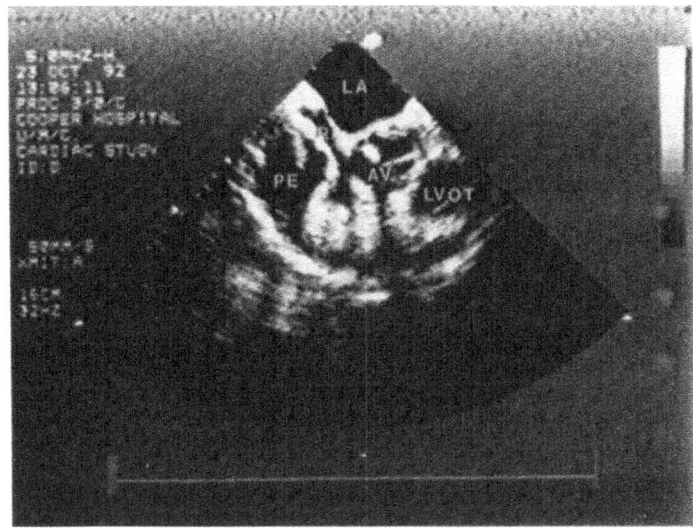

Figure 9. Modified horizontal plane four-chamber view in case 1, documenting the presence of pericardial tamponade as evidenced by diastolic collapse of the right atrium (RA). PE = pericardial effusion; LA = left atrium; AV = aortic valve; LVOT = left ventricular outflow tract.

The more posterior structures (the left atrium and right atrium) are now closest to the transducer and therefore appear at the top of the screen. As in all horizontal plane TEE images, structures to the patient's left (such as the left atrium) appear towards the right side of the screen.

Figure 9 is a horizontal plane four-chamber TEE view in case number 1, the patient with acute myocardial infarction, ventricular septal defect and pericardial tamponade. The TEE probe is located at a level slightly superior in the esophagus compared to the anatomic section of Figure 8, allowing visualization of more of the atria, and less of the ventricles. The large pericardial effusion (PE) can be seen to be indenting or compressing the normally convex posterior wall of the right atrium (RA). This diastolic collapse of the right atrium is an echocardiographic manifestation of pericardial tamponade. Tamponade was diagnosed in this extremely ill patient by emergency TEE in the catheterization laboratory even before the right heart catheters could be inserted to confirm the diagnosis. As you can see in Figure 9, the right atrium is so compressed by the elevated pressure in the pericardial space that there is barely enough room to put a label on it in the figure. When the Swan-Ganz catheter was inserted shortly after these images were obtained, cardiogenic shock secondary to pericardial tamponade was confirmed.

This emergency TEE study also demonstrated the cause of pericardial tamponade in this patient. Left ventricular segmental wall motion showed evidence of acute inferior myocardial infarction, with left ventricular rupture causing the tense, bloody pericardial effusion. Color-flow Doppler immediately demonstrated a ventricular septal defect in the region of the infarction, with significant left-to-right shunt as shown in Figure 6B above. Once the left heart catheters were in place, coronary angiography demonstrated an occluded right coronary artery.

The patient was taken emergently to the operating room. Bloody pericardial tamponade was relieved, and a patch was placed over the ventricular septal defect. TEE imaging was continued intra-operatively to assess both the adequacy of relief of tamponade, and the success of closure of the ventricular septal defect. Figure 10 is the post-operative horizontal plane four-chamber TEE view in this patient. This image can be compared to a similar pre-operative view seen in Figure 9. We see that the large pericardial effusion present pre-operatively is no longer present. The right atrium (RA) is no longer collapsed, but shows a normal rounded shape, documenting relief of pericardial tamponade. In this same view, we can see the bright white echo returns from the patch over the ventricular septal defect at the base of the interventricular septum (SEP), just below the tricuspid valve (TV) and mitral valve (MV) level. With activation of the color-flow Doppler function, the area of the patch was interrogated for the presence of residual left-to-right shunt flow. None could be found, indicating successful operative closure of the ventricular septal defect.

Figure 11A is a modified horizontal plane four-chamber view taken from the second case, a patient with a flail anterior mitral leaflet and chorda tendinea. The transverse imaging plane in this instance has been rotated to the patient's left in order to focus on the mitral valve plane. We see the left atrium (LA) at the top of the screen, closest to the transducer, and the left ventricle in the far-field, towards the bottom of the screen. The right atrium and right ventricle are off the screen to the left. The mitral valve (MV) can be

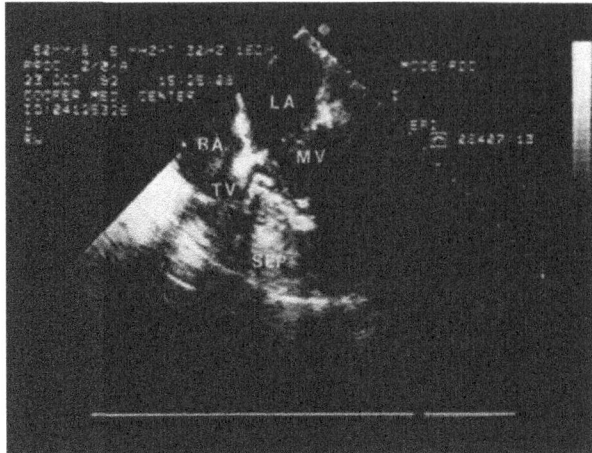

Figure 10. Post-operative horizontal plane four-chamber view in case 1. Note that the large pericardial effusion previously seen in Figure 9 is no longer present. The right atrium (RA) has returned to its normal convex shape following relief of tamponade. At the base of the interventricular septum (SEP), just below the annulus of the tricuspid valve (TV) and mitral valve (MV) plane, dense white echo returns from the patch over the ventricular septal defect can be seen. LA = left atrium.

seen in a close-up view between the left atrium and left ventricle. The anterior leaflet (AL) is on the left of the screen, and the posterior leaflet (PL) is on the right. The white linear echo labelled "FC" is a flail chorda tendinea of the mitral valve, which can be seen to prolapse posteriorly (upwards) into the left atrium in this systolic frame. The flail chord was readily identified by TEE as the cause of severe mitral regurgitation in this patient. One can also appreciate in this view the upwards or posterior "bowing" of the mitral valve anterior leaflet (AL) into the left atrium consistent with mitral valve prolapse, in a

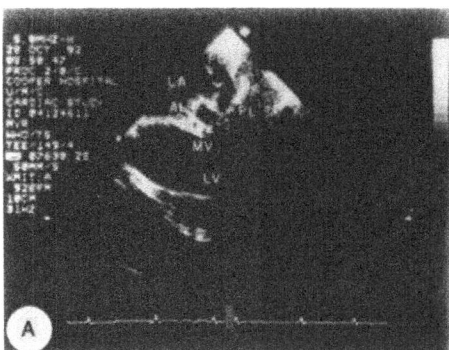
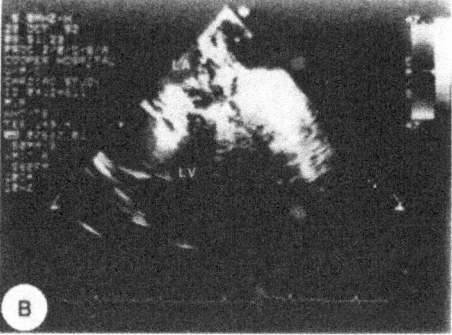

Figure 11. A. Modified horizontal four-chamber view of the mitral valve in case 2 with flail mitral chorda tendinea (FC). LA = left atrium; LV = left ventricle; AL = anterior leaflet and PL = posterior leaflet of the mitral valve (MV). B. The same view with color-flow Doppler activated. Note the turquoise jet of turbulence originating at the gap between the mitral leaflets, at the site of the flail chord, and directed laterally (to the right) into the left atrium.

thickened, myxomatous-appearing mitral valve. The anterior leaflet can also be seen to prolapse back beyond the margin of the posterior leaflet resulting in a visible gap between the two leaflets. One can predict, even before pushing the button to activate color-flow Doppler, that the jet of mitral regurgitation will originate at this gap, and be deflected laterally, which is towards the right in this view. Figure 11B is the exact same view as in Figure 11A, but with the color-flow Doppler function activated. The left atrium (LA) and left ventricle (LV) are again labelled for orientation. As expected, the bright turquoise color-flow jet of mitral regurgitation can be seen to originate at the gap between the mitral leaflets, and is directed to the right of the image, which is towards the lateral portion of the left atrium.

Figure 12 is taken from the same patient, and demonstrates an example of the use of another Doppler modality: pulsed-wave Doppler. Pulsed-wave Doppler is used in this case to demonstrate pulmonary venous systolic flow reversal, a marker of severe mitral regurgitation. This finding is the Doppler correlate of 5+ mitral regurgitation by left ventriculography, where contrast injected into the left ventricle not only regurgitates back into the left atrium, but refluxes into the pulmonary veins. The pulsed-wave Doppler modality allows us to place a "sample volume," indicated on the screen by a small circle, over an area of interest, and sample blood flow information from this one small area only. In this case we are interested in flow in the pulmonary veins, so the sample volume is placed in one of the left pulmonary veins at the point where it enters the left atrium. In Figure 12, the location of the Doppler sample volume is indicated by a small circle in the 2–D image at the upper right corner of the screen. This small ultrasound sector is a smaller version of the same view of the left atrium and mitral valve we saw in Figure 11A. The lower half of Figure 12 shows the pulsed-wave Doppler flow signal

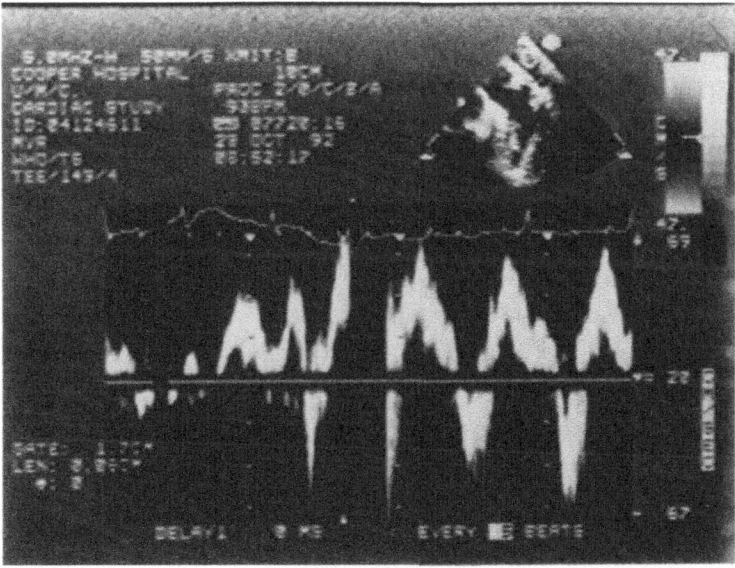

Figure 12. Pulse-wave Doppler documenting pulmonary venous systolic flow reversal in case 2. (see text for details).

obtained from this site in the pulmonary vein. A simultaneous ECG signal is displayed just above the flow signal, to allow timing of systolic versus diastolic flow. In the center of the flow signal is a white horizontal baseline. Flow towards the transducer, or into the left atrium, is displayed as an upward signal above the baseline. Normal pulmonary venous flow is always upwards, or above the baseline, throughout the cardiac cycle. In severe mitral regurgitation, however, there is reversal of pulmonary venous flow, indicated by a negative flow signal (below the baseline) during systole. This indicates reflux of blood back into the pulmonary veins, caused by the severe systolic mitral regurgitation. We see this negative systolic flow signal shortly after the QRS on the ECG documenting systolic pulmonary venous flow reversal, and therefore severe mitral regurgitation. Pulsed-wave Doppler can be used to identify this sign pre-operatively to help document the need for mitral valve surgery. The disappearance of this finding by TEE intra-operatively and post-operatively can be used to help document the adequacy of mitral valve repair. In this patient, repair was successful and pulmonary venous systolic flow reversal was no longer present on TEE imaging immediately after coming off cardiopulmonary bypass. Doppler can also be employed intra-operatively, as it was in this patient, to ensure that no significant stenosis is created in the process of repairing the mitral valve.

Figure 13 is another pre-operative view of this same patient with severe mitral regurgitation, but now using the vertical imaging transducer of a biplane probe. Starting in the horizontal plane four-chamber TEE view of the mitral valve (Figure 11), the vertical plane transducer is activated. This produces the left ventricular inflow view of the mitral valve, as illustrated previously in Figure 7B. This provides another perspective of the mitral valve leaflets and chordal apparatus, in a plane perpendicular to the horizontal view. This is obtained with the probe in the same position in the esophagus, and is acquired by simply activating the vertical rather than the horizontal imaging transducer. The vertical plane often affords more detail of the papillary muscles and mitral subchordal apparatus, and provides important additional information on the suitability of the valve for repair. In this patient, we see another view of the flail chorda tendinea prolapsing into the left atrium.

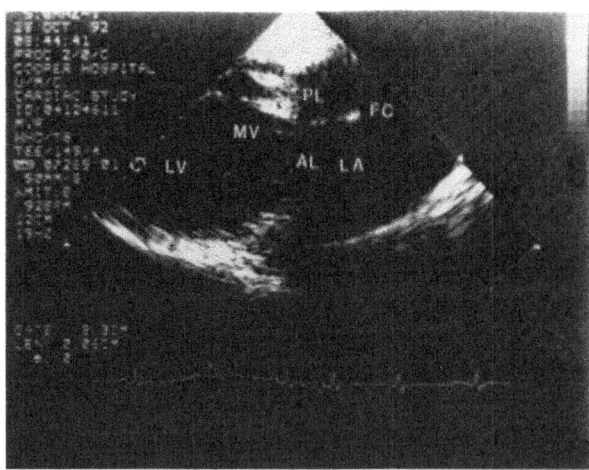

Figure 13. Vertical plane left ventricular inflow view in case 2, showing flail mitral chorda tendinea (FC). LV = left ventricle; AL = anterior leaflet; and PL = posterior leaflet of mitral valve (MV); LA = left atrium.

For orientation, remember that in this longitudinal plane, superior structures are displayed towards the right of the screen. The flail chord (FC) of the mitral valve is therefore seen pointing towards the right (superiorly) in this image.

Figure 14 is a horizontal plane, short axis "doughnut" TEE view of the left ventricle at the level of the mitral valve annulus. Here we are looking right down the barrel of the mitral orifice in this same patient with a flail chord. The color-flow Doppler function has been activated, and the turquoise jet of severe mitral regurgitation (MR) is again easily appreciated in this pre-operative image. To review the orientation, the posterior wall (POST) of the left ventricle is at the top of the screen, nearest to the TEE probe. The anterior wall (ANT) is in the far-field, at the bottom of the screen. Leftward structures in the patient are towards the right of the screen, so the lateral wall (LAT) of the left ventricle is on the right. We can see again in this view that the eccentric jet of mitral regurgitation (the turquoise color-flow signal) is directed laterally, towards the right of the screen.

Figure 15 is taken from the same case 2 with the flail mitral valve chord, as the patient is coming off cardiopulmonary bypass. The horizontal plane close-up four-chamber TEE view of the left atrium (LA) is shown with the mitral valve (MV) and a small portion of the left ventricular outflow tract (LVOT). The multiple white echogenic spots seen in the left atrium and LVOT are the typical appearance of microbubbles of air moving through the heart as cardiopulmonary bypass is being terminated. In real-time, these bright echoes show random motion reminiscent of a swarm of fireflies. Imaging by TEE intra-operatively can be used to assure adequate de-airing of the heart. In addition, we can see that prolapse of the anterior mitral valve leaflet into the left atrium is no longer present following operative repair of the mitral valve. The gap between the mitral leaflets, which was seen on the pre-operative images, is also no longer present.

Figure 16 shows the same view with the patient completely off cardiopulmonary bypass, and with color-flow Doppler activated. The jet of mitral regurgitation is now only a small red central plume, rather than the large

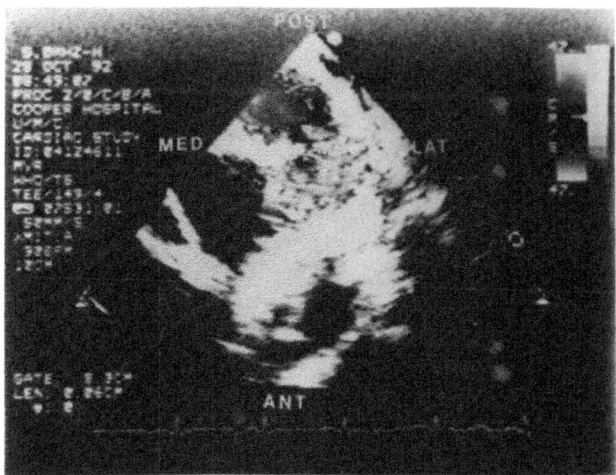

Figure 14. Horizontal plane short-axis view of the left ventricle obtained with the TEE probe in the stomach in case 2. Color-flow Doppler is activated to show the turquoise-colored turbulent jet of severe mitral regurgitation (MR) directed laterally (LAT). MED = medial; POST = posterior; ANT = anterior.

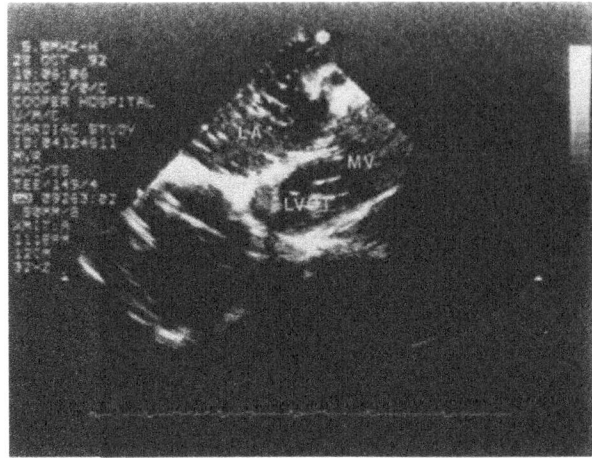

Figure 15. Modified horizontal plane four-chamber view focusing on the mitral valve (MV) in case 2. This is the same view as the pre-operative image shown in Figure 11 above. LA = left atrium; LVOT = left ventricular outflow tract. As the patient is weaned from cardiopulmonary bypass, multiple bright white echoes in the LA and LVOT indicate microbubbles passing through the heart. Note also that the flail mitral chord and anterior leaflet prolapse seen in Figure 11 are no longer present following mitral valve repair.

turquoise turbulent signal of severe mitral regurgitation seen on the pre-operative TEE images. This indicates a successful mitral valve repair.

Figure 17 shows the vertical plane long-axis view of the repaired mitral valve obtained by switching to the vertical transducer of a biplane probe, with the probe in the same position in the patient. In this orientation, remember superior structures are displayed to the right of the screen, therefore the left atrium (LA) appears to the right. This view is similar to the pre-operative view shown in Figure 13, although now obtained from a slightly superior position in the esophagus. Comparing these two figures we can see that the flail chord

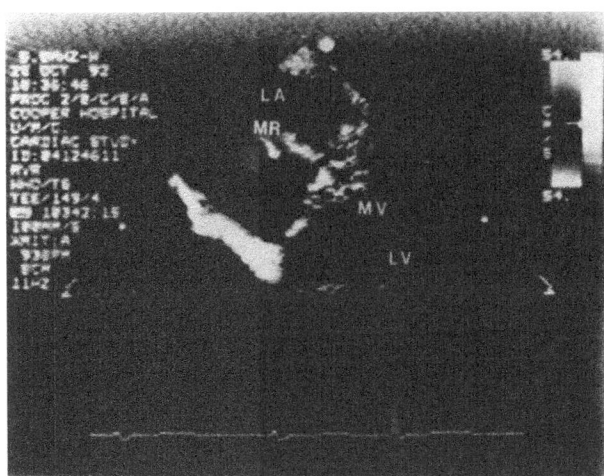

Figure 16. Modified horizontal plane four-chamber view of the mitral valve (MV) in case 2, following operative repair. LA = left atrium; LV = left ventricle. Only a small red plume of residual mitral regurgitation (MR) could be identified by color-flow Doppler.

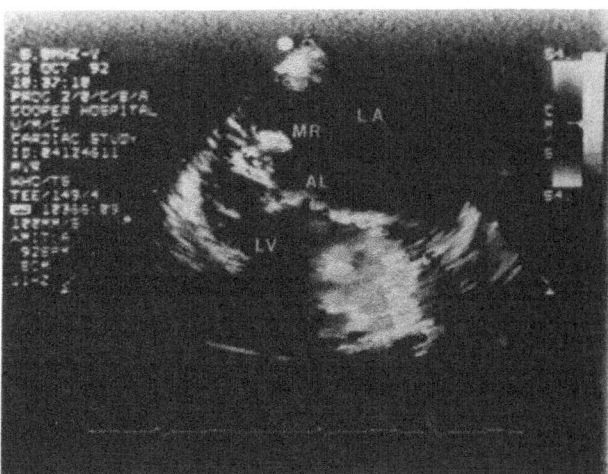

Figure 17. Vertical plane left ventricular inflow view of the repaired mitral valve in case 2. Only a small reddish-yellow plume of residual mitral regurgitation (MR) could be identified by color-flow Doppler in this view, perpendicular to the plane of Figure 16. LA = left atrium; LV = left ventricle; AL = anterior leaflet of the mitral valve.

is no longer present. And with activation of color-flow Doppler we see, in another plane, that only a small reddish-yellow jet of mitral regurgitation (MR) remains following repair.

One note of caution regarding assessment of the severity of mitral regurgitation immediately upon coming off cardiopulmonary bypass; make note of the systolic blood pressure. If the pressure is quite low, one may not obtain an accurate assessment of the success of the repair. In some cases it may be necessary to raise the systolic pressure and afterload with an intravenous pressor agent in order to be sure that significant residual mitral regurgitation will not be present at normal post-operative blood pressures. If significant residual mitral regurgitation is judged to persist following repair, further attempts at repair, or the placement of a mitral prosthesis, may be indicated.

Figure 18 is a post-operative short-axis or doughnut view of the left ventricle at the level of the repaired mitral valve. With color-flow Doppler

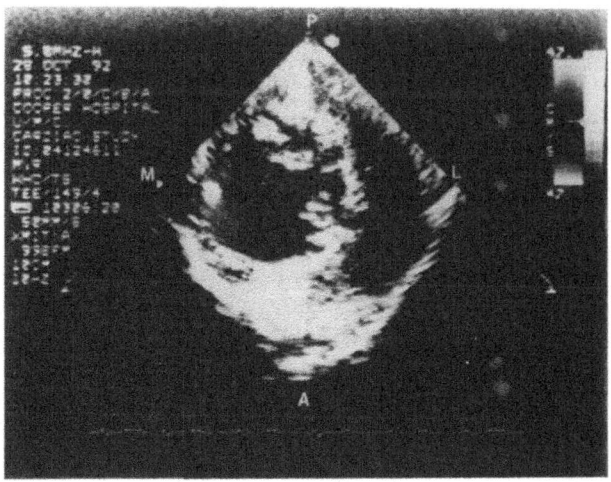

Figure 18. Horizontal plane short-axis view of the left ventricle at the mitral valve plane in case 2. In this post-operative systolic image with color-flow Doppler activated we see no residual mitral regurgitation. The dark blue color seen represents normal, non-turbulent blood flow in the region of the repaired mitral valve. A = anterior; L = lateral; M = medial. (Compare to a similar preoperative view shown in Figure 14 above.)

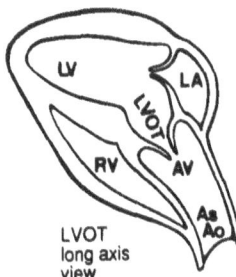

LVOT
long axis
view

Figure 19. Illustration of standard vertical plane left ventricular outflow tract (LVOT) view. LV = left ventricle; LA = left atrium; AV = aortic valve; AsAo = ascending aorta; RV = right ventricle.

activated, we now see only a dark blue signal indicating normal, non-turbulent blood flow velocities in the region of the repaired mitral valve. The bright turquoise color flow signal of severe mitral regurgitation seen in the similar pre-operative TEE image of Figure 14 is no longer present.

The final standard TEE imaging plane that I would like to present is another vertical or long-axis view of the left ventricle. This is the left ventricular outflow tract (LVOT) view, which is in a slightly different vertical plane from the left ventricular inflow view described previously, as shown in Figure 7.

Whereas the LV inflow view focuses on the left atrium and mitral valve, the LVOT view focuses on the outflow portion of the left ventricle, including the aortic valve and proximal aortic root. This view, which is obtained with the vertical imaging transducer of a biplane TEE probe, represents another area of significant advantage of biplane over monoplane probes. With the single horizontal imaging plane of a monoplane probe, it is often impossible to align the Doppler ultrasound beam optimally for evaluation of the aortic valve for either aortic stenosis or aortic regurgitation. With a biplane (or multiplane) probe, however, the vertical imaging transducer can be used to acquire the left ventricular outflow tract (LVOT) long-axis view, as shown diagrammatically in Figure 19. In this view, the left ventricle is closest to the transducer, since the TEE probe has been advanced from the esophagus down into the fundus of the stomach. The posterior wall of the left ventricle therefore appears at the top of the screen. A portion of the left atrium (LA) and mitral valve apparatus are also seen. The plane of ultrasound is directed parallel to the left ventricular outflow tract (LVOT) and aortic valve (AV). The ascending aorta (AsAo) is seen in the far field towards the bottom of the diagram.

Figure 20 shows an example of this vertical plane left ventricular outflow tract view. This image is from case 3, a patient with suspected malfunction of a porcine bioprosthetic aortic valve. It is a "close-up" or higher magnification view than the diagram in Figure 19, to allow closer examination of prosthetic aortic valve leaflets, sewing ring and stents. A small segment of the basal left ventricle is seen at the top left of the ultrasound sector. The ascending aorta is (As Ao) is seen in the far field, towards the bottom right of the screen. Between these two structures, in the center of the ultrasound sector, we see one of the three stents (STENT) of the bioprosthetic aortic valve, as well as the prosthetic leaflets (L), which appear as a thin white linear echo. This figure demonstrates the fine detail one can obtain by TEE imaging of the prosthetic valve leaflets and stents, which appear entirely normal in this patient. If the leaflets were significantly thickened, torn, failed to coat

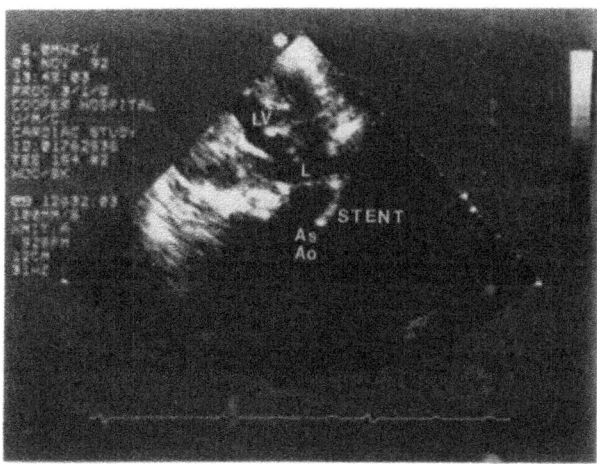

Figure 20. Vertical plane left ventricular outflow tract (LVOT) view in case 3 with a porcine bioprosthetic aortic valve. LV = left ventricle; AsAo = ascending aorta; L =prosthetic leaflets and STENT = stent of prosthetic valve. Note the fine detail of the prosthetic stent and leaflets that is provided by TEE.

properly, or had attached vegetations or thrombus, TEE represents one of the most sensitive imaging modalities for identification of these abnormalities. Dehiscence of the sewing ring, as evidenced by abnormal rocking motion during the cardiac cycle, can also be readily appreciated. With the use of color-flow Doppler, paravalvular versus valvular regurgitation can be distinguished and quantified.

For evaluation of valvular stenosis, including stenosis of prosthetic heart valves, the continuous-wave (CW) Doppler modality is the most useful. Continuous-wave Doppler, which is available on most biplane and multiplane TEE probes, directs a single line of ultrasound parallel to the area of suspected stenotic flow. In the case of a native or prosthetic aortic valve, this is usually best accomplished in the LVOT long-axis view just described. Figure 21 shows the use of CW Doppler to interrogate the aortic valve in this same patient with a porcine bioprosthetic aortic valve. The display is quite similar to that shown in Figure 12 for pulsed-wave (PW) Doppler in the discussion of systolic pulmonary venous flow reversal in severe mitral regurgitation. In Figure 21

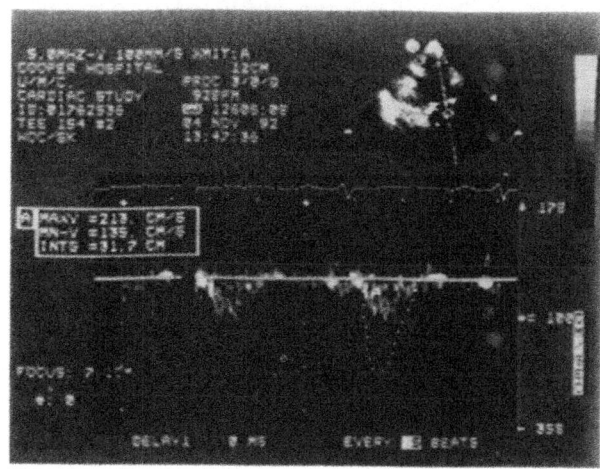

Figure 21. Continuous-wave (CW) Doppler evaluation of the bioprosthetic aortic valve in case 3, to evaluate possible aortic stenosis. The same vertical plane left ventricular outflow tract view of Figure 20 can be seen in the upper right-hand corner, with a white line indicating the orientation of the CW Doppler beam. No stenosis is demonstrated in this case (see text for details).

we again see a small ultrasound sector in the upper right corner of the monitor screen. In this case, the imaging sector shows the same LVOT view of the aortic valve prosthesis seen in Figure 20. A single white line is seen originating from the apex of ultrasound sector, directed through the center of the aortic valve prosthesis. This line represents the continuous-wave Doppler ultrasound beam, and shows that it is aimed to measure the velocity of blood as it passes through the orifice of the prosthesis into the aortic root and ascending aorta. In the lower half of the screen, the CW Doppler signal is displayed, again with a simultaneous ECG tracing for timing of systole versus diastole. A horizontal white line through the center of the display again represents the baseline or zero flow-velocity line. Immediately following the QRS on the ECG tracing, flow below the baseline can be seen. By convention, flow away from the ultrasound transducer is shown as a negative velocity, below the baseline. In this view, therefore, flow through the aortic prosthesis is directed away from the TEE transducer, and is displayed as a negative signal. The peak of this velocity profile can be used to calculate the maximum pressure gradient across the valve, and can be used to indicate the degree of stenosis present. In this particular patient, no stenosis was demonstrated and the TEE study was able to document a normally-functioning prosthetic valve.

Figure 22 shows a transverse plane short axis view of the same aortic valve prosthesis. The left atrium (LA) is seen at the top of the screen, with the three bright white echoes just below it indicating the three stents of the porcine bioprosthesis, viewed in cross-section. A thin white line of echoes in the center of the three stents is the point of coaptation of the prosthetic aortic leaflets. If significant leaflet thickening, calcification or vegetations are present on prosthetic leaflets or stents, these abnormalities are usually readily-identified by TEE. This is particularly true when the valve can be examined in numerous imaging planes, as is most easily done with a biplane or multiplane probe.

Case 4 is an example of thoracic aortic disruption diagnosed by TEE in a young woman injured in a motor vehicle accident. She had suffered extensive abdominal trauma and was hypotensive despite vigorous blood

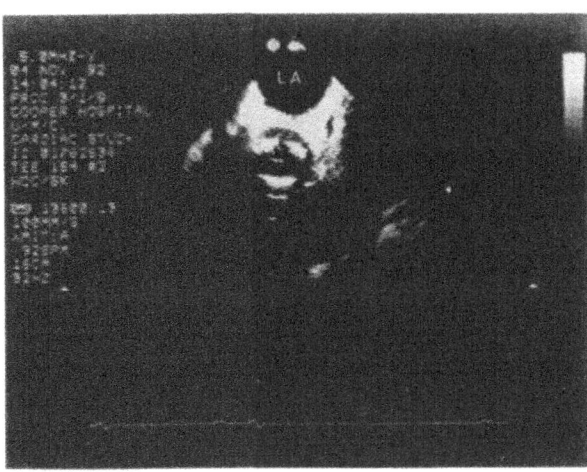

Figure 22. Horizontal plane short-axis view at the level of the aortic valve in case 3, with a bioprosthetic aortic valve. LA = left atrium. Note the three round white echoes just below the LA in this view representing the three stents of the bioprosthetic valve. A single white linear echo at the center of the 3 stents is the point of coaptation of the bioprosthetic leaflets.

Descending Thoracic Aorta

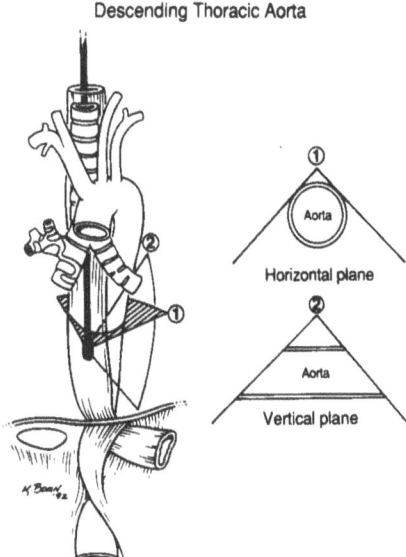

Figure 23. Illustration of the standard biplane TEE imaging planes of the descending thoracic aorta. On the left, a TEE probe is shown in the esophagus, rotated posteriorly to view the descending aorta. The orientation of the horizontal (1) and vertical (2) imaging planes can be seen as they intersect the aorta, with the corresponding images of the aorta shown at the right of the diagram.

transfusion. As she was being transported to the operating room for repair of intra-abdominal injuries, an emergency transesophageal echocardiogram was performed. This showed a previously unsuspected aortic disruption. Figure 23 is a diagram of the standard TEE imaging planes of the aorta. To image the descending thoracic aorta from the esophagus, the TEE probe is rotated posteriorly, as shown in the diagram. With a biplane probe directed towards the aorta, one can activate the horizontal transducer element to obtain a short-axis view of the aorta (plane 1 in Figure 23). Switching to the vertical transducer element from the same probe position produces a long-axis view of the same segment of the aorta (plane 2 in Figure 23).

Figure 24 shows a horizontal plane view of the descending thoracic aorta (AO) at a level just distal to the aortic arch in this patient with traumatic aortic rupture (RUP). The linear white echoes protruding from the top and

Figure 24. Horizontal plane view of the descending thoracic aorta (Ao) in case 4 with aortic disruption. The site of rupture (RUP) is towards the left of the image into an area of walled-off hematoma. The white linear echos protruding from the top and bottom of the aorta are retracted portions of the wall at the site of aortic disruption.

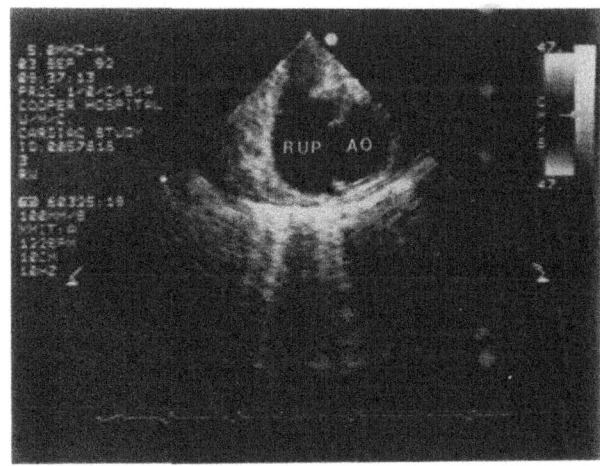

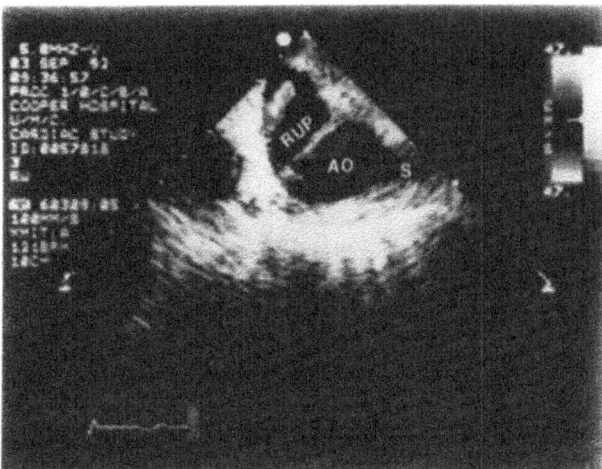

Figure 25. Vertical plane view of descending thoracic aorta in the region of the aortic arch in case 4 with aortic disruption. With color-flow Doppler activated, flow can be seen from the aorta (AO) into the area of walled-off rupture (RUP) as a red signal. At the right margin of the sector the origin of the left subclavian artery (S) can be seen.

bottom of the aorta are echoes from the retracted portions of the aortic walls at the site of disruption.

Figure 25 is the image obtained from the same probe position with the vertical imaging transducer activated. Because the probe is in the region of the aortic arch, the vertical plane transducer in this case still produces a circular image of the aorta, rather than a tube-like one. In this plane we can again image the lumen of the aorta (AO), as well as the walled-off hematoma in the region of rupture (RUP). In this frame we have also activated the color-flow Doppler function. We see a red color-flow signal indicating flow from the aorta into the area of walled-off rupture. In this vertical plane we can also see the origin of the subclavian artery (S), which courses off to the right of the screen, which is superiorly in this view. This site just distal to the origin of the left subclavian artery is a typical site for aortic disruption. Based on the findings on TEE, the chest was opened in the operating room and aortic rupture was confirmed and repaired with placement of a graft.

The final case (case 5) is a patient who was involved in a motor vehicle accident and suffered a fractured femur which required pinning. On the first post-operative day he developed sudden hypotension. He had also suffered

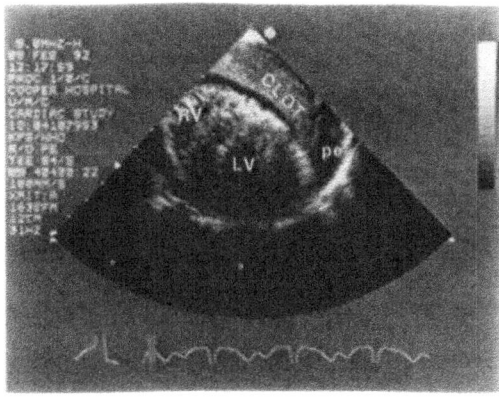

Figure 26. Horizontal plane short-axis view of left ventricle (LV) and right ventricle (RV) in case 5, with large bloody pericardial effusion (pe) with a mass of clotted blood (CLOT) within the effusion.

chest wall trauma at the time of the accident, but had no significant abnormalities on chest X-ray or ECG. We were called urgently to the bedside in the trauma intensive care unit for an emergency TEE to help identify the cause of sudden unexplained hypotension. Figure 26 is the horizontal plane short-axis view obtained from the transgastric probe position. The left ventricle (LV) and right ventricle (RV) are seen in cross-section. The grayish material surrounding the heart is a cap of clotted blood (CLOT) in a large bloody pericardial effusion (pe), which is the black echo-free space the clot is contained within.

From the standard transgastric TEE probe position, it is sometimes helpful to insert the probe even deeper into the stomach and flex the probe tip (and therefore the plane of imaging) upwards by clockwise rotation on the large control wheel. This produces a deep transgastric horizontal plane four-chamber view from the apex of the heart. This TEE view is virtually identical to that obtained from the apical chest wall echocardiographic window, since in both cases the transducer is located near the apex of the left ventricle. Chest wall imaging, however, is often quite technically limited an acutely ill patient such as this, and is also difficult to perform without interfering with the subxiphoid pericardiocentesis. From this TEE view, as shown in Figure 27, we were able to guide the pericardiocentesis needle (N) from the subxiphoid insertion site into the pericardial space, to allow withdrawal of the bloody fluid and relief of the pericardial tamponade. The needle appears as a bright echogenic linear structure entering the image from the left margin of the image, and passing into the pericardial effusion (pe) adjacent to the right ventricle (RV). Clotted blood (CLOT) can still be seen in the pericardial space in this view. This case is another example of the use of TEE to guide the placement of various catheters into and around the heart. The patient's systolic blood pressure had dropped to about 60 mm Hg despite high-dose intravenous epinephrine just prior to the emergency needle pericadiocentesis. Immediately after withdrawal of the bloody fluid, the arterial pressure began to rise and marked sinus tachycardia began to diminish. Incidentally noted in Figure 27 is a bright white echo return in the right ventricular chamber from a Swan-Ganz (s-g) catheter.

The patient was taken directly to the operating room for a subxiphoid pericardiotomy, to remove residual pericardial blood and clot, and to attempt

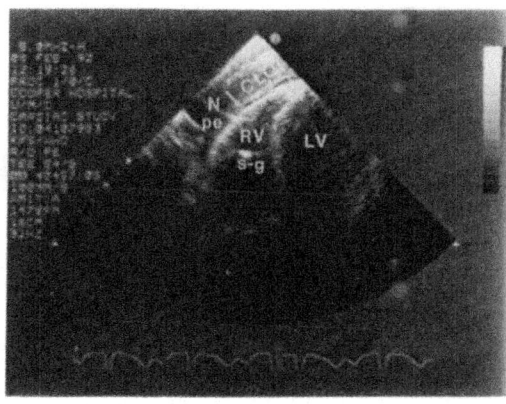

Figure 27. Deep transgastric horizontal plane four-chamber view of the heart in case 5, showing TEE-guided needle pericardiocentesis. pe = pericardial effusion; N = pericardiocentesis needle; RV = right ventricle; LV = left ventricle. A Swan-Ganz catheter (s-g) can also be seen in the right ventricle.

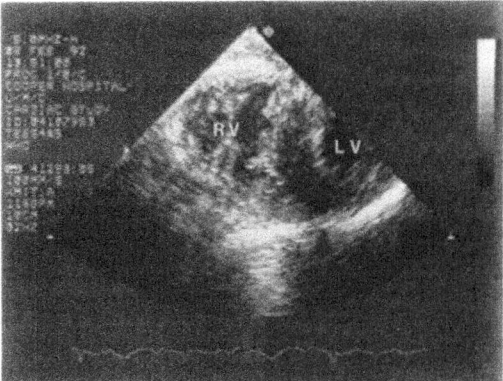

Figure 28. Horizontal plane transgastric short-axis view of the left ventricle (LV) and right ventricle (RV) in case 5. Note that the large pericardial effusion and clot previously seen in the pre-operative image of Figure 26 is no longer present. The right ventricle can be seen to be dilated compared to the left ventricle. Real-time imaging also showed severe hypokinesis of the walls of the right ventricle, consistent with contusion.

to define the source of the bloody pericardial effusion. TEE imaging was continued intra-operatively to help identify the source of bleeding into the pericardial space. Figure 28 shows the findings on intra-operative TEE in the standard transgastric horizontal plane short-axis view of the ventricles. Blood and clot are no longer seen in the pericardial space following surgical removal. A careful search was made by TEE imaging and color-flow Doppler for a residual source of bleeding into the pericardium, such as a tear in one of the great vessels, or in the atria. What was found instead by intra-operative TEE was a dilated, hypokinetic right ventricle. As can be appreciated from the still-frame image of Figure 28, the right ventricular chamber (RV) is significantly larger than the left ventricular chamber (LV). In the real-time images recorded in the operating room, the left ventricle showed vigorous segmental wall motion and normal ejection fraction once tamponade had been relieved. The right ventricle, on the other hand, showed severe hypokinesis as well as dilatation, particularly in its apical portion. Based on these findings, and in the absence of any other apparent source of pericardial bleeding by operative exploration or by intra-operative TEE, our presumptive diagnosis was that the patient had suffered a right ventricular contusion at the time of initial trauma. Blood had presumably oozed into the pericardial space from the contused right ventricular myocardium over the first 24 hours, resulting in

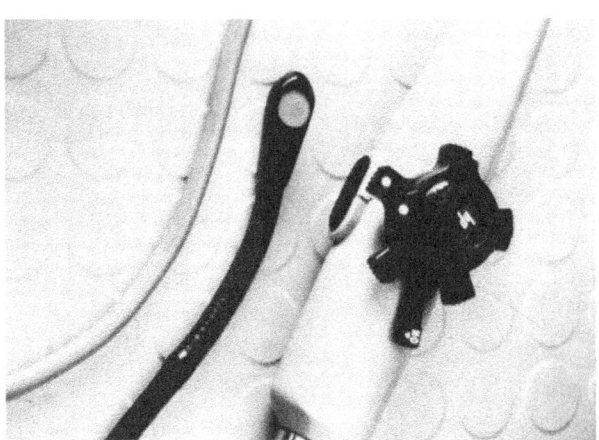

Figure 29. Multiplane TEE probe. The proximal end of the probe has two control wheels, similar to those of standard monoplane or biplane probe, used for tip manipulation. In addition, there is a switch located near these control wheels (black oval in this model) which rotates the sector of ultrasound around its central axis to obtain a virtually unlimited number of imaging planes.

progressive sinus tachycardia and eventually profound unexplained hypotension secondary to pericardial tamponade. Urgent bedside TEE was able to quickly establish the reason for hypotension, guide the placement of the pericardiocentesis needle to reverse it, and establish the presumed reason for the development of tamponade by intra-operative TEE imaging. The patient recovered uneventfully thereafter, and a follow-up TEE was obtained several weeks later. The right ventricle showed significant recovery, returning to nearly normal size and systolic function, as is often the case following right ventricular contusion.

I hope that the above brief overview and case presentations have provided some appreciation of the many uses of transesophageal echocardiography in cardiac surgery patients, for pre-operative, intra-operative and early post-operative applications.

I would also like to mention some future directions in TEE. One new direction that I mentioned earlier is the development of multiplane TEE probes. Just as the addition of biplane capability extended the power of TEE imaging beyond that possible with monoplane transducers, multiplane probes promise to extend the technique even further. Figure 30 shows the configuration of a typical multiplane or omniplane TEE probe. An additional control button, which is a small black oval located near the control wheels in this model, is used to rotate the plane of imaging. The transducer element at the distal tip of the probe is circular, allowing the sector of ultrasound to be rotated counterclockwise around its central (z) axis as shown in Figure 30. The ultrasound imaging sector starts out at 0 degrees, which is the orientation of the single horizontal plane of a monoplane TEE probe. In a multiplane probe, the imaging plane can be rotated to obtain vertical plane views at 90 degrees of rotation. Further rotation of up to 180 degrees provides even greater versatility of imaging planes. In addition, all intermediate planes can be utilized producing a continuous "sweep" through structures of interest. This sweep often provides an appreciation of anatomic relationships that is difficult or impossible to obtain with a single plane, or even by alternate activation of the two orthogonal planes of a biplane probe. And with a multiplane probe, these multiple imaging planes can be obtained without the need for extensive manipulation of the probe tip, which is time-consuming and sometimes uncomfortable for the awake patient.

One final future direction has to do with the increased interaction between the cardiac surgeon, anesthesiologist and cardiologist that the use

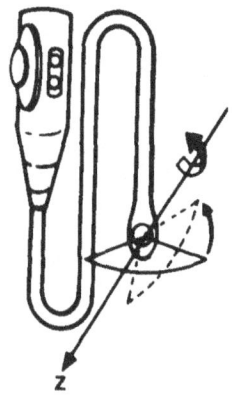

Figure 30. Multiplane TEE probe—Diagram of imaging plane rotation. The sector of ultrasound is initially oriented in the horizontal plane (0°) of a standard monoplane probe. A control button is depressed to rotate the plane of imaging around its central axis (z) in a counterclockwise direction through 90° (the standard vertical plane) and through all intermediate angles of imaging to 180°.

of transesophageal echocardiography fosters. This increased use of a multi-disciplinary approach to the evaluation and treatment of cardiac surgery patients is likely to have significant benefits in quality of care.

BIBLIOGRAPHY

Aronson S Lee B Wiencek J et al: Assessment of myocardial perfusion during CABG surgery with two-dimensional transesophageal contrast echocardiography. Anesthesiology 1991; 75:433–440.

Barzilai B Marshall WG Saffitz JE et al: Avoidance of embolic complications by ultrasonic characterization of the ascending aorta. Circulation 1989; 80(suppl 1):277–279.

Chan KL: Transesophageal echocardiography for assessing cause of hypotension after cardiac surgery. Am J Cardiol 1988; 62:1142–43.

Clements FM deBruijn NP: Perioperative evaluation of regional wall motion by transesophageal two-dimensional echocardiography. Anesth Analg 1987; 66:249–261.

Daniel WC Mugge A Martin R et al: Improvement in the diagnosis of abscesses associated with endocarditis by transesophageal echocardiography. N Engl J Med 1991; 324:795–800.

Davison M Burstow DJ: Transesophageal echocardiography in the assessment of hemolytic anemia following mitral valve surgery (abstract). J Am Soc Echocardiogr 1990; 3:221.

Erbel R Rohmann S Drexler et al: Improved diagnostic value of echocardiography inpatients with infective endocarditis by transesophageal approach. A prospective study. Eur Heart J 1988; 9:43–53.

Karalis DG Chandrasekaran K Victor M et al: Recognition and embolic potential of intraaortic atherosclerotic debris. J Am Coll Cardio 1991; 17:73–78.

Kochar GS Jacobs LE Kotler MN: Right atrial compression in postoperative cardiac patients: Detection by transesophageal echocardiography. J Am Coll Cardiol 1990; 16:511–516.

Kreindel MS Schiavone WA Lever HM et al: Systolic anterior motion of the mitral valve after Carpentier ring valvuloplasty for mitral valve prolapse. Am J Cardio 1986; 57:408–412.

Leung JM O'Kelly B Browner WS et al: Prognostic importance of postbypass regional wall-motion abnormalities in patients undergoing coronary artery bypass graft surgery. Anesthesiology 1989; 71:16–25.

Marwick T Obarski T Salcedo E et al: Transesophageal echo evaluation of mitral stenosis may underestimate "splitability score" (abstract). J Am Coll Cardiol 1990; 3:211.

Marwick T Stewart WJ: Intraoperative echocardiography guides extent of myectomy in hypertrophic cardiomyopathy (abstract). Circulation 1989; 80(suppl 2):268.

Marwick T Currie PJ Stewart WJ et al: Echocardiographic evaluation of immediate and late failed mitral valve repair (abstract). J Am Coll Cardiol 1989; 3:114.

Matsuzaki M Toma Y Kusukawa R: Clinical applications of transesophageal echocardiography. Circulation 1990; 82:709–722.

Mauere G Czer L: Intraoperative color Doppler assessment of mitral and tricuspid valve repair in Echocardiography and Doppler in Cardiac Surgery. New York Igaku-Shoin Medical publishers Inc. 1989:243–257.

Mihaileanu S Marino JP Chauvaud S et al: Left ventricular outflow obstruction after mitral valve repair (Carpentier's technique). Circulation 1988; 78(suppl 1):78–84.

Mohr-Kahaly S Kupferwasser I Erbel R et al: Regurgitant flow in apparently normal valve prostheses: Improved detection and semiquantitative analysis by transesophageal two-dimensional color-coded Doppler echocardiography. J Am Soc Echocardiogr 1990; 3:187–195.

Nellessen U Schnittger I Appleton C et al: Transesophageal two-dimensional echocardiography and color Doppler flow velocity mapping in the evaluation of cardiac valve prostheses. Circulation 1988; 78:848–855.

Salcedo EE Stewart WJ Klein AL et al: Evolution of transesophageal and epicardial echocardiography for intraoperative decision-making (abstract). J Am Soc Echocardiogr 1990; 3:219.

Sheikh KH deBruijn NP Rankin JS et al: The utility of transesophageal echocardiography and Doppler color flow imaging in patients undergoing cardiac valve surgery. J Am Coll Cardiol 1990; 15:363–372.

Stewart WJ Salcedo EE Cosgrove DM: The value of echocardiography in mitral valve repair. Cleve Clin J Med 1991; 57:177–183.

Stewart WJ Currie PJ Salcedo EE et al: Intraoperative Doppler color flow mapping for decision-making in valve repair for mitral regurgitation. Circulation 1990; 81:556–566.

Stewart WJ Agler DA Homa DA et al: Predicting the mechanism of mitral regurgitation prior to repair: A system using leaflet motion and color Doppler jet direction (abstract). Circulation 1990; 82(suppl 3):551.

Stewart WJ Currie PJ Salcedo EE et al: Jet direction by color flow mapping accurately depicts the mechanism of mitral regurgitation. (abstract). Circulation 1988; 78(suppl 2):434.

VanDaele ME Sutherland GR Mitchell MM et al: Do changes in pulmonary capillary wedge pressure adequately reflect myocardial ischemia during anesthesia: A correlative preoperative hemodynamic electrocardiographic and transesophageal echocardiographic study. Circulation 1990; 81:865–871.

THE USE OF CIRCULATORY SUPPORT IN CARDIAC SURGERY

R. L. Kormos, M.D.

University of Pittsburgh School of Medicine
Pittsburgh, Pennsylvania

The principal goal of mechanical circulatory support is to provide physiologic blood flow to the body's end organs in the situation where the natural heart fails to do so. The scenarios under which cardiac surgeons will encounter the need for mechanical circulatory support occur in one of two settings, i.e., the post-cardiotomy failure or in patients facing hemodynamic deterioration while awaiting cardiac transplantation. {1,2}

Despite improvements in surgical technique and perioperative myocardial preservation, a proportion of patients undergoing cardiac surgery are at risk of developing postoperative low output syndrome. Approximately 1 to 1.5 percent of patients undergoing cardiac surgery cannot be weaned from cardiopulmonary bypass despite adequate volume loading, metabolic stabilization, physiologic pacing, and full inotropic or intra-aortic balloon support. In addition, 10 to 15 percent of patients with acute myocardial infarction and subsequent cardiogenic shock and up to 20 percent of patients awaiting cardiac transplantation may be candidates for more extensive circulatory support. {3,4} This may be instituted for true ventricular "assistance" for postcardiotomy cardiogenic shock or as a "bridge" to cardiac transplantation when a donor heart is not immediately available. In the former case, the patient's ventricle is expected to recover and in the latter, it is not.

MECHANICAL CIRCULATORY SUPPORT FOR POST-CARDIOTOMY FAILURE

Most hospitals undertaking cardiac surgery have encountered the need to provide support to patients with refractory post-cardiotomy cardiogenic shock. The successful use of mechanical circulatory support under this circumstance is based on the premise that temporary ventricular support will allow the heart to recover from a potentially reversible injury. Circulatory support is provided by decompressing the left atrium or ventricle and returning blood to the aorta for left ventricular support. Decompressing the right atrium and returning the blood to the pulmonary artery provides right ventricular support. The mechanical link is provided by either an electrically or pneumatically driven pump. These pumps are either the bladder type containing prosthetic valves for an inlet and outlet or centrifugal pumps which produce continuous flow. The goals of mechanical circulatory support for post-cardiotomy heart failure include: 1) To provide adequate perfusion to the vital organs, 2) to reduce the left or right ventricular wall tension, 3) to allow recovery from myocardial injury, and 4) to provide circulatory support to allow time for diagnosis and/or therapy. Recovery may occur in the border zone of myocardial ischemia around established infarction if the self-perpetuating cycle of ischemia, low cardiac output, progressive, and irreversible myocardial damage, and shock can be halted. [5,6] The etiology of ischemic injury after cardiopulmonary bypass is usually attributed to poor myocardial protection. Ischemic injury may also result from overdistension of the ventricle, metabolic abnormalities, incomplete revascularization, coronary spasm, and embolism of air or particulate matter into coronary arteries. Such insults result in an imbalance between myocardial oxygen supply and demand with a subsequent depletion of adenosine triphosphate (ATP) stores. [7] Washout of nucleotide precursors during reperfusion may also lead to fluid extravasation, cellular and interstitial edema, increased regional wall stiffness, and ventricular dysfunction. Recovery of cardiac function occurs as myocardial edema is relieved, coronary spasm is resolved, and/or ATP stores are replenished. The ATP stores necessary for maintaining cellular membrane integrity take up to 3 to 4 days to be replenished and functional recovery may lag behind by as much as one week. One tactic in maintaining the balance between oxygen supply and demand is to reduce myocardial oxygen consumption (VO_2). The principal determinant of myocardial VO_2 is ventricular pressure work; volume work, preload and heart rate are less important. [8] Graham et al. demonstrated that myocardial VO_2 depends primarily on left ventricular peak wall stress and the intrinsic contractility of the muscle. [9] Because contractility is already depressed in the low output syndrome, one can only reasonably reduce the myocardial VO_2 by decreasing the peak ventricular wall stress.

The principles of ventricular support include reducing ventricular afterload, preload, and ventricular wall stress, and ultimately myocardial VO_2, augmenting myocardial perfusion, and maintaining a physiologic systemic cardiac output. The more complete the reduction in afterload and ventricular tension-time index, the greater the reduction in myocardial VO_2 and, therefore, infarct size. This approach is more physiologic than the administration of inotropic drugs, which increases contractility, cardiac output, and mean blood pressure at the expense of increasing myocardial VO_2. Some physicians argue that these goals are achieved with the use of the intra-aortic balloon. Indeed, as many as 50 percent of patients who initially cannot be weaned from cardiopulmonary bypass can be helped with conventional medical therapy, including the use of the intra-aortic balloon. The intra-aortic balloon pump provides afterload reduction for the failing left ventricle, augments coronary perfusion during diastole, and indirectly reduces left ventricular end–diastolic pressure. However, subendocardial perfusion is not maintained and infarct size is not reduced by the intra-aortic balloon because it is able to reduce myocardial VO_2 by only 50 percent of that achieved by left ventricular assistance. Also, the intra-aortic balloon can support a ventricle only if that ventricle is functioning at least marginally. {10–12} By supporting the failing ventricle with a left ventricular assist device, the physician can arrest the cycle of low output and ischemia and allow for functional recovery in areas not totally infarcted while supporting the systemic circulation. There is ample evidence that myocardial infarct size can be limited and myocardial function can be restored by supporting the ventricle with an external pumping device for a period of several hours to days.

Indications for Ventricular Assistance

Although many potential candidates are assessed for circulatory support, most are not suitable for the rigors of long-term ventricular bypass. The successful use of a ventricular assist device (VAD) depends on careful patient selection.

In general, patients are candidates for mechanical circulatory support following post-cardiotomy failure if they satisfy the following criteria: They have undergone technically successful cardiac surgery, they fail traditional methods to wean for cardiopulmonary bypass, they fulfill specific hemodynamic and/or clinical criteria, and have been on no greater than 4–5 hours of cardiopulmonary bypass. Patients who are over the age of 70, have had technically unsuccessful surgery, are suffering from an uncontrolled bleeding diathesis, have active sepsis or fever, or have other major chronic debilitating diseases should be excluded from mechanical circulatory support. At the end of cardiac surgery, several distinct interventions should be carried out if a problem in weaning from cardiopulmonary bypass is experienced and before the decision to insert a VAD is made. A circulatory support system should be implanted as soon as the failure to wean is detected by traditional means. However, the surgeon should not deviate from the normal progression of less invasive therapies that are available. The medical therapy of refractory ventricular failure after cardiac surgery involves correction of electrolyte, acid-base and metabolic abnormalities, adequate volume loading, treatment of dysrhythmias and atrioventricular sequential (physiologic) pacing. While these corrections are being made, a 10 to 20 minute period of reperfusion on cardiopulmonary bypass is advisable and often may permit weaning from bypass. Inotropic agents, such as calcium, epinephrine, dopamine, or dobutamine, may be required but may also induce ventricular irritability. Finally, the presence of residual surgically correctable abnormalities such as incomplete revascularization, valvular defects, or septal defects should be corrected.

Indications for Left Ventricular Assistance

Failure to wean from bypass because of left ventricular failure is defined by the presence of a cardiac index below 1.8 L/min/m^2 and urine output below 20 ml/hr in the presence of a left atrial pressure (LAP) above 25 mg Hg, and a central venous pressure (CVP) less than 20 mm Hg with a systolic blood pressure less than 90 mm Hg or a mean blood pressure less than 60 mm Hg. These criteria for failure to wean remain the same at each increasingly invasive stage of intervention during the weaning process (Figure 1). Patients with persistent severe cardiac dysfunction, despite volume loading and pharmacologic support, are eligible for insertion of the intra-aortic balloon for counterpulsation. This will decrease the left ventricular afterload and increase myocardial perfusion, which in turn will increase the cardiac index by about 0.8 L/min/m^2. Patients with normal acid-base balance and electrolyte concentrations who remain in cardiac failure despite intra-aortic balloon counterpulsation are candidates for a left ventricular assist device (LVAD).

Indications for Right Ventricular Assistance

Right ventricular failure occurs either primarily, as a result of poor myocardial protection during cardiopulmonary bypass or incomplete myocardial revascularization, or secondary to severe left ventricular failure. Isolated right ventricular failure is unusual but can be characterized by a cardiac index of less than 1.8 L/min/m^2, a systolic blood pressure less than 90 mm Hg (mean less than 60 mm Hg), and a CVP above 25 to 30 mm Hg in conjunction with a LAP below 10 to 15 mm Hg. The physician is unable to raise the LAP above 10 to 15 mm Hg with volume, despite an elevated CVP (25 to 30 mm Hg). The medical therapy of isolated right ventricular failure is usually limited because of the dysrhythmias (including tachycardia) secondary to the high doses of inotropic agents. Occasionally, right ventricular failure may occur during the use of left ventricular support and is characterized by an inability to provide adequate LVAD flow because of low left atrial filling pressure in association with a high CVP. The treatment options leading to right ventricular support are similar to those for left ventricular support and include treatment of associated left ventricular failure, volume loading, physiologic pacing, inotrope support, and intra-aortic balloon counterpulsation, which reduces pulmonary artery pressure indirectly by reducing left atrial pressure. In addition, counterpulsation improves right ventricular function by improving coronary perfusion. In some patients, isoproterenol reduces pulmonary vascular resistance and increases right ventricular contractility. Severe reactive pulmonary vascular hypertension may be reduced by the use of prostaglandin E$_1$. {13,14} More recently, a pulmonary artery balloon has been developed for counterpulsation and has been shown experimentally to be efficacious in the treatment of severe right ventricular failure; unfortunately it has been slow to gain clinical acceptance. {15}

Indications for Biventricular Assistance

The maximum output of the LVAD is directly dependent on the maximum flow achieved by the right ventricle. In some patients, passive flow through the pulmonary vascular bed may be accomplished by increasing the CVP and by using inotropic agents, such as isoproterenol. However, this therapy can lead to peripheral venous hypertension and edema formation. Mild right ventricular failure can be managed by pharmacologic agents and volume loading, but if the CVP is persistently higher than 25 mm Hg and the LVAD flow rates are below 1.8 L/min/M^2, a biventricular device or the addition of a right ventricular assist device (RVAD) is indicated.

Devices for Ventricular Assistance

Since the introduction of the cardiopulmonary bypass system in cardiac surgery by Gibbon in 1953, many full or partial bypass systems relying on left atrial or left ventricular decompression and aortic or femoral artery return have been developed for mechanical circulatory support. {16–19} Clinical evidence for the usefulness of a VAD was initially anecdotal. Patients who could not be weaned from cardiopulmonary bypass recovered after additional periods of bypass. As early as 1958, veno-arterial bypass was proposed for acute cardiogenic shock. {20} The need for systemic heparinization and the degree of trauma to blood elements produced by the presence of a bubble oxygenator prompted the search for better methods of circulatory support.

The concept of arterial counterpulsation was first proposed in 1961 by Clauss et al., who developed a pump that could withdraw blood from the arterial circuit during systole and return it during diastole. {16} This system, however, failed to provide adequate circulatory support, especially in the presence of profound hypotension. The need for an oxygenator was eliminated by using a transatrial septal approach to the left atrium from the jugular vein, which allowed partial decompression of the left atrium and returned oxygenated blood to the femoral artery. {17} This system required full heparinization and was very traumatic to the blood elements because a roller pump was used. Therefore, a cup was developed by Anstadt et al. in 1966; this cup fit around the ventricles and functioned as a mechanical form of cardiac compression. {21} However, the cup proved too damaging to the myocardium, especially in hearts with prosthetic valves, or aortocoronary bypass grafts. Similarly, the intraventricular balloon was too invasive and traumatic to the ventricle. {22} Although noninvasive, an external counterpulsation device, which was worn around the lower part of the body {23}, increased both preload and afterload and resulted in severe leg pain and cranial venous congestion after several hours of use.

The systems designed around a roller pump required a reservoir and anticoagulation and resulted in damage to pump tubing and blood elements. The occlusive nature of the roller pump on pump tubing permitted the entrance of air under conditions of low preload or ruptured lines when pumping against high afterload. The intra-aortic balloon has the advantage of being less invasive but fails to provide adequate cardiac unloading for reduction of myocardial work.

Most of the available systems are able to provide a wide range of required flows by decompressing the left atrium or ventricle. With the exception of the roller pump, these systems have been designed to produce minimal trauma to the blood elements and require minimal or no heparin administration postoperatively. Two major categories of VAD systems have been used clinically with significant success in the United States: 1) extracorporeal bypass pump systems (roller pump, centrifugal pump, and membrane oxygenator systems), and 2) pneumatic or electrically driven paracorporeal or implantable systems.

Centrifugal Bypass Systems

The Biomedicus (Biomedicus Inc., Minnetonke, MI) centrifugal pump requires $300 in disposable pump parts per case and is relatively simple to apply. This latter system has been used extensively by Magovern et al. for patients with both univentricular and biventricular failure. {24} The Biomedicus pump consists of rotating cones that impart a centrifugal force to the blood, moving it through a constrained vortex. Its non-occlusive nature is purported to result in less trauma to blood elements and tubing. Because of the unique shape and negative charge of the internal surfaces of the rotating cones, the pump has been reportedly used with minimal or no heparin. More recently, methods of bonding heparin to bypass pump tubing have been successfully used in these Biomedicus centrifugal pump heads. One disadvantage to this system is that the pump head does require changing every 24–48 hours as dictated by the regulatory restrictions on its use. This is in part due to potential bearing wear and overheating but also to the fact that even with anticoagulation, small amounts of thrombi are known to collect beneath the rotor and along its internal struts. Nevertheless, this device holds the most attraction for many centers where patients with medically refractory low output syndromes require treatment. This is primarily because of its cost effectiveness and ease of implantation. The pump adjusts automatically by reducing its output in the presence of an increased afterload resulting from arterial outflow obstruction even though the pump continues to rotate. A reservoir and heat exchanger are not required.

CANNULATION TECHNIQUES FOR CENTRIFUGAL PUMPS

The atrial cannulation site for an LVAD is determined by the desired degree of ventricular decompression and ease of insertion. Several experimental animal studies suggest that true reduction of infarct size necessitates full decompression of the left ventricle, which is achieved only through ventricular apical cannulation; but other studies have achieved ventricular function via left atrial decompression. [25,26] Ventricular cannulation is more invasive, immobilizes the heart and increases the risk of postoperative bleeding and ventricular outflow tract obstruction and high flow rates into the device. [27] Finally, ventricular cannula removal is traumatic to the marginally functioning left ventricle. These considerations are not important, however, when the device is used to support a patient before cardiac transplantation and the recovery of the native heart is not expected. Also, in this situation atrial cannulation may be difficult because of the immense size of the heart and the risk of thrombus formation increases. Although there are no specific cannula designed for the use with these systems, a variety of venous cannula from sizes 32 to 34 French can be placed either through the left atrial appendage, the right lateral wall of the left atrium posterior to the interatrial groove at the junction of the right superior pulmonary vein or through the roof of the left atrium between the aorta and superior vena cava caudate to the right pulmonary artery. Left atrial cannulation behind the interatrial groove tends to rotate the cannula tip into the atrial appendage where tissue can collapse around it and produce poor atrial decompression and low flow. The cannula may also rotate against the native or prosthetic mitral valve. Finally, thrombus formation more commonly will occur at the insertion site near the superior pulmonary vein. Using the left atrial appendage can be dangerous because of its inherent friability. Furthermore, in this position, a circumflex coronary artery graft may be prone to compression by the cannula. For these reasons, a more optimal position is the roof of the left atrium between the right pulmonary artery, aorta and superior vena cava. A venous cannula which is flexible and long enough should be chosen that can be advanced through the mitral valve into the main chamber of the left ventricle. Theoretical concerns about interfering with the function of the mitral valve are not realized and, indeed, when attempting to wean the patient from left ventricular support, the mitral valve is found to be competent. This, then, is the optimal position for a cannula that will take blood flow to the pump.

Arterial blood from the pump should be returned to the ascending aorta. Femoral artery cannulation presents a risk of femoral artery thrombosis unless full anticoagulation is employed or complex cannulation techniques for proximal and distal flows are used. In general, a site on the right lateral wall of the ascending aorta in a position proximal and lateral to the existing cardiopulmonary bypass cannula should be chosen. Should the aorta be too friable, small or short, the existing aortic perfusion cannula could be left in place. This is less desirable because this cannula has to be brought through the top of the incision which is an open path for infection, and inflexibility of the cannula leads to aortic erosion during long-term perfusion.

When cannulating the right heart for bypass, the cannula is usually placed through the right atrial appendage into the right ventricle and arterial return is to the main pulmonary artery. Important points to consider when using this type of system are that the cannulae should be tunneled sub-costally to allow for full closure of the sternum. This will reduce the amount of bleeding which is a major complication with the use of any type of ventricular assist device. Similarly, double purse-string techniques should always be used with pledgeted sutures at all cannulation sites to again reduce the risk of postoperative bleeding. In this way, virtually all bleeding can be controlled.

PNEUMATIC PARACORPOREAL SYSTEMS

The most common type of pneumatic paracorporeal system used for ventricular assistance is the Pierce–Donachy type pump (Thoratec Laboratories, Berkeley, CA). This pump employs a pneumatically activated polyure-thane pumping chamber and a polycarbonate housing. {28,29} The chamber has Bjork-Shiley (Shiley Inc., Irvine, CA) inlet and outlet valves and has a stroke volume of 65 ml. It can operate at either a fixed rate which is determined by the user, a fill to empty mode by which the heart ejects when a switch is tripped by the pumping chamber being filled, or a mode synchro-nized to the R wave of the ECG. This device lies outside the abdominal wall; two percutaneous cannulae drain the left atrium and return blood to the aorta. The device can be used either for left, right, or biventricular support with the use of two pumps. The inflow cannula to the pump is sewn directly to the left ventricular apex and arterial return is through a Dacron conduit sewn in an end-to-side fashion to the ascending aorta. A second type of inflow cannula has been designed to be placed through the left atrial appendage. In most cases for post-cardiotomy failure, the left atrial cannula is chosen usually because of space considerations on the ascending aorta where venous grafts have been sewn. These devices are FDA regulated and are expensive and therefore, require a considerable amount of technical and engineering expertise to be used. These more complex pumps have a larger role to play, both as investigational therapeutic tools and also as a bridge to cardiac transplantation.

RESULTS OF CIRCULATORY SUPPORT: POST CARDIOTOMY FAILURE

The combined ASAIO/ISHLT registry for mechanical ventricular assist pumps reveals that about 50 percent of patients can be weaned from mechanical support following post-cardiotomy failure. The overall hospital discharge rate, however, has remained at 25 percent, irrespective of whether simple centrifugal pumps or more complex pneumatic pumps are used (Table 1). The average length of support appears to be somewhere between 3–5 days during which time a rational decision can be made about the weanability of the device. The decision as to whether a left or right ventricular device can be removed is one which is usually based on a combination of weaning trials while hemodynamic indices are recorded. More recently, transesophageal echo has been used as a guide in measuring ventricular ejection fraction while an LVAD is weaned. A ventricle shows potential recoverability and a device may be considered appropriately discontinued when the native thermodilution output increases as the LVAD pump flow is decreased. In concert with this, an increase in LV shortening fraction on transesophageal echo indicates potential weanability.

The most important factors influencing outcome following ventricular support for post-cardiotomy failure include delay in insertion of the device, the presence or development of biventricular failure and the presence of completed myocardial infarction at the time of insertion of the device. {30-32} The most commonly occurring complications include bleeding, renal failure, and biventricular failure (Table 2). Bleeding remains a vexing complication of all mechanical circulatory support and often relates to the use of antiplatelet agents or anticoagulants prior to cardiac surgery and to the presence of hepatic dysfunction in patients with acute cardiogenic shock. The length of time spent on cardiopulmonary bypass during cardiac surgery prior to device implantation will also influence outcome significantly. Finally, technical factors such as insuring that suture sites and cannula insertion areas have been adequately secured and that the sternum has been fully closed following device implantation are all important factors in reducing blood loss.

The cause of death in patients undergoing ventricular support is most commonly persistent ventricular failure, renal failure, respiratory failure or bleeding. Because of the short term of support, infection and mechanical failure have less of a role to play in causing patient mortality. It should also be kept in mind that the rates of survival following support after post-cardiotomy failure are the highest in those patients who enter cardiac surgery with relatively normal left ventricular ejection fractions and have a sudden and unpredicted complication during surgery. Patients who enter cardiac surgery with ejection fractions of 20 percent or less and are not weanable from cardiopulmonary bypass rarely will recover with more extended periods of left ventricular support. If they do, they ultimately rarely survive to hospital

Table 1. Combined Registry: Post-cardiotomy Cardiogenic Shock; Overall Results

	# Pts	Weaned	Discharged
Centrifugal	863	399 (46.2%)	219 (25.4%)
Pneumatic	322	144 (44.7%)	79 (24.5%)
All others	38	10 (26.3%)	5 (13.2%)
Total	1223	553 (45.2%)	303 (24.8%)

Table 2. Post-cardiotomy Cardiogenic Shock

Complication*	Centrifugal (n=863)%	Pneumatic (n=322)%
Bleeding/DIC	55	40
BV Failure/Low Cardiac output	38	34
Renal Failure	31	37
Infection	11	23
Neurologic	12	11
Thrombus/Emboli	11	14
Hemolysis	5	10
Technical Problems	3	7

*Some patients presented with multiple complications.

discharge. Therefore, careful patient selection even in this critically ill group of patients is of utmost importance.

MECHANICAL SUPPORT AS A BRIDGE TO CARDIAC TRANSPLANTATION

The future of replacement therapy for end-stage heart disease has, until now, rested on cardiac transplantation. Improvements in postoperative care and immunosuppressive therapy have led to increasing success with progressive reduction in perioperative mortality and improved five-year actuarial survival of near 75 percent. Unfortunately, inevitable expansion of the recipient pool has not been met by similar growth in the donor heart pool. Faced with longer lists, transplant centers needed to provide a viable alternative for patients who are dying of sudden death or multiorgan failure. Thus, pneumatically driven artificial hearts[33] and more recently, electrically activated ventricular assist devices[34] are being employed in protocols to "bridge" critically ill patients to cardiac transplantation with mechanical circulatory support. This technology was initially applied with the belief in mind that transplantation would occur as soon as possible. However, the average waiting time for a donor heart is increasing, and surgeons are faced with transplant candidates who have the potential of requiring prolonged mechanical circulatory support. [35] Previous experience has shown that mortally ill candidates supported on inotropic drugs and/or the intra-aortic balloon pump enjoy equally good five year actuarial survival as those who undergo elective transplantation, given that a donor heart becomes available before multiorgan failure occurs. [36] Unfortunately, as waiting lists have increased, a larger percentage of these patients on inotropic support ultimately required an intra-aortic balloon pump and these patients, in turn, succumbed to the complications of immobility, lack of nutrition, and potential line sepsis from indwelling catheters. In unpublished data from the University of Pittsburgh, the thirty-day mortality of transplantation in a patient supported by an intra-aortic balloon pump is 21 percent compared to the mortality of a patient supported on inotropic agents of 12 percent and of a patient undergoing elective transplantation of 7 percent.

Indications for Circulatory Support as a Bridge to Transplantation

Although the goals for mechanical support in a patient being bridged to transplantation are comparable to that in a patient being supported with post-cardiotomy failure with respect to providing adequate perfusion for the vital organs, heart transplantation imposes new goals which are more demanding than those of post-cardiotomy support. For a transplant candidate, not only is the goal to provide a physiologic state compatible with life to allow a patient to survive to transplantation but it is important to realize that such devices should allow for physical rehabilitation, improve the patient's quality of life and ultimately reduce the mortality of transplantation. Inherent in these goals is the fact that a bridge to transplantation may require support for periods extending as long as six months to a year whereas in post-cardiotomy failure if recovery has not been seen within 7–14 days, the patient needs to be ultimately weaned from the device.

The stimulus for increasingly more invasive forms of circulatory intervention in a transplant candidate are primarily driven by increasing symptoms of congestive heart failure and evidence of reduced perfusion to the end organs such as kidney, liver, and brain. Initial therapies are directed to the use of vasodilators, digitalis, and diuretics. Ultimately more frequent hospital admissions with increasing symptoms of heart failure result in institution of inotropic agents such as dopamine, dobutamine, inocor, and enoximone. At this point, frequent right heart catheterizations, gated nuclear scans, and echocardiograms all are employed looking for evidence of decreased myocardial contractility and ventricular chamber dilatation. Confirmatory evidence of reduced end-organ perfusion is gained from renal and hepatic indices. However, a more sensitive measure of a failing heart and its effect on overall perfusion may be gained from measurement of the mixed venous oxygen saturation both at rest and with minimal exercise. Specific indications for the insertion of an intra-aortic balloon pump are center-specific but, in general, include changes in mental status, reduction in the mixed venous oxygen saturation (SvO_2) below 50 percent, a widening othe arterial-venous oxygen content difference [$C(a-v)O_2$], an elevation of the total serum bilirubin above 3 µg/kg/dL, and a rise in the serum creatinine above 2.5 m/kg/dL. Often, the onset of ventricular or atrial arrhythmias may also herald severe ventricular decompensation.

Initial success with the use of a intra-aortic balloon pump confirmed its potential in halting the progressive acidosis and initial hepatic or renal failure caused by low output syndrome. It may even be possible to wean the intra-aortic balloon pump after short periods of support. However, evidence suggests that the mortality of a patient who has required intra-aortic balloon pump support will be as high as 50 percent in the subsequent period awaiting cardiac transplantation if further measures are not instituted. As mentioned earlier, the long-term complications of immobility and infection imposed by the intra-aortic balloon pump prohibit use beyond periods of longer than 2–3 weeks.

Indications for the Use of Ventricular Assist Devices or the Total Artificial Heart as a Bridge to Cardiac Transplantation

When optimal medical management and/or intra-aortic balloon support fail to provide adequate cardiac output for adequate tissue perfusion and life in a cardiac transplant candidate, more aggressive mechanical assistance must be employed. The decision to insert a mechanical support system depends on clinical signs and symptoms of inadequate end-organ perfusion; namely, confusion, cool extremities, congestive heart failure, and reduced urine output. Ultimately, the decision to proceed with a ventricular assist device or total artificial heart (TAH) will depend on the availability of these devices at a particular center, as well as the consent of the individual patient or their relatives. As most of the available devices are regulated by the FDA for investigational use, the majority of centers will have limited access to them. Also, because of the investigational nature of these devices, certain other general criteria for inclusion must be met. In most cases, criteria for insertion of mechanical circulatory support is based upon a combination of either the total amount of required support including the level of inotropic agents and/or the intra-aortic balloon pump or evidence of hemodynamic deterioration as evidenced by a cardiac index below either 1.8 L/min/m^2 or 2.0 L/min/m^2, depending on the particular device used. Contraindications to the use of mechanical support in a patient awaiting cardiac transplantation include active infection, renal or hepatic failure, other debilitating systemic diseases, a panel reactive antibody level greater than 20 percent, and patients whose size by either body surface area or age are too small for the particular device used. In addition, most device protocols restrict the use of these experimental devices to patients under the age of 65. It is important to realize that because of the experimental nature of these devices, careful patient selection is of the utmost importance and that, in general, any patient who is not a good transplant candidate at the time of contemplated device insertion is by definition not a candidate for mechanical support as a bridge to transplantation.

As a transplant candidate begins to deteriorate, the greatest challenge is in designating the optimum time for intervention with these more invasive devices. The risks of infection, bleeding, thromboembolism, and multiorgan failure provoke a conservative approach; however, results of bridging will be diminished if one waits until a patient develops significant renal or hepatic failure. Once again, data from the University of Pittsburgh reveals that the risks of infection following the use of mechanical circulatory support are related to the peak total bilirubin prior to device implantation and to the number of days of intra-aortic balloon pump or inotropic support prior to contemplated device insertion. [37] These data support a more aggressive approach for device implantation in order to achieve successful support until transplantation.

Besides deciding on the appropriate patient for mechanical support prior to transplantation and the timing of that intervention, one must next choose the type of device for mechanical support. Currently, there are three devices which are considered experimental but are available for use under FDA guidelines as a bridge to cardiac transplantation.

The first of these is the Thoratec, or Pierce–Donachy, type pneumatic system previously described above for use in cases of post-cardiotomy failure. This system can be used for either univentricular support on the left side or as a biventricular assist device in appropriate circumstances. Two other devices are designed solely for left ventricular support and these are the Novacor left ventricular assist system, which is an electrically driven system, and the Thermedics pneumatic pump. Both of these pumps operate on a pusher-plate principal whereby either an electromagnet or air is used to compress a flexible bladder. Finally, experience has been gained with the Jarvik-7 total artificial heart which orthotopically replaces the native right and left ventricle. The decision to use univentricular or biventricular support is guided by the hemodynamics and measurement of the right ventricular ejection fraction at the time of device implantation. Patients with a right ventricular ejection fraction greater than 20 percent will survive univentricular support without significant difficulty. On the other hand, patients with right ventricular ejection fractions less than 20 percent will ultimately require large doses of inotropic support and/or a right ventricular assist device for the right ventricle in approximately 30–40 percent of the cases. The 60 percent who do survive univentricular support show progressive recovery of the right ventricle following LVAD implantation. Whether or not a patient develops right ventricular failure on a left ventricular assist device as a bridge to transplantation depends on the balance between several factors: The inherent preoperative right ventricular failure, relative right ventricular ischemia, mechanical effects of the LVAD on the interventricular septum and on right ventricular performance, and finally, the preoperative state of the patient. Any factors impeding pulmonary flow such as the need for increased blood transfusions and their effect on the pulmonary microvasculature, imminent multi-organ failure or severe biventricular dysfunction at the end stages of congestive heart failure may all affect outcome on univentricular support. Obviously, controlled trials will have to be performed in the future to see whether a patient is better served by the total artificial heart or two ventricular assist devices in situations of biventricular failure.

Results of Circulatory Support: Bridge to Transplantation

Overall results of bridge to transplantation with LVAD support only are presented in Table 3. Approximately 60–70 percent of patients supported with either centrifugal, electric or pneumatic devices will reach cardiac transplantation while approximately 60–70 percent will eventually be discharged. Results with centrifugal pumps are somewhat limited however because of the short periods of support available with this type of device. At the University of Pittsburgh, our initial results with bridge-to-transplantation using the total artificial heart were somewhat disappointing. Of 20 patients receiving implants, although 17 were ultimately transplanted, only 9 ultimately could be discharged from the hospital. Six of these nine died from infection during support periods which ranged between 2–48 days and averaged nine days of support. [37] This led to an ultimate bridge success of 45 percent. The ultimate cause of death in these patients was unrecognized infection, most commonly mediastinitis, which in most cases developed after transplantation. Approximately 20 percent of total artificial heart-supported patients had an infection before implant compared with 18 percent of patients using the Novacor left ventricular assist device. During the implant period 15 percent of patients bridged with a total artificial heart had an infection, and 100 percent of these patients died. On the other hand, 27 percent of the LVAD patients developed an infection during the support period, but the mortality rate was only 14 percent. Finally, 41 percent of the total artificial heart

Table 3. Bridge-to-Transplant Combined Registry; LVAD Only

	# Pts	Transplanted	Discharged
Centrifugal	22	16 (72.7%)	13 (59.1%)
Electrical	64	44 (68.8%)	40 (62.5%)
Pneumatic	80	59 (73.8%)	54 (67.5%)

patients had an infection after transplantation, and 85 percent of these patients died. The incidence of infection after transplant in the LVAD patients was 22 percent with no mortality. The experience with the total artificial heart has been less severe at other centers which report only minor infections with an incidence of only 42 percent. However, the average period of support in these patients was only nine days, and 42 percent were bridged to transplantation as a result of post-cardiotomy failure. [38] In this setting, patients were not subjected to the effects of chronic low output syndrome in an intensive care unit awaiting transplantation. It is interesting to note that in total artificial heart patients infection was related to either the peak or implant bilirubin and to the days on inotropic support and total hospital days prior to device implantation. Similarly, infections in the LVAD patients appeared to be related to the number of days on an intra-aortic balloon pump support appeared to correlate with subsequent device infection. Current results with the Novacor LVAD in 35 patients at the University of Pittsburgh show that approximately 75 percent of patients will ultimately reach transplantation and that 90 percent of these patients will be successfully discharged following transplantation. The superior survival appears to be related to improved patient selection using more rigorous guidelines. Patients on high doses of alpha agents with elevated white blood cell counts or signs of vasoactivity are considered very high risk for device support and are considered infected or imminent multiorgan failure unless otherwise proven.

From the joint ASAIO/ISHLT circulatory support database, the most common complications following bridge to transplantation using left ventricular assist devices are listed in Table 4.

Similarly, the most common causes of death relate to bleeding, renal failure, infection and embolism.

Perhaps a more important issue to deal with is the potential chronicity being seen with mechanical support for bridge to transplantation. As transplant waiting lists increase and more Status 1 patients are added, the waiting periods approach 6–8 months in some centers. As we learn more about the

Table 4. Bridge to Transplant

Complications	LVAD (n=161)	Causes of Death	LVAD (n=54)
Bleeding	29%	Bleeding	24%
Infection	24%	Renal Failure	22%
Embolus	14%	Infection	18%
Renal Failure	12%	Embolus	17%
Neurologic, not embolic	8%	Respiratory Failure	13%
Respiratory Failure	8%	Mechanical Failure	2%

effects of chronic support, the realization that this form of support will allow patients to recover from the effects of chronic low output syndrome has led to the development of programs focusing on the rehabilitation of patients. The potential for outpatient care has been recently acknowledged with the discharge of two patients on the TCI Heartmate device and three patients on the Novacor left ventricular assist device at the University of Pittsburgh. {39} The effects of this outpatient care are seen not only in the reduction of the total hospital charges and costs but also in improved quality of life for the patient and family. {40} Chronic support also provides the ability for patients to participate in an active exercise rehabilitation program which has shown that patients who participate in these programs have peak heart rates, mean exercise tolerance, and achieve peak work rates which approach those of transplant patients who have been discharged from hospital and been at home for at least 30 to 60 days. Therefore, we now have the potential of converting a patient in chronic heart failure to one with a physiologic state approaching that of a patient following transplantation. Ultimately, this will reduce the risk of heart transplantation and allow for quicker recovery and discharge from the hospital.

The future of mechanical circulatory support as a means to bridge a patient to transplantation will ultimately lie in totally implantable devices. Hopefully, these will include more biologically lined components, potentially valveless axial flow pumps, and wider application of univentricular support in carefully selected patients. More extensive physiologic control systems will have to be developed and ultimately, this technology will have to be applicable to home-based care.

CONCLUSION

Clearly, we have seen the evolution of mechanical circulatory support for two major uses, i.e., the post-cardiotomy failure and for chronic support as a bridge to cardiac transplantation. The technological needs in both these cases are vastly different, and issues relating to patient selection are important in both cases. While the success of these devices in post-cardiotomy failure relies mainly on the appropriate timing of implantation and careful patient selection, the success of bridge to transplantation will rely upon more biologically compatible devices which allow complete patient mobility and adaptability in the community.

REFERENCES

1. McGee MG Zillgitt SL Trono R et al: Retrospective analysis of the need for mechanical circulatory support (intra-aortic balloon pump/abdominal left ventricular assist device or partial artificial heart) after cardiopulmonary bypass: A 44 month study of 14,168 patients. Am J Cardiol 1980; 46:135.

2. The working group on mechanical circulatory support of the National Heart Lung and Blood Institute: artificial heart and assist devices: directions needs costs societal and ethical issues. May 1985.

3. Pae WE Pierce WS: Temporary left ventricular assistance in acute myocardial and cardiogenic shock: rationale and criteria for utilization. Chest 1981; 79:692.

4. Copeland JG Emery RW Levinson MM et al: The role of mechanical support and transplantation in the treatment of patients with end-stage cardiomyopathy. Circulation 1985; 72:II-7.

5. Ellis SG Henschke CI Sandor T et al: Biochemical and functional recovery of subepicardial border zone salvaged by reperfusion (abstr.) Am J Cardiol 1982; 49:1046.

6. Braunwald E Kloner RA: The stunned myocardium - prolonged post-ischemic ventricular dysfunction. Circulation 1982; 66:1146.

7. Reimer KA hill ML Jennings RB: Prolonged depletion of ATP and of the adenine nucleotide pool due to delayed resynthesis of adenine nucleotides following reversible myocardial ischemic injury in dogs. J Mol Cell Cardiol 1981; 13:229.

8. Sarnoff SJ Braunwald E Welch GH et al: Hemodynamic determinants of oxygen consumption of the heart with special reference to the tension-time index. Am J Physiol 1958; 192:148.

9. Pennock JL Pierce WS Prophet GA et al: Myocardial oxygen utilization during left heart bypass: Effect of varying percentage of bypass flow rate. Arch Surg 1974; 109:635.

10. Takanashi Y Campbell CD Laas J et al: Reduction of myocardial infarct size in swine: a comparative study of intra-aortic balloon pumping and transapical left ventricular bypass. Ann Thorac Surg 1981; 32:474.

11. LeGal YM Rideout SC: Reduction of myocardial infarct size: a comparison of the effectiveness of intra-aortic balloon pumping and transapical left ventricular bypass. Trans Am Soc Artif Intern Organs 1983; 29:593.

12. McDonnell MA Kralios AC Tsargaris TJ et al: Comparative effects of counterpulsation and bypass on left ventricular myocardial oxygen consumption and dynamics before and after coronary occlusion. Am Heart J 1979; 97:78.

13. D Ambra MN LaRara PJ Philbin DM et al: Prostaglandin E: a new therapy for refractory right heart failure and pulmonary hypertension after mitral valve replacement. J Thorac Cardiovasc Surg 1985; 89:567.

14. Fonger JD Borkow AM Baumbgartner WA et al: Acute right ventricular failure following heart transplantation; improvement with prostaglandin E and right ventricular assist. Heart Transplantation 1986; 5:317.

15. Spense PA Weisel RD Easdown JA et al: The hemodynamic effects and mechanism of action of pulmonary artery balloon counterpulsation in the treatment of right ventricular failure during left heart bypass. Ann Thoracic Surg 1985; 39:329.

16. Clauss RH Birtwell WC Albertal G et al: Assisted circulation. I. The arterial counterpulsator. J Thorac Cardiovasc Surg 1961; 41:447.

17. Dennis C Hall DP Morena JR et al: Reduction of the oxygen utilization of the heart by left heart bypass. Circ Res 1962; 10:298.

18. Debakey ME: Left ventricular bypass pump for cardiac assistance. Clinical experience. Am J Cardiol 1971; 27:3.

19. Stuckey JH Newman MM Dennis C et al: The use of the heart-lung machine in selected cases of acute myocardial infarction. Surgical Forum 1957; 8:342.

20. Connolly JE Bacaner MB Bruns EL et al: Mechanical support of the circulation in acute heart failure. Surgery 1958; 44:225.

21. Anstadt GL Schiff D Baue AE: Prolonged circulatory support by direct mechanical ventricular assistance. Trans Am Soc Artif Intern organs 1966; 12:72.

22. Donald DE Bove AA McGoon DC: Sustained circulation by a left ventricular balloon pump after severe myocardial damage in dogs. J Thorac Cardiovasc Surg 1972; 63:681.

23. Soroff HS Birtwell WC Giron F et al: Support of the systemic circulation and left ventricular assist by synchronous pulsation of extramural pressure. Surgical Forum 1965; 16:148.

24. Magovern GJ Park SB Maher TD: Use of the centrifugal pump without anticoagulants for postoperative left ventricular assist. World J Surg 1985; 9:25.

25. Pennock JL Pae WE Jr Pierce WS et al: Reduction of myocardial infarct size: Comparison between left atrial and left ventricular bypass. Circulation 1979; 59:275.

26. Ruf W Smith GT Geary G et al: The effect of left ventricular-to-aortic bypass on infarct size and infarct microcirculation in baboons. J Thorac Cardiovasc Surg 1981; 81:408.

27. Cox JL Pass HI Anderson RW et al: Augmentation of coronary collateral blood flow in acute myocardial infarction. Surgical Forum 1975; 26:238.

28. Pierce WS Rosenberg G Donachy JH et al: Postoperative cardiac support with a pulsatile assist pump: Techniques and results. Artif Organs 1987; 11:247.

29. Pennington DG Samuels LD Williams G et al: Experience with the Pierce–Donachy ventricular assist device in post-cardiotomy patients with cardiogenic shock. World J Surg 1985; 9:37.

30. Bernhard WF Berger RL Stetz JP et al: Temporary left ventricular bypass: factors affecting patient survival. Circulation 1979; 60:131.

31. Pennock JL Pierce WS Wisman CB et al: Survival and complications following ventricular assist pumping for cardiogenic shock. Ann Surg 1983; 198:469.

32. Pennington DG Merjavy JP Swartz MT et al: The importance of biventricular failure in patients with postoperative cardiogenic shock. Ann Thorac Surg 1985; 39:16.

33. Griffith BP Hardesty RL Kormos RL et al: Temporary use of the Jarvik-7 artificial heart prior to transplantation. New Eng J Med 1987; 316:130–4.

34. Kormos RL Borovetz HS Gasior T et al: Experience with univentricular support in mortally ill cardiac transplant candidates. Ann Thor Surg 1990; 49(2):261–71.

35. Kormos RL Borovetz HS Armitage JM et al: Evolving experience with mechanical circulatory support. Ann Surg 1991; 214(4):471–7.

36. Hardesty RL Griffith BP Trento A et al: Mortally ill patients and excellent survival following cardiac transplantation. Ann Thorac Surg 1986; 41:126.

37. Kawai A Kormos RL Griffith BP: Management of infections in mechanical circulatory support devices. In: Cardiac Surgery State of the Art Reviews: Mechanical Cardiac Assist Ott RA Gutfinger DE Gazzaniga AB (eds). Hanley and Belfus Inc. Philadelphia PA 1993:413–424.

38. Pifarre R Sullivan H Montoya A et al: The use of the Jarvik-7 total artificial heart and Symbion ventricular assist device as a bridge to transplantation. Surgery 1990; 108:681–685.

39. Kormos RL Murali S Dew MA et al. : Chronic mechanical circulatory support: Rehabilitation low morbidity and superior survival. Ann Thor Surg (in press).

40. Dew MA Kormos RL Roth LH et al: Life quality in the era of bridging to cardiac transplantation: Bridge patients in an outpatient setting. ASAIO Journal 1993; 39:145–152.

BLOOD TRANSFUSION PRACTICES IN CARDIOVASCULAR SURGERY

Richard K. Spence, M.D. Aurel C. Cernaianu, M.D., and
Anthony J. DelRossi, M.D.

University of Medicine and Dentistry of New Jersey
Robert Wood Johnson Medical School
Camden, New Jersey

Blood transfusion has made cardiovascular surgery possible. Without
the ability to prime the heart lung machine or to replace losses encountered
during aortic procedures, cardiovascular surgery would not exist as we know
it today. As cardiovascular procedures became more prevalent, the amount
of blood transfused increased. It was not uncommon in the recent past to
type and cross patients for 20 or more units of blood for a major cardiovascular procedure. The widespread use of large amounts of blood was justified
by the belief that transfusion was innocuous, carrying little risk beyond the
rare reaction and the occasional case of hepatitis. This sense of security
disappeared abruptly in the 1980's when transfusion-related acquired immune deficiency syndrome (AIDS) surfaced. Although the incidence of post-
transfusion AIDS was, and still is, very low, the fact that the disease is
uniformly fatal was enough to cause cardiovascular surgeons to reassess
their transfusion practices and to look for alternatives to homologous blood.

If we are to eliminate the risks associated with homologous blood
transfusion, our ultimate goal should be to perform cardiovascular surgery
using only the patient's own blood. Current maximum surgical blood ordering
schedules (MSBOS) recommend typing and crossing three to five units of
homologous blood for major cardiovascular procedures. [1-3] Both autologous predonation of blood and perioperative autotransfusion have significantly reduced the need for homologous transfusion, but neither approach
has completely eliminated its use. Moreover, these modalities are not always
available to or advisable for cardiovascular surgical patients. Anemic patients
and those with symptomatic disease cannot safely donate their own blood
preoperatively; reinfusion of shed blood presents risks of its own.

Our interest in bloodless cardiovascular surgery developed as part of a
program designed to provide surgical care to Jehovah's Witness patients who
refuse both homologous and autologous predonated blood transfusion. [4]
Our success in performing major abdominal procedures without transfusion

Cardiac Surgery: Current Issues 2, Edited by A. C. Cernaianu and A. J. DelRossi,
Plenum Press, New York, 1993

prompted us to examine our results in cardiovascular surgery to determine 1) if homologous blood use could be eliminated safely and 2) if autologous predonation of blood was necessary.

MATERIALS AND METHODS

We examined the hospital course and outcome of 59 patients who underwent 63 elective cardiovascular procedures at our institution between the years 1984 1nd 1991. Procedures are defined in Table 1. Elective major vascular procedures were defined as those involving the great vessels or for which the risk of bleeding was high and/or perioperative transfusion was considered likely according to prior experience and maximum surgical blood ordering schedules (MSBOS). All procedures were performed by the authors. Regional anesthesia was used in vascular cases where appropriate. All patients were monitored noninvasively during surgery with pulse oximetry. Those undergoing cardiac and aortic procedures, as well as those with anemia, were monitored perioperatively with pulmonary artery flow directed catheters and peripheral arterial catheters. Patient characteristics are described in Table 2. All were Jehovah's Witnesses who refused homologous blood transfusion and autologous predonation of blood on religious grounds. These patients accepted the use of a modified version of a washed-cell autotransfusion device (Electromedics, Englewood, CO) that was constructed to provide an unbroken circuit between the patient and the autotransfusion machine. Intraoperative autotransfusion was not used in the 13 patients who underwent lower extremity bypass grafting, amputation, or infected graft excision.

The preoperative hemoglobin (Hb) averaged 11.6 g/dL and ranged between 5.2 and 14.8 g/dL. The majority of our vascular patients (16 of 23 70 percent) were anemic preoperatively with an average Hb level of 10.1 g/dL. Three severely anemic (average Hb 6.3 g/dL) patients were treated with a perioperative infusion of Fluosol (Green Cross, Osaka, Japan) a perfluorocarbon compound, as part of a clinical trial of this product's safety and efficacy in the treatment of anemia. Three other patients were treated with recombinant erythropoietin injections (Ortho Biotech, Raritan, NJ) postoperatively as part of a clinical trial of this drug's role in the treatment of acute, perioperative anemia.

Table 1. Operative Procedures

Procedure	No.	Preoperative Hb (g/dL)	Postoperative Hb (g/dL)	Blood loss (cc)
Coronary artery bypass graft	27	12.8 (9.4–14.8)	7.3 (5.8–9.2)	800
Aortic valve replacement	8	12.1 (8.4–14.5)	7.0 (6.3–8.4)	1000
Abdominal aortic aneurysm repair	11	12.6 (9.4–14.8)	8.9 (7.3–10.5)	950
Leg bypass	5	11.5 (9.7–12.7)	10.5 (9.1–12.2)	150
Portocaval shunt	4	5.9 (5.6–6.1)	5.0 (3.5–58)	1600
Other*	8	9.6 (5.2–12.8)	8.4 (2.7–12.2)	475

*Excision infected graft (1), revision of femoral popliteal graft (3), amputation (4); parentheses represents range.

Table 2. Patient Characteristics

Variables	
Gender (F/M)	31/28
Age (yrs)	63 (41–79)
Preoperative Hb (g/dL)	11.6 (5.2–14.8)
Postoperative Hb (g/dL)	7.4 (2.7–14.5)
Estimated blood loss (cc)	900 (250–2500)

Data presented as mean; parentheses represent ranges.

RESULTS

Three of fifty-nine patients died (5.1 percent); two post aortic valve replacement, and one post portacaval shunt. Only one patient who underwent aortic valve replacement died as a result of operative bleeding. The second patient died on the 30th postoperative day from an unexpected arrhythmia following aortic valve replacement. The third patient died eight days after a portocaval shunt when he apparently occluded his shunt and exsanguinated from variceal bleeding. There was no cardiac morbidity in the remaining patients.

Estimated blood loss (EBL) was similar for both the cardiac and vascular patient groups: cardiac EBL = 800 cc average, 300–2000 cc range; vascular EBL = 955 cc average, 50–2500 cc range. The decrease in hemoglobin level was twice as great in the cardiac group (average Hb drop 5 g/dL) compared to the vascular group (average Hb drop 2.2 g/dL). Blood loss was substantially less in those patients who underwent lower extremity bypass (150 cc average) when compared to the remaining vascular and/or cardiac patients. The average amount of reinfused autologous blood was 360 cc (range: 250–1000 cc).

DISCUSSION

Techniques designed to limit the use of homologous blood transfusion in cardiovascular surgery can be divided conveniently into preoperative, intraoperative and postoperative measures, with the understanding that there is some overlap in each of these areas. (Table 3) Of the preoperative measures, autologous predonation of blood has had the greatest impact. In a study of 271 consecutive patients undergoing elective open heart surgery, Owings and colleagues showed that autologous predonation eliminated the need for homologous blood use in 73 percent of the group. [5] This information is even more compelling when one considers that 82 percent of those who did not predonate required banked blood. The amount of homologous blood given to the predonation group was significantly lower 0.8 + 1.5 units vs. 3.7 + 3.6 units. Similar results have been reported by others. [6–8]

The success of autologous predonation depends on a number of factors, including time, hemoglobin level, patient disease, and cooperation, both from the patient and the physician. Successful autologous predonation requires intervention by the cardiologist or surgeon at least one month before sched-

Table 3. Approach to Bloodless Surgery

Surgical phase	Measures
Preoperative	Check Hb/Hct, iron stores, nutritional status
	Iron replacement
	Erythropoietin
	Limit blood drawing
	Schedule autologous predonation
	Erythropoietin
Intraoperative	Hemodilution
	Autotransfusion
	Platlet pheresis
	Halstedian principles
	Blood substitutes/alternatives
	Pharmacologic support
	Heparin/protamine
	Desmopressin
	Aprotinin
	Fibrin glue
	Lower transfusion trigger
Postoperative	Autotransfusion
	Limit blood drawing
	Restore red cell mass
	Nutritional support
	Iron replacement
	Erythropoietin
	Lower transfusion trigger

uled surgery. The average donor can give 3 to 4 units of blood in this time frame with collection continuing up to 72 hours before surgery. {5,8} Because time is critical, it is essential that the surgeon consider predonation as early as possible. The amount of blood needed for cardiovascular surgery varies according to the operation. Maximum surgical blood ordering schedules based on reviews of large numbers of patients call for a minimum of three units for open heart and major vascular surgery. {1} More than one month may be needed for predonation if patients are to attain the level of five units recommended by Axelrod et al in his study of transfusion requirements for cardiac surgery. {2}

Unfortunately, the amount of time required for successful predonation often creates major problems. The interval from the time of catheterization until surgery is less than one month for many patients who undergo coronary artery bypass grafting. Approximately one-half of Owings' patients fell into this category and could not predonate. {5} Since many patients do not meet their surgeons until a few days before surgery, predonation must be initiated early by the referring cardiologist if adequate amounts of blood are to be obtained. A preoperative delay of one month may not be possible or advisable for some patients, especially those with symptomatic or large aneurysms and those with esophageal varices and a history of recent bleeding. Autologous predonation is not an option for Jehovah's Witnesses.

Preoperative anemia may eliminate a patient from consideration for autologous predonation. The American Association of Blood Banks has defined 11 g/dL as the lowest acceptable hemoglobin level for predonation.

{9} Using this limitation, 15 to 20 percent of patients are unable to donate. Women tend to be anemic more often than men and donate on average one unit less. {5} Patients should be evaluated preoperatively for iron-deficiency anemia and treated with oral iron preparations to promote recovery of red cell mass. If possible, surgery can be postponed until adequate hemoglobin levels have been reached to allow predonation. Preoperative administration of erythropoietin has been shown to increase the number of units donated from 4.1 to 5.4 in a prospective, randomized study of patients scheduled for orthopedic surgery, but this drug is not available for widespread use at present. {10}

Predonation is contraindicated in patients with critical aortic stenosis or symptomatic coronary artery disease. {9} Vascular surgeons should add to this list the precautions noted above. The majority of patients who are candidates for major vascular surgery also have coronary artery disease. Although Owings reported that autologous predonation was safe in a group of patients with known coronary artery disease, i.e., those scheduled for coronary artery bypass surgery, a small percentage of patients had hypotensive responses to blood withdrawal. Symptoms can be minimized in this group by infusing saline during phlebotomy and by limiting the total amount of blood collected at each session to 500 cc. {5}

Even with these precautions, the incidence of reactions may be higher than initially thought. Spiess et al recently reported a significant incidence of hemodynamic reactions in a group of 123 high-risk patients who donated blood preoperatively. {11} Over thirty percent had a 20 percent or greater decrease in either systolic or diastolic blood pressure. 5.4 percent had tachycardia; 3.1 percent had serious dysrhythmias. The characteristics of the high-risk patient in this group will sound very familiar to the cardiovascular surgeon. Criteria included: a history of myocardial infarction, angina, dysrhythmia, hypertension requiring two or more medications, congestive heart failure, valvular or congenital heart disease, seizure disorder, cerebral vascular insufficiency, or a previous cerebral vascular accident. Since most patients scheduled for elective cardiovascular surgery will fit into one or more of these categories, it would appear that autologous predonation is a high-risk endeavor in this group. In response to Spiess's conclusions, Sandler and Sacher recommended that autologous predonation be approached conservatively in this group of patients. {12}

Although physician acceptance of autologous predonation is increasing, many physicians are either unaware of the existence of such programs or are unfamiliar with how to arrange for their patients to predonate blood. A nationwide study of autologous predonation published in 1987 estmated that only 10 percent of eligible patients actually gave blood before surgery. {7} Although this finding may be due in part to lack of patient compliance, physicians must also bear some responsibility for the poor response to autologous predonation. Goodnough found that this option was not offered to any open-heart patients in one of two hospitals he surveyed in spite of the fact that the hospital had an active autologous program for other procedures. {8}

If the patient cannot or will not donate blood before hospitalization, the next best option is to collect and reinfuse the blood in the perioperative period, i.e., autotransfusion. Intraoperative autotransfusion can be performed safely with systems that either collect and reinfuse shed blood directly or more sophisticated devices that wash the blood before reinfusion. Each approach has its advantages and disadvantages. Systems that wash blood eliminate the risk of reinfusion of free hemoglobin, coagulation byproducts and contaminants contained in plasma, but they are expensive, time-consuming and require technical expertise when compared to simpler, direct reinfusion devices. Both have been used successfully to reduce the need for homologous blood transfusion in major vascular surgery. [13–17] However, to our knowledge, autotransfusion by itself has never been shown to completely eliminate homologous transfusion.

Our Jehovah's Witness patients generally accept a modified form of intraoperative autotransfusion. We prefer to use a system that collects, washes, and reinfuses shed blood via a continuous circuit from the patient to the machine and back to the patient constructed from intravenous tubing and Y-connectors. Our success with this adjunct is demonstrated in our ability to reinfuse most of the shed blood we collect. The average estimated blood loss was approximately 900 cc; the average amount of reinfused blood was 360 cc in this group. If one considers that the hematocrit of washed, reinfused blood is approximately 45–50 percent, our actual blood loss was less than 50 percent of our estimates. The calculated difference between average preoperative and postoperative hemoglobin levels of 2.0 g/dL in our vascular patients reinforces the value of autotransfusion in reducing absolute operative blood loss.

Autotransfusion was not used in thirteen patients who underwent lower extremity bypass, amputation or removal of an infected bypass graft. In the latter two groups, we chose not to use this modality because of difficulties salvaging blood and the desire not to reinfuse stagnant or contaminated blood. The five extremity bypasses, although done in anemic patients, resulted in very little drop in hemoglobin levels (11.5 g/dL preop to 10.5 g/dL postop). Estimated blood loss was only 150 cc. Even if homologous blood transfusion had been acceptable to these patients, it would not have been necessary. We believe that maximum surgical blood ordering schedules should be reduced to zero for the majority of lower extremity bypasses.

Acute normovolemic hemodilution became an integral part of cardiac surgery when crystalloid solutions replaced blood as the pump prime. [18–20] In their excellent review of the subject, Stehling and Zauder discuss the success of hemodilution in reducing the need for homologous transfusion in a wide variety of surgical procedures, including both cardiac and vascular cases. [21] In a randomized trial comparing autologous predonation to acute normovolemic hemodilution in patients who underwent radical retropubic prostatectomy, Ness et al. reported that hemodilution was successful both in replacing autologous predonation and in eliminating homologous blood use. [22] The authors correctly state that the results of this randomized trial can be applied to any procedure in which a blood loss of 1000 mL or greater is anticipated. We have used hemodilution techniques successfully during open heart surgery in Jehovah's Witness patients as long as the hemodilution occurs via the heart lung machine. Our vascular patients have refused the actual removal of blood that is required for hemodilution. Moreover, the majority of our vascular patients in this study were anemic, precluding acute normovolemic hemodilution as an option.

Hemodilution theoretically offers an advantage over autotransfusion in the form of a better blood product. Phlebotomy and temporary storage of a unit or more of whole blood as is done in hemodilution does not diminish or activate plasma clotting factors or platelets as does suctioning blood through a collection wand or circulating it through the heart lung machine. Reinfusing the latter type of blood product without washing or filtering may be hazardous if large quantities are given. Washing shed blood before reinfusion solves this problem, but at the expense of eliminating desirable clotting factors and platelets. The advantages of both approaches have been combined in the form of platelet sequestration.

Platelet sequestration has been shown to reduce both blood loss and the need for homologous transfusion in cardiac surgery. [23,24] A unit of whole blood is withdrawn from a large-bore intravenous line prior to heparinization and is replaced with crystalloid, thereby hemodiluting the patient. The whole blood is separated into packed cells and a platelet-rich plasma component using a centrifuge-based autotransfusion device or, if available, by hemofiltration. The packed red cells are reinfused as needed during the case. The platelet-rich plasma, which has avoided exposure to both heparin and the heart-lung machine, is reinfused when coming off bypass. This provides the patient with both active platelets and clotting factors at a time when both may be decreased. This technology can be applied not only to cases where extracorporeal circulation is required but also to vascular procedures in which autotransfusion is used.

Blood loss can also be reduced by careful attention to operative detail. [25,26] We prefer to use a midline approach for abdominal aortic surgery because it is avascular and minimizes incisional bleeding. Comparisons of the midline to the retroperitoneal approach have shown that blood loss is similar regardless of which is employed. [27] The key to preventing blood loss lies more in incorporating Halstedian principles into the approach most familiar to the surgeon, rather than in unquestioning adoption of unfamiliar procedures. Dissection should be done along avascular planes using cautery when possible. All potentially vascular structures sholud be clipped or tied before being cut. This is essential in the patient with portal hypertension if massive bleeding from disrupted, engorged veins is to be avoided. An intravenous infusion of vasopressin started before making an incision in portacaval shunt cases helps to constrict these dilated vessels. If prosthetic material is required for aortic replacement, woven Dacron offers the advantage of less blood loss over more porous knitted grafts. [28] Gelatin-sealed and polytetrafluoroethylene materials may offer similar advantages. [28,29]

Pharmacologic prevention of blood loss holds promise for the future. Monitoring of heparin levels and reversal with protamine is standard practice in cardiac surgery and does not interfere with other blood conservation techniques. Although we have not used desmopressin or aprotinin, these drugs have been shown to reduce the amount of blood loss in cardiac surgery and, consequently, the need for homologous transfusion. [30–36] We treated three of our severly anemic (hemoglobin less than 7.0 g/dL) patients with infusions of Fluosol DA-20 percent as part of a clinical trial of the safety and efficacy of this product in the treatment of acute anemia. [37] Fluosol significantly increases dissolved oxygen content, but this addition appears to have little clinical effect on overall outcome. Disappointing results with

Fluosol are a result of its low concentration of perfluorocarbon and its rapid elimination from the circulation. Future formulations that address these problems may be more useful. We believe that perfluorocarbons will have a definite but limited role in future bloodless surgery as hemodilution agents, modifiers of reperfusion injury or as temporary support in patients with well defined critical oxygen deficits.

Erythropoietin holds much greater promise as an adjunct in bloodless surgery. Goodnough et al. have shown that erythropoietin administered preoperatively can significantly increase the number of units of blood obtained through autologous predonation. {10} It follows from this finding that the time required for predonation can be decreased, thereby reducing the potential risk to patients with critical vascular lesions. Three of our patients recieved erythropoietin as part of a clinical trial of its usefulness in treating perioperative anemia. (Unpublished data) Each received an initial dose of 300 units/kg intravenously or subcutaneously on a Monday-Wednesday-Friday schedule followed by a similar dosage regimen using 150 units/kg. Overall results are preliminary but encouraging in that hematocrits were significantly higher in those treated with erythropoietin when compared to a group of similar, untreated patients. Erythropoietin appears to accelerate recovery of hematocrit in the anemic, postoperative patient. We believe that perioperative administration of erythropoietin will have a significant impact on future bloodless cardiovascular surgery.

Postoperative blood conservation measures are primarily continuations of those steps taken pre and intraoperatively. These include nutrition, iron restoration and erythropoietin to stimulate red cell mass replacement. Mediastinal blood can be collected and reinfused in the immediate postoperative period if the patient will accept this process. Although this process appears to be safe if time limitations are imposed, its overall benefit in reducing the need for homologous blood transfusion has been questioned. Desmopressin and aprotinin may be useful in the postoperative period to control blood loss. However, none of the above adjuncts should substitute for early re–exploration in a patient who is bleeding actively. {38–41}

We have become our own worst enemies in the intensive care unit. After having performed high quality surgery using blood conservation techniques, we bleed our patients repeatedly by using cookbook order sheets that include standing orders for frequent, often unnecessary lab tests. Smoller and Kruskall measured daily blood losses of 41.5 mL in ICU patients, which totals approximately a one unit blood loss per week. {40} Blood samples should be limited to essential studies and determinations that cannot be made through other monitoring systems. By using pediatric collection tubes and returning flush solutions from arterial and central venous lines, blood wastage can be eliminated. Now that postoperative hemoglobin levels of 7, 8, and 9 g/dL are routinely accepted, few patients can tolerate repeated, unecessary blood sampling.

An absolutely essential component of a bloodless surgery program is the willingness to accept a lower transfusion trigger, i.e., a perioperative hemoglobin level less than 10 g/dL. Our previous work has shown that patients can safely undergo elective surgery with preoperative hemoglobin levels as low as 6 g/dL. {4} The average preoperative hemoglobin level in this group of patients was 11.6 g/dL with somewhat lower levels in the vascular patients

(Hb 10.1 g/dL). There were no intraoperative problems, deaths or myocardial events from ischemia caused by a low hemoglobin preoperative level. The one patient who died during surgery could not be weaned from the heart lung machine following redo coronary bypass surgery because of poor ventricular function. Her blood loss was a contributing factor. Our study results support the premise that survival in the anemic surgical patient depends more on the amount of blood lost during surgery than on the starting hemoglobin. By collecting and reinfusing shed blood, both absolute blood loss and mortality can be reduced.

Our results show that major cardiovascular procedures can be done safely without the use of either homologous blood transfusion or autologous predonation. We realize that this group of Jehovah's Witness patients is unique in refusing to accept both homologous blood transfusion and autologous predonation and in the restrictions they place on the use of intraoperative autotransfusion. Our success, however, should not be attributed to any uniqueness inherent in the group, since these patients do not differ from those treated routinely by cardiovascular surgeons around the country. Our ability to perform major cardiovascular surgery with the above restrictions is a result of the systematic application of blood conservation techniques available to all.

Not all patients will refuse homologous transfusion as do Jehovah's Witnesses. Nonetheless, the risks of disease transmission and immunomodulation present compelling arguments for finding alternatives for all of our patients. We believe that bloodless cardiovascular surgery can be offered to the majority of patients if surgeons adopt the principles and employ the techniques outlined above. The willingness to accept a lower transfusion trigger by basing the decision to transfuse on the patient's overall clinical condition, not on a hemoglobin value alone, is essential. Coupling this acceptance with the use of multiple, effective blood conservation techniques tailored to the individual patient's needs will allow us to attain our goal of eliminating unnecessary homologous transfusion.

REFERENCES

1. Lowery TA Clark JA: Successful Implementation of a Maximum Surgical Blood Ordering Schedule. J Med Assoc Ga 1989; 78(3):155–8.

2. Axelrod FB Pepkowitz SH Goldfinger D: Establishment of a schedule of optimal preoperative collection of blood. Transfusion 1989; 29:677–80.

3. Cosgrove DM Loop FD Lytle BN et al: Determinants of Blood Utilization during Myocardial Revascularization. Ann Thorac Surg 1985; 40:380–84.

4. Spence RK Carson JA Poses R et al: Elective surgery without transfusion: influence of preoperative hemoglobin level and blood loss on mortality. Am J Surg 1990; 159:320–4.

5. Owings DV Kruskall MS Thurer RL et al: Autologous blood donations prior to elective cardiac surgery. JAMA 1989; 262(14):1963–68.

6. Britton LW Eastlund DT Dziuban SW et al: Predonate autologous blood use in elective cardiac surgery. Ann Thorac Surg 1989; 47:529–32.

7. Toy PTCY Strauss RG Stehling LG et al: Predeposited autologous blood for elective surgery: a national multicenter study. N Engl J Med 1987; 316(9):517–20.

8. Goodnough LT Johnston MFM Toy PTCY et al: The variability of transfusion practice in coronary artery bypass surgery. JAMA 1991; 265(1):86–90.

9. The National Blood Resource Education Program Expert Panel. The use of autologous blood. JAMA 1990; 263:414–47.

10. Goodnough LT: Erythropoietin as a pharmacologic alternative to blood transfusion in the surgical patient. Transf Med Rev 1990; IV(4):299–296.

11. Spiess BD Sassetti R McCarthy RJ et al: Autologous blood donation: hemodynamics in a high-risk patient population. Transfusion 1992; 32:17–22.

12. Sandler SG Sacher RA: Preoperative autologous blood donation by high-risk patients. Transfusion 1992; 32:1–2.

13. Hallet JW Jr: Minimizing the use of homologous blood products during repair of abdominal aortic aneurysms. Surg Clinics N Amer 1989; 69(4):817–26.

14. Brewster DC Ambrosion JJ Darling RC et al: Intraoperative autotransfusion in major vascular surgery. Am J Surg 1979; 137:507–13.

15. Boldt J Kling D von Bormann B et al: Blood conservation in cardiac operations: Cell separation versus hemofiltration. J Thorac Cardiovasc Surg 1989; 97:832–40.

16. Dietrich W Barankay A Dilthey G et al: Autotranfusion and hemoseparation in cardiac surgery. What can be saved in cardiac reoperations and operations of thoracic aortic aneurysms? Thorac Cardiovasc Surg 1989; 37:84–8.

17. Pittman RD Inahra T: Eliminating homologous blood trasnfusions during abdominal aortic aneurysm repair. Am J Surg 1990; 159:522–4.

18. Cooley DA Crawford ES Howell JF et al: Open heart surgery in Jehovah's Witnesses. Am J Cardiol 1964; 13:779–81.

19. Beall AC Yow EM Bloodwell MJ et al: Open heart surgery without blood transfusion. Arch Surg 1967; 94:567–70.

20. Hallowell P Bland JHL Buckley MJ et al: Transfusion of fresh autologous blood in open-heart surgery. A method for reducing bank blood requirements. J Thorac Cardiovasc Surg 1972; 64:941–8.

21. Stehling L Zauder HL: Acute normovolemic hemodilution. Transfusion 1991; 31(9):857–69.

22. Ness PM Bourke DL Walsh PC: A randomized trial of perioperative hemodilution versus transfusion of preoperatively deposited autologous blood in elective surgery. Transfusion 1991; 31(9):226–40.

23. DelRossi AJ Cernaianu AC Vertrees RA et al: Platelet-rich plasma reduces postoperative blood loss after cardiopulmonary bypass. J Thorac Cardiovasc Surg 1990; 100(2):281–6.

24. Giordano GF Sr Girodano GF Jr Rivers SL et al: Determinants of homologous blood usage utilizing autologous platelet-rich plasma in cardiac operations. Ann Thorac Surg 1989; 47:897–902.

25. Pearlman NW Stiegmann GV Vance V et al: A prospective study of incisional time blood loss pain and healing with carbon dioxide laser scalpel and electrosurgery. Arch Surg 1991; 126:1018–20.

26. Spence RK: The status of bloodless surgery. Trans Med Rev 1991; V(4),274–86.

27. Cambria RP Brewster DC Abbot WM et al: Transperitoneal versus retroperitoneal approach to aortic reconstruction: A prospective study. J Vasc Surg 1990; 11:314–25.

28. Fisher JB Dennis RC Valeri CR et al: Effect of graft material on loss of erythrocytes after aortic operations. SGO 1991; 173:131–6.

29. Reid DB Pollock JG: A prospective study of 100 gelatin-sealed aortic grafts. Ann Vasc Surg 1991; 5:320–24.

30. Salzman EW Weinstein MJ Wientraub RM et al: Treatment with desmopressin acetate to reduce blood loss after cardiac surgery: a double blind randomized trial. N Engl J Med 1986; 314:1402–6.

31. Rocha E Llorens R Paramo JA et al: Does desmopressin acetate reduce blood loss after surgery in patients on cardiopulmonary bypass? Circulation 1988; 77:1319–1323.

32. Hackman T Gascoyne RD Naiman SC et al: A trial of desmopressin (1–desamino-8–D-Arginine Vasopressin) to reduce blood loss in uncomplicated cardiac surgery. N Engl J Med 1989; 321:1437–1443.

33. D'Ambra MN Risk SC: Aprotinin erythropoietin and blood substitutes. Int Anesthes Clin 1990; 28(4):237–240.

34. Wildevuur RH Eijsman L Gu YJ et al: Aprotinin reduces bleeding during cardiopulmonary bypass in aspirin treated patients. J Cadiovasc Surg 1990; 31:34.

35. Royston D Bidstrup BP Taylor KM et al: Effect of Aprotinin on need for transfusion after repeat Open Heart Surgery. Lancet 1987; 2:1289–91.

36. Czer LSC Bateman Gray RJ et al: Treatment of svere platelet dysfunction and hemorrhage after cardiopulmonary bypass: Reduction in blood product usage with Desmopressin. J Am Coll Cardiol 1987; 9:1139–47.

37. Spence RK McCoy S Costabile J et al: Fluosol DA-20 in the treatment of severe anemia: randomized controlled study of 46 patients. Crit Care Med 1990; 18(11):1227–30.

38. Adan A Brutel de la Riviere A Haas F et al: Autotransfusion of Drained Mediastinal Blood after Cardiac Surgery: a reappraisal. Thorac Cardiovasc Surg 1988; 36:10–14.

39. Roberts SR Early GL Brown B et al: Autotransfusion of unwashed shed mediastinal blood fails to decrease banked blood requirements in patients undergoing aortocoronary bypass surgery. Am J Surg 1991; 162:477–80.

40. Smoller BR Kruskall MS: Phlebotomy for diagnostic laboratory tests in adults: pattern of use and effect on transfusion requirements. N Eng J Med 1986; 314:1233–5.

41. Welch HG Meehan KR Goodnough LT: Prudent strategies for elective red blood cell transfusion. Ann of Int Med 1992; 116(5):393–402.

BLEEDING, THROMBOSIS AND THE DEFENSE REACTION DURING CARDIOPULMONARY BYPASS

L. Henry Edmunds, Jr., M.D.

University of Pennsylvania School of Medicine
Philadelphia, Pennsylvania

Cardiopulmonary bypass (CPB) causes bleeding, thrombotic complications, and triggers the body's defense systems to initiate a general inflammatory response. These reactions are caused by activation of blood constituents by contact with the synthetic surfaces of the heart-lung machine. Bleeding results from heparin, fibrinolysis, and loss of platelet numbers and function. Thrombosis generates emboli. Production of vasoactive substances alters cardiac function, vascular tone and capillary permeability. Massive fluid retention and temporary dysfunction of nearly every organ system results. The major complications of CPB due to blood activation are listed in Table 1.

CPB also produces other changes that contribute to morbidity. In addition to the physiologic stresses of anesthesia and surgery, CPB dilutes blood constituents and produces a pulseless circulation. Pulseless bypass does not significantly alter distribution of blood flows[1] or cause ill effects, [2] but crystalloid dilution of blood constituents reduces plasma colloid osmotic pressure and increases interstitial edema. The combination of increased capillary permeability, reduced colloid osmotic pressure and increased venous pressures causes massive fluid retention. The accumulated fluid affects cardiac loading, burdens the kidneys, reduces pulmonary compliance, and increases alveolar-arterial oxygen differences. [3]

The embolization produced by CPB is presented in Table 2. [4] Platelet and neutrophil emboli are produced by blood activation and red cell debris

Table 1. Complications of CPB Attributed to Activation of Blood Constituents

---

- Fever
- Bleeding (heparin, fibrinolytic, platelet loss)
- Emboli (fibrin, fat, platelet aggregates, red cell debris, gas, clot, foreign material)
- Fluid retention (increased capillary permeability, decreased colloid osmotic pressure, increased venous pressures)
- Temporary organ dysfunction (heart, lungs, kidneys, liver, etc.)

Cardiac Surgery: Current Issues 2, Edited by A. C. Cernaianu and A. J. DelRossi,
Plenum Press, New York, 1994

is produced by destruction from shear and osmotic forces. Fat emboli develop from denaturation of lipoproteins, coalescence of chylomicrons, and circulation of free fat droplets. CPB produces fibrin emboli and introduces foreign emboli aspirated from the operative field by the cardiotomy sucker system. Aspirated tissue debris, calcium, clots and other foreign material may escape filtration and enter the circulation. If roller pumps are used, spallation of bits of tubing compressed by the roller may circulate.

CPB Also produces gas emboli. Air may enter the perfusion circuit from the sucker system, poorly secured venous cannulas, the heart, an open stopcock, or any break in the system. Oxygen bubbles may also enter from the oxygenator. Hypothermia, particularly deep hypothermia, produces gas emboli if cooling is too rapid. Cooling increases the solubility of gas in plasma, thus when cold blood reaches the warm body, gas may come out of solution. Because nitrogen is poorly soluble, air is the most important gas embolus. Arterial line filters remove large solid emboli but do not remove all gas emboli or particles below the minimum pore size of 25 microns.

CPB is not possible without heparin. Blood contact with the synthetic surfaces of the extracorporeal perfusion circuit produces a massive throm-

Table 2. Emboli Produced during CPB

• Platelet aggregates	• Fat (free fat, chylomurons, denatured lipoproteins)
• Leukocyte aggregates	• Gas
• Red cell debris	• Foreign material
• Fibrin	• Spallation

botic stimulus that requires large doses of heparin to suppress. The doses required are much larger than those needed to prevent intravascular thrombosis without CPB, yet fibrin is still produced. (5) A priori heparin contributes to bleeding problems associated with CPB, but since the drug acts near the end of the coagulation cascade, it fails to suppress the defense reaction triggered by CPB. The body's defense reaction, which is initiated by key plasma proteins and blood cells, produces a "whole body inflammatory response"{6} that is responsible for much of the morbidity associated with CPB.

Heparin accelerates the rate of antithrombin III (ATIII) binding to thrombin and factor Xa, the activated form of coagulation factor X. Antithrombin III (molecular weight 58,000 daltons) is a serine protease inhibitor that is present in relatively high concentration in plasma. Antithrombin III forms tight covalent bonds with thrombin and factor Xa and therefore is consumed when these substrates are produced. Heparin, however, dissociates from ATIII after substrate binding and is available to catalyze another reaction. It is important to note that heparin does not prevent the formation of thrombin or factor Xa; the drug only inhibits the two serine proteases after they are formed. Therefore, during CPB minute quantities of thrombin may circulate and possibly stimulate platelets, endothelial cells and other blood elements.

When heparinized blood first contacts a synthetic, non-endothelial cell surface, plasma proteins adsorb onto the surface. Within seconds, a protein layer up to 200 angstroms thick is produced, but the composition and surface geography of the proteins varies between materials[7] and is not predictable. The amounts of adsorbed proteins differ from their concentrations in plasma and are influenced by the chemical and physical characteristics of the surface material. Fibrinogen is selectively adsorbed but albumin is not. Hydrophobic surfaces adsorb more fibrinogen and albumin than hydrophilic surfaces. Other plasma proteins including factor XII, prekallikrein, high molecular weight kininogen, hemoglobin, von Willebrand Factor, fibronectin, thrombospondin and immunoglobulin G are also adsorbed. [8]

The composition of surface proteins varies over time. Adsorbed fibrinogen is rapidly displaced by high molecular weight kininogen[9] but little is known about protein flux beyond the first few minutes in extracorporeal perfusion systems. Most likely surface adsorbed proteins interact with circulating blood elements and influence subsequent reactions in circulating blood.

During CPB, four plasma protein systems and four blood "cells" are activated (Table 3). The complex reactions that follow change plasma concentrations of more than 25 different vasoactive substances. [10] These compounds, defined as those that alter cardiac, endothelial cell or vascular smooth muscle contractions, affect myocardial contractility, vascular tone, hydrostatic pressures and capillary permeability, and significantly contribute to the organ dysfunction and fluid retention associated with CPB.

Blood contact with non-endothelial cell surfaces activates the contact system of plasma proteins (Table 4). On negatively charged, non-endothelial

Table 3. Blood Constituents Activated during CPB

Plasma Protein Systems	"Cells"
• Contact	• Neutrophils
• Coagulation	• Monocytes
• Complement	• Endothelium
• Fibrinolytic	• Platelets

cell surfaces, coagulation factor XII (Hageman factor) in the presence of prekallikrein and high molecular weight kininogen (HK) is cleaved into factor XIIa and factor XII fragments (XIIf). Factor XIIa activates the fourth protein of the contact system, factor XI, to initiate the coagulation cascade via the intrinsic pathway. The chain of reactions that follow amplify and accelerate a cascade that eventually produces thrombin. Thrombin, in turn, cleaves fibrinogen to form fibrin.

Table 4. Contact System Primary Proteins

• Factor XII (Hageman Factor)
• Prekallikrein
• High molecular weight kininogen
• Factor XI

Factor XIIa also cleaves prekallikrein to form kallikrein and cleaves HK to form bradykinin, a powerful vasodilator with a short half-life. Kallikrein accelerates the cleavage of factor XII and thus amplifies all of the reactions that are initiated by activating contact system proteins.

Recent studies indicate that coagulation may also be initiated during prolonged CPB by the extrinsic pathway of coagulation. During recirculation of fresh heparinized human blood, Kappelmayer and colleagues found that progressively increasing numbers of monocytes express tissue factor (thromboplastin) as recirculation continues. [11] Expression of tissue factor correlates closely with procoagulant activity of monocytes. Thus during CPB, coagulation proceeds by both the intrinsic and extrinsic pathways of coagulation.

The third plasma protein system activated by CPB is complement. Factor XIIa activates C1, the first component of complement. Activated C1 proceeds by the classical pathway (through C2 and C4)[12] and probably also by the alternative pathway (properdin)[13] to form C3a, the activated form of C3. C3a increases progressively during CPB[14] and causes activation of C5 and the remaining complement proteins (C6–9) that form the cell "membrane attack complex." C3a, C4a and C5a are all anaphylatoxins and have powerful vasoactive properties. Complement proteins are also activated by the heparin-protamine complex which is formed when protamine is given to neutralize heparin after CPB. [15]

Activated complement (C5a), kallikrein and factor XIIa stimulate neutrophils. Activated neutrophils, guardians against foreign invaders and noxious substances, contain a host of cytotoxic enzymes and chemicals, including free oxygen radicals. Normally chemotactic substances direct activated neutrophils to specific locations; however, during CPB neutrophils release powerful enzymes and chemicals into the circulation. [16] Capillary permeability of virtually all organs increases; interstitial fluid increases proportionately.

The third cell activated by CPB does not circulate but nevertheless is in constant contact with the perfusate. The endothelial cell is the only cell blood normally "sees" within the body and covers a vast surface area estimated to be between 1000 and 5000 M^2 in adults. Endothelial cells maintain the fluidity of blood by active metabolic processes. Endothelial cells produce prostacyclin, which inhibits platelets; heparan, a form of heparin; protein S, which activates the natural anticoagulant, protein C; and LACI, an inhibitor of the extrinsic pathway of coagulation. Endothelial cells bind thrombin and remove it from the circulation. Endothelial cells also produce tissue plasminogen activator (t-PA) which cleaves circulating plasminogen to plasmin. During CPB, t-PA increases; [17] plasmin is produced and fibrinolysis occurs. Thus activation of the fourth plasma protein system—the fibrinolytic—during CPB increases the likelihood of bleeding.

The fourth "cell" activated during CPB is the platelet, which for lack of a nucleus is not a cell at all. During CPB, platelets are immediately activated and rapidly adhere to surface adsorbed fibrinogen. The mechanism by which platelets are activated is not known, but circulation of minute quantities of thrombin that escape Antithrombin III or release of ADP (adenosine diphosphate) from lysed red cells are possibilities. Platelets adhere to binding sites located in the alpha chain and also in the C terminal domain of the gamma chain of surface adsorbed fibrinogen. [18] The platelet GPIIb/IIIa receptor complex, which is exposed by activation, is responsible for platelet adhesion to the fibrinogen binding site (18,19) (Figure 1). The GPIb receptor, which participates in the formation of the hemostatic plug in vivo, is not involved. (19)

Within a few minutes, platelet adhesion appears complete. The surface no longer binds platelets. Antibody to fibrinogen no longer reacts with surface adsorbed fibrinogen by high molecular weight kininogen—the Vroman effect. (9) The surface becomes "passivated" to platelets in that platelets no longer appear to react and adhere to the surface. (21)

Consequences of the initial few minutes of blood-surface contact, however, cause the thrombocytopenia and loss of platelet function that are associated with CPB. Some of the activated platelets aggregate and circulate as microemboli. Both surface adherent and aggregated platelets release granule contents and synthesize thromboxane A_2, a powerful platelet agonist and vasoconstrictor. Platelet dense granules release ADP, ATP, calcium and serotonin. Alpha granules release coagulation proteins, including fibrinogen, thrombospondin, fibronectin and factor Va and VIII, albumin, beta thromboglobulin, platelet factor 4, neutrophil activating protein (22) and several cationic proteins. (23) Lysosomes release several acid hydrolases. (24) Some platelets do not release granule contents, some partially release, and others completely release to become attached or circulating platelet ghosts.

Some adherent platelets detach from the surface and leave bits of platelet membrane behind. The average number of platelet GPIIb/IIIa and adrenergic receptors for circulating platelets decreases during CPB. (25) Fragments of platelet membrane also circulate. (26) New platelets enter the circulation from the bone marrow. (27) The resulting mixture is a heterogeneous population of young platelets, intact platelets, platelets with shape change, partially and completely degranulated platelets, and platelet fragments. Platelet count is reduced more than can be attributed to dilution; platelet function is impaired.

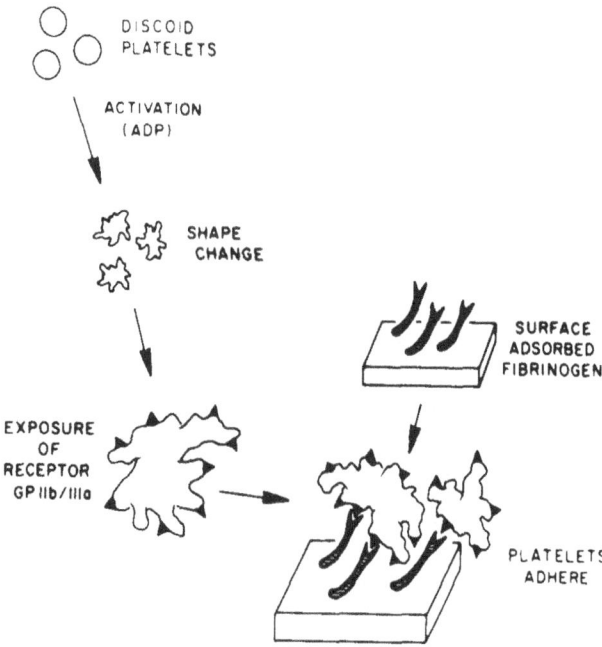

Figure 1. Mechanism by which platelets adhere to non-endothelial cell synthetic materials. During CPB fibrinogen adsorbs onto the surface and discoid platelets are activated to expose GPIIb/IIIa receptors. Activated platelets attach to specific fibrinogen binding sites on the alpha and gamma chains of adsorbed fibrinogen. (Reprinted from *Cardiac Chronicles*, Vol. 5, No. 10, pp. 1–8, 1992, with permission.)

Template bleeding times, a measure of overall platelet function, increases[28] and remains increased several hours after bypass ends.

The combined stresses of anesthesia and surgery, the hemodynamic and dilutional changes of CPB, and the consequences of activating four plasma protein systems and four blood cells produces a host of circulating vasoactive hormones, autocoids and cytokines[10] Table 5. These vasoactive substances constitute the body's defense reaction. Most autacoids and cytokines are not designed to circulate; however, during CPB these local mediators do circulate and have been identified in plasma. [10] Thus, exposure of blood to the huge synthetic surfaces of the perfusion circuit triggers an explosive release of vasoactive substances that are widely circulated by the mechanical pump to produce a "whole body inflammatory response."[6]

Attempts to produce a non-thrombogenic synthetic material have failed. Although some materials initiate coagulation more slowly than others and are termed "thromboresistant,"[29] none are non-thrombogenic. The living endothelial cell is the only known non-thrombogenic surface.

Recent attempts to develop a non-thrombogenic surface attach heparin by ionic or covalent bonds to the synthetic material. The Duraflo II (Baxter Laboratories Inc.) and Carmeda (Medtronic Inc.) processes are two proprietary methods of binding heparin to various synthetic materials by strong bonds. [30] There is evidence that the Duraflo II process involves some ionic binding and slow desorption of heparin from the surface occurs. [31]

Animal studies using functional assays of coagulation activity[32] and anecdotal human experience support the claim that Carmeda heparin surfaces are thromboresistant. The surface has thrombin inhibitory activity when known amounts of thrombin are added. Using chromogenic assays, the Carmeda surface appears to partially inhibit factor Xa (when antithrombin III is present)[33] and also surface adsorption and activation of factor XII. [34] In vitro studies further suggest that the Carmeda heparin surface inhibits platelet release of beta thromboglobulin and synthesis of thromboxane A^2. [35] Other studies suggest that the Carmeda heparin surface also attenuates complement and neutrophil activation. [36] Although constrained by methodologic limitations, evidence suggests that the Carmeda heparin surface may be a unique thromboresistant synthetic surface. There are no claims that the surface is nonthrombogenic, however. When employed in patients, systemic

Table 5. Vasoactive Substances Altered during Extracorporeal Perfusion

"Hormone"	"Autacoids"
• Epinephrine, Norepinephrine	• Platelet Activating Factor
• Renin, Angiotensin II	• PGI2, Thromboxane A2, PGE2
• Vasopressin, Aldosterone	• Endothelin-1, Nitric Oxide
• Atrial Natriuretic Factor	• Serotonin, Histamine
• Bradykinin	• Leukotrienes LTB4, LTC4, LTD4
• Glucagon	• Proteases
• Thyroid: T3, T4	• Free Oxygen Radicals
• Complement: C3a, C4a, C5a	• Lysosomal Enzymes
• Electrolytes: Ca^{++}, Mg^{++}, K^+	

heparin is required to prevent thrombosis, as evidence by generation of fibrinopeptide A during perfusions. (37)

An alternative to the development of an artificial endothelial cell is to selectively inhibit those blood elements that are initially activated by contact with synthetic material. (29) Surface contact clearly activates the contact proteins, which activate the intrinsic pathway of coagulation, complement and neutrophils. Platelets may be directly activated by surface contact or may be indirectly activated by minute quantities of circulating thrombin. Thrombin probably activates endothelial cells to produce t-PA. (38) Thus, it is possible that complete inhibition of factor XII activation can inhibit all of the reactions that occur in blood during CPB except for generation of tissue factor from wounds and monocytes. Because of tissue factor, an anticoagulant at the level of factor X (common coagulation pathway) is needed. However, discovery of an effective inhibitor of factor XII offers the prospect of suppressing most of the defense reaction during CPB.

In 1989, Bidistrup and colleagues reported that high doses of aprotinin, an inhibitor of plasmin and kallikrein, reduced bleeding after open heart surgery by approximately 50 percent. (39) They further observed that the drug attenuated the postoperative bleeding time but did not improve platelet count.

Subsequent studies show that aprotinin attenuates platelet alpha granule release and loss of platelet function by mechanisms that are not yet clear(40) Aprotinin also reduces neutrophil activation and release by inhibiting kallikrein and decreasing complement activation. (41). Because aprotinin inhibits plasmin, the drug inhibits postoperative fibrinolysis and prevents bleeding from that cause. By decreasing neutrophil activation and release, aprotinin also may modulate the "whole body inflammatory response." This happy possibility is difficult to quantify, and as yet is not proven.

Nearly all of the active (enzymatic) proteins of the contact, complement, coagulation and fibrinolytic systems are serine proteases. This large class of proteases shares a serine–195 residue at the active site of peptide bond hydrolysis. A substantial number of inhibitors of serine proteases exist (Table 6); aprotinin is only one. The various inhibitors of factor XIIa, factor XII fragments, factor XIa, factor Xa, kallikrein, $C1_s$, t-PA, plasmin, thrombin and neutrophil elastase have different binding and rate constants for each serine protease. Both reversible and irreversible inhibitors are known. One or more of these serine protease inhibitors may prove more useful than aprotinin in controlling the defense response to CPB.

Thrombin, produced by activation of both the intrinsic and extrinsic coagulation pathways during CPB, is the likely mediator of platelet and

Table 6. Some Inhibitors of Serine Proteases

• Arg 15 Aprotinin	• Corn Trypsin Inhibitor, Soybean Trypsin Inhibitor
• Ala 357 Arg358 alpha 1-antitrypsin	
• Nafamostat mesilate (Porton)	• Eglin
• Kunitz serine protease inhibitor (Scios)	• R-hirudin and derivatives
• Boroarginine Peptide Thrombin Inhibitor (Du Pont)	• Antistasin (Merck)
• Boroarginine Peptide Kallikrein Inhibitor (Du Pont)	• Tick Anticoagulant Peptide

endothelial cell activation. As such, prevention of thrombin formation or complete inhibition of circulating and cell-bound thrombin has high priority in the strategy of selectively inhibiting activation of blood elements by CPB. Heparin, of course, inhibits both thrombin and factor Xa. Low molecular weight heparins are better inhibitors of factor Xa than standard heparin, but inhibit thrombin less well. {42} Hirudin, a 65 amino acid, tight-binding thrombin inhibitor found in medicinal leeches, is now produced by recombinant technology. {43} Smaller peptides that contain the active site of the parent hirudin have also been developed. {44} Boroarginine peptides, which are small molecules, also reversibly inhibit thrombin and other proteases. {45} Chloromethylketones are chemical, irreversible inhibitors of thrombin. {46}

Two new peptides isolated from leeches and ticks inhibit factor Xa. Factor Xa catalyzes the formation of prothrombinase, which cleaves prothrombin to form thrombin. Antistasin (Merck) and tick anticoagulant peptide (TAP) are two promising factor Xa inhibitors. {48} Other more potent or more useful analogs may be developed. These inhibitors offer the prospect of suppressing thrombin formation, which may be much more effective than inhibiting thrombin after it is formed.

Reversible platelet inhibitors are also available or in the pipeline. Dipyridamole is a weak platelet inhibitor that raises platelet cyclic AMP by inhibiting phosphodiesterase, the enzyme that metabolizes cyclic AMP. {48} The drug is minimally or ineffective in concentrations that patients can tolerate{48} but has been used successfully to protect platelets during clinical CPB. {49} The drug has a long half-life in plasma (100 minutes) and therefore is not quickly reversible after bypass ends.

The prostanoids, PGI_2 (prostacyclin) and iloprost (an analog of PGI_2) also raise cyclic AMP and reversibly inhibit platelets. Both drugs are given by constant infusion but cause hypotension at doses that are sufficient to protect platelets. {50} PGI_2 is rapidly metabolized in plasma and is therefore easily reversed by stopping the infusion. Iloprost is more potent that PGI_2 and causes less vasodilation at effective doses. The half-life is somewhat longer but the effects of the drug are gone within an hour after stopping the drug. Iloprost is still an investigational drug, but has been used successfully with substantial doses of phenylephrine during open heart surgery in patients with heparin-induced thrombosis. {51}

The disintegrins are a new class of reversible platelet inhibitors that are derived from snake venom. These peptides contain an RGD sequence and inhibit the platelet GPIIb/IIIa receptor which mediates platelet aggregation and adhesion to synthetic surfaces. During simulated extracorporeal perfusion, various disintegrins prevent or attenuate platelet adhesion and alpha granule release. {52} During long-term perfusion in sheep, a single dose of bitistatin, a disintegrin, attenuates platelet loss and alpha granule release for 12 to 16 hours. {53} Recent data suggest that the prostanoids and disintegrins, which inhibit platelets by different mechanisms, act synergistically. This may reduce the undesirable side effects of using either drug alone.

An understanding of the complex reactions that result from activation of the four plasma protein systems and four blood "cells" during CPB begins to explain the bleeding, thrombotic and defense reactions associated with this technology. Control of the adverse consequences of extracorporeal perfusion is likely to reduce the morbidity of open heart surgery and to increase the applications of extracorporeal circulatory and respiratory support. Because the endothelial call maintains the fluidity of blood by active metabolic processes, development of a synthetic non-thrombogenic surface is not likely soon. Nevertheless, development of better thromboresistant surfaces, such as the Carmeda surface-bound heparin process, may quantitatively reduce activation of some blood elements. The further development of specific serine protease inhibitors to prevent or control key reactions within CPB-activated blood offers realistic, near term prospects for controlling the adverse consequences of short and long-term cardiopulmonary bypass.

REFERENCES

1. Eoucher JK, Rudy LW, Edmunds LH Jr: Organ blood flow during pulsatile cardiopulmonary bypass. J Appl Physiol 1974; 36:86–90.

2. Edmunds LH Jr: Pulseless cardiopulmonary bypass. J Thor Cardiovasc Surg 1982; 84:800–804.

3. Parker DJ, Karp RB, Kirklin JW, Bedard P: Lung water and alveolar and capillary volumes after intracardiac surgery. Circulation 1972; 45(Suppl I):139–146.

4. Edmunds LH Jr, Williams W: Microemboli and the use of filters during cardiopulmonary bypass. In Utley, J. R. (Ed) Pathophysiology and Techniques of Cardiopulmonary Bypass, Vol II, Williams and Wilkins, Baltimore 1983:101–114.

5. Davies GC, Salzman EW, Sobel M: Elevated fibrinopeptide A and Thromboxane A2 levels during cardiopulmonary bypass. Circulation 1980; 61:808-814.

6. Blackstone EH, Kirklin JW, Stewart RW, Chenoweth, DE: The damaging effects of cardiopulmonary bypass. In Wu, K. K. and Roxy, E. C. (editors), Prostaglandins in Clinical Medicine: Cardiovascular and Thrombotic Disorders. Chicago, IL. : Yearbook Medical Publishers Inc. 1982:355–369.

7. Uniyal S, Brash JL: Patterns of adsorption of proteins from human plasma onto foreign surfaces. Thrombosis and Haemostat 1982; 47:285–290.

8. Ziats NP, Pankowsky DA, Tierney BP, et al: Adsorption of Hageman Factor (Factor XII) and other human plasma proteins to biomedical polymers. J Lab Clin Med 1990; 116:687–696.

9. Brash JL, Scott CF, ten Hove P, Wojciechowski P, Colman RW: Mechanism of transient adsorption of fibrinogen from plasma to solid surfaces: role of the contact and fibrinolytic systems. Blood 1988; 71:932–939.

10. Downing SW, Edmunds LH Jr: Release of vasoactive substances during cardiopulmonary bypass. Ann Thorac Surg 1992; 54:1236-1243.

11. Kappelmayer J, Bernabei A, Edmunds LH Jr, Edgington TS, Colman RW: Tissue factor is expressed on monocytes during simulated extracorporeal circulation. Circ Res 1993; 72:1075–1081.

12. Wachtfogel YT, Harpel PC, Edmunds LH Jr, Colman RW: Formation of C1s-C1-inhibitor, kallikrein-C1-inhibitor and plasmin-alpha 2-plasmin inhibitor complexes during cardiopulmonary bypass. Blood 1989; 73:468–471.

13. Collett B, Alhaq A, Abdullah NB, Korjtsas L, Waree RJ, Dodd NJ, Alimo E, Ponte J, Vergani D: Pathways to complement activation during cardiopulmonary bypass. Br Med J 1984:289:1251.

14. Chenoweth DE, Cooper SW, Hugli TE, Stewart RW, Blackstone EH, Kirklin JW: Complement activation during cardiopulmonary bypass: evidence for generation of C3a and C5a anaphylatoxins. N Engl J Med 1981; 304:497-503.

15. Kirklin JK, Chenoweth DE, Naftel DC, Blackstone EH, Kirklin JW, Bitran DD, Curd JG, Reves JG, Samuelson PN: Effects of protamine administration after cardiopulmonary

bypass on complement, blood elements and the hemodynamic state. Ann Thorac Surg 1986; 41:193–199.

16. Wachtfogel YT, Kucich U, Greenplate J, Gluszko P, Abrams W, Weinbaum G, Wenger RK, Rucinski B, Niewiarowski S, Edmunds LH Jr, Colman RW: Human neutrophil degranulation during extracorporeal circulation. Blood 1987; 69:324–330.

17. Stibbe J, Kluft C, Brommer EJP, Gomes M, de Jong DS, Nauta J: Enhanced fibrinolytic activity during cardiopulmonary bypass in open-heart surgery in man is caused by extrinsic (tissue-type) plasminogen activator. Eur J Clin Invest 1984; 14:375–382.

18. Gluszko P, Rucinski B, Musial J, Wenger RK, Schmaier AH, Colman RW, Edmunds LH Jr, Niewiarowski S: Fibrinogen receptors in platelet adhesion to surfaces of extracorporeal circuit. Am J Physiol 1987; 252:H615–621.

19. Sheppeck RA, Bentz M, Dickson C, Hribar S, White J, Janosky J, Bercelil SA, Borovetz HS, Johnson PC: Examination of the roles of glycoprotein Ib and Glycoprotein IIb/IIIa in platelet deposition on an artificial surface using clinical antiplatelet agents and monoclonal antibody blockade. Blood 1991; 78:673–680.

20. Vroman L, Adams AL, Klings M, Fischer GC: Fibrinogen, globulins, albumin and plasma at interfaces. Adv Chem Ser 1975; 145:255-

21. Shigeta O, Gluszko P, Downing SW, Lu W, Niewiarowski S, Edmunds LH Jr: Protection of platelets during long-term extracorporeal membrane oxygenation in sheep with a single dose of disintegrin. Circulation 1992; 86(suppl II):II-398-II-404.

22. Holt JC, Zhanqing Y, Lu W, Stewart GJ, Niewiarowski S: Isolation, characterization, and immunological detection of neutrophil-activating peptide 2; a proteolytic degradation product of platelet basic protein. Proc Soc Exp Biol Med 1992; 199:171–177.

23. Zilla P, Fasol R, Groscurth P, Klepetko W, Reichenspurner H, Wolner E: Blood platelets in cardiopulmonary bypass operations. J Thorac Cardiovasc Surg 1989; 97:379–388.

24. Addonizio VP Jr, Strauss JF III, Chang LF, Fisher CA, Colman RW, Edmunds LH Jr: Release of lysosomal hydrolases during simulated extracorporeal circulation. J Thorac Cardiovasc Surg 1982; 84:28–34.

25. Wenger RK, Lukasiewicz H, Mikuta BS, Niewarowski S, Edmunds LH Jr: Loss of platelet fibrinogen receptors during clinical cardiopulmonary bypass. J Thorac Cardiovasc Surg 1989; 967:235–239.

26. George JN, Thoi LL, McManus LM, Reimann TA: Isolation of human platelet membrane microparticles from plasma and serum. Blood 1982; 60:834-840.

27. Laufer N, Merin G, Grover NB, Pessachowicz B, Borman JB: The influence of cardiopulmonary bypass on the size of human platelets. J Thorac Cardiovasc Surg 1975; 70:727–731.

28. Edmunds LH Jr, Ellison N, Colman RW, Niewiarowski S, Rao AK, Addonizio VP Jr, Stephenson LW, Edie RN: Platelet function during open heart surgery: comparison of the membrane and bubble oxygenators. J Thorac Cardiovasc Surg 1982; 83:805–812.

29. Edmunds LH Jr: The Sangreal. J Thorac Cardiovas Surg 1985; 90:1-6.

30. Larm O, Larsson R, Olsson P: A new non-thrombogenic surface prepared by selective covalent binding of heparin via a modified reducing terminal residue. Biomat Med Dev Art Org 1983; 11:161–173.

31. Pradhan MJ, Fleming JS, Nkere UU, Arnold J, Wildevuur Ch RH, Taylor KM: Clinical experience with heparin-coated cardiopulmonary bypass circuits. Perfusion 1991; 6:235–242.

32. Toomasian JM, Hsu L-C, Hirschl RB, Heiss KF, Hultquist KA, Bartlett RH: Evaluation of Duraflow II heparin coating in prolonged extracorporeal membrane oxygenation. Trans Am Soc Artif Intern Organs 1988; 34; 410–414.

33. Kodama K, Pasche B, Olsson P, Swedenborg J, Adolfsson L, Larm O, Riesenfeld J: Antithrombin III binding to surface immobilized heparin and its relation to factor Xa inhibition. Thromb Haemost 1987; 58(4): 1064–1067.

34. Elgue G, Blomback, Olsson P, Riesenfled J: On the mechanism of coagulation inhibition on surfaces with endpoint immobilized heparin. Thromb Haemost 1993; 70:289–293.

35. Stenach N, Korn RL, Fisher CA, Jeevanandam V, Addonizio VP: The effects of heparin bound surface modification (Carmeda Bioactive Surface) on human platelet alterations during simulated extracorporeal circulation. J Am Soc Extracorpor Technol 1992; 24:97–106.

36. Videm V, Svennevig JL, Fosse E, Semb G, Osterud A, Mollnes TE: Reduced complement activation with heparin-coated oxygenator and tubings in coronary bypass operations. J Thorac Cardiovasc Surg 1992; 103; 806–813.

37. Bindslev L, Gouda I, Inacio J, Kodama K, Lagergren H, Larm O, Nilsson E, Olsson P: Extracorporeal elimination of carbon dioxide using a surface-heparinized veno-venous bypass system. Trans Am Soc Artif Intern Organs 1986; 32; 530–533.

38. Levin EG, Marzec U, Anderson J, Harker LA: Thrombin stimulates tissue plasminogen activator release from cultured human endothelial cells. J Clin Invest 1984; 74:1988–1995.

39. Bidistrup BP, Royston D, Sapsford RN, Taylor KM: Reduction in blood loss and blood use after cardiopulmonary bypass with high dose aprotinin (Trasylol). J Thorac Cardiovasc Surg 1989; 967:364–372.

40. Baluhut B, Gross C, Necek S, Doran JE, Spath P, Lundsgaardhansen P: Effects of high-dose aprotinin on blood loss, platelet function, fibrinolysis, complement, and renal function after cardiopulmonary bypass. J Thorac Cardiovasc Surg 1991; 101:958–967.

41. Wachtfogel Y, Kucich U, Hack CE, Niewarowski S, Colman RW, Edmunds LH Jr: Aprotinin partially inhibits the contact and platelet activation systems during extracorporeal perfusion. In press. J Thorac Cardiovasc Surg.

42. Harenberg J: Pharmacology of low molecular weight heparins. Semin Thromb Hemost 1990; 16:12–34.

43. Lindhout T, Blezer R, Hemker HC: The anticoagulant mechanism of action of recombinant hirudin (CGP 39393) in plasma. Thromb Haemost 1990; 64:464–468.

44. Maraganore JM, Chao B, Joseph ML, Jablonski J, Ramachandran KL: Anticoagulant activity of synthetic hirudin peptides. J Biol Chem 1989; 264:8692–8698.

45. Kettner C, Mersinger L, Knabb R: The selective inhibition of thrombin by peptides of borarginine. J Biol Chem 1990; 265:18289–18297.

46. Hanson SR, Harker LA: Interruption of acute platelet-dependent thrombosis by the synthetic antithrombin D-phenylalanyl-L-prolyl-L-arginyl chloromethyl ketone. Proc Natl Acad Sci 1988; 85:3184–3188.

47. Vlasuk GP, Ramjit D, Fujita T, Dunwiddie CT, Nutt EM, Smith DE, Shebuski RJ: Comparison of the in vivo anticoagulant properties of standard heparin and the highly selective Factor Xa inhibitors antistats in and tick anticoagulant peptide (TAP) in a rabbit model of venous thrombosis. Thromb & Haemost 1991; 65:257–262.

48. FitzGerald GA: Dipyridamole. N Eng J Med 1987; 316:1247–1257.

49. Teoh KH, Christakis GT, Wwisel RD, Wong PY, Mee AV, Ivanov J, Madonik M, Levitt DS, Reilly PA, Rosenfield JM, Glynn MFX: Dipyridamole preserved platelets and reduced blood loss after cardiopulmonary bypass. J Thorac Cardiovasc Surg 1988; 96:332–341.

50. Malpass TW, Armory DW, Harker LA, Ivey PD, Williams DB: The effects of prostacyclin infusion on platelet hemostatic function in patients undergoing cardiopulmonary bypass. J Thorac Cardiovasc Surg 1984; 87:550–555.

51. Kappa JR, Fisher CA, Bell P, Campbell FW, Ellison N, Addonizio VP: Intraoperative management of patients with heparin-induced thrombocytopenia. Ann Thorac Surg 1990; 49:713–723.

52. Musial J, Niewiarowski S, Rucinski B, Williams JA, Steward GJ, Edmunds LH Jr: Inhibition of platelet adhesion to surfaces of extracorporeal circuit by disintegrins: RGD containing peptides from viper venoms. Circulation 1990; 82:261–273.

53. Shigeta C, Gluszko P, Downing SW, Lu W, Niewiarowski S, Edmunds LH Jr: Protection of platelets during long-term extracorporeal membrane oxygenation in sheep with a single dose of disintegrin. Circulation 1992; 86(suppl II):II-398-II-404.

HOMOLOGOUS BLOOD, SALVAGED BLOOD, OR NO TRANSFUSION?

The Choices Facing Cardiac Surgeons

Brian S. Bull, M.D.

Loma Linda University Medical Center
Loma Linda University School of Medicine
Loma Linda, California

THE PHYSIOLOGICAL ADVANTAGES OF POSTOPERATIVE ANEMIA

The question of whether to transfuse at all comes before the question of whether to use autologous versus homologous blood. Until recently, a hemoglobin level of 10 g/dL was considered the lowest acceptable level for a patient undergoing surgery. [1] There is now good evidence that this "action level" is too high. Indeed, oxygen delivery to the tissues is enhanced by a modest degree of anemia provided the patient can maintain an increased cardiac output. This is because the viscosity of whole blood is largely dependent upon the volume of red cells that it contains. High hematocrit blood can deliver increased oxygen to the tissues only if it can be moved swiftly through the microcirculation; and the high viscosity of such blood guarantees a prolonged circulation time. Why then does Mother Nature equip us with a hematocrit of 45 when there are so many physiological advantages that accrue when the hematocrit drops to 25? The answer is that most of us are upright and exercising large muscle groups most of the time. We are not resting quietly, lying in bed following major surgery. During vigorous physical activity a reserve capacity for oxygen transport is very helpful. Some athletes have received a one or two unit transfusion of their own blood just before competition for this very reason. Other athletes practice their sport at high altitude to achieve the same result.

Postoperatively, however, there is good evidence that hemoglobin levels of 7 or 8 g/dL are well tolerated. [2,3] The NIH Consensus Conference on Perioperative Red Blood Cell Transfusion recommends that clinical judgement (can the patient maintain the elevated cardiac output?) be substituted for previous "action limits" in this matter. [4] But what of those patients whose surgical blood loss drops their hematocrit below even these limits and cardiovascular decompensation sets in? Under these circumstances a blood transfusion is clearly needed. Assuming that autologous blood is available,

Cardiac Surgery: Current Issues 2, Edited by A. C. Cernaianu and A. J. DelRossi,
Plenum Press, New York, 1994

is the risk-benefit ratio always overwhelmingly on the side of autologous transfusion?

THE RISK-BENEFIT RATIO OF AUTOLOGOUS VERSUS HOMOLOGOUS BLOOD

The transfusion of homologous blood exposes the recipient to several risks. The one most feared by patients is that the blood will infect them with one of the viral agents responsible for AIDS, or hepatitis B or C. The risk of acquiring AIDS has now dropped to approximately 1:250,000. [5] Recent estimates of acquiring hepatitis B are of about the same order of magnitude. [5] The hazard of acquiring hepatitis C from homologous blood is higher as testing has shown that the incidence of anti-HCV antibody in the U. S. donor pool is about 1 percent. [6] Fortunately, hepatitis C in patients with normal immunity is usually a relatively mild disease. With routine screening of donors for antibodies to HCV now in place, it is reasonable to expect a marked drop in the transmission of hepatitis C by transfusion.

There are, however, other risks of homologous transfusion. In immuno-compromised patients the cytomegalovirus poses a significant risk, as does graft versus host disease. In addition, homologous blood transfusion typically induces a state of mild immunosuppression in the recipient. This increases the likelihood of postoperative infection and, in some studies on cancer patients, shortens survival time. Finally, there is a rare occurrence of some clerical or technical error which leads to a transfusion of the wrong ABO type and a hemolytic transfusion reaction.

Autologous (i.e., the patient's own) blood will avoid all of the above hazards. However, if the autologous blood has been salvaged from the operative field it poses a novel and very serious threat to the recipients health. The novel threat occurs because the patient may be exposed to an infusion that contains large numbers of activated white cells and platelets. Once these cells are returned to the circulation in an activated state they may damage the microcirculation of the lungs and other body organs as well as precipitate disseminated intravascular coagulation. The symptom complex that results has been termed the Salvaged Blood Syndrome (SBS). [7] The spate of recent publicity emphasizing the benefits of mild anemia in the perioperative patient has, inadvertently, made SBS more likely. The pathophysiology of the disorder and its relationship to hematocrit levels perioperatively is now partially understood. The matter is well worth exploring. While SBS is presently relatively rare following cardiac surgery the rarity is happenstance and changes in surgery protocols have the potential to place many more cardiac surgery patients at risk.

HYDRAULICS OF THE BOWL FILLING CYCLE

Typical blood salvage devices wash the red cells free of plasma and other contaminating substances, such as hemoglobin from lysed red cells. The critical part of the device is a small, rapidly spinning polycarbonate bowl, This bowl relies on centrifugal force to separate cells from the suspending medium. The separation takes place because cellular elements are more dense and thus separate quickly under a high g force. The density of red cells is approximately 1.10 g/mL, white cells, approximately 1.07–1.08 g/mL, and platelets, approximately 1.065 g/mL. In contrast, the density of plasma is much less at approximately 1.026 and normal saline is even less dense at approximately 1.01. {8} At a typical hematocrit of 45 percent, whole blood will have a density of about 1.06 and will thus be 0.034 g/mL (1.06 minus plasma density of 1.026 = 0.034) heavier than the plasma which has been separated from blood aspirated earlier and which now fills the center of the centrifuge bowl. This density difference is acted upon by the g field of the spinning bowl. A typical bowl exerts more than 1500 g at its lower outer rim when rotating at design speed. This g force is more than adequate to separate incoming blood into cells (which stay in the outer portions of the bowl) and plasma which "floats" towards the center and then travels up to the exit port. Thus, design parameters assumed in normal centrifuge operation include a density difference between incoming blood and the already separated plasma of 0.034 g/mL and a force field on the order of 1500 g.

As blood is diluted, either with its own plasma or with saline, its density decreases. Half of the density difference assumed in the design of the salvage equipment disappears as the hematocrit of salvaged blood drops from 44 to 22. As a result of a decreased density difference, the separation process slows and becomes increasingly inefficient. Incoming blood, instead of separating into cells and plasma almost immediately upon entry, travels much further up and into the core of the spinning bowl along the path normally followed by plasma. As a result, cells in the incoming blood, when finally separated from suspension, will strike the bowl wall higher than usual. Often this point of contact is well above any cushioning red cell layer. When this happens, contact with the hard polycarbonate surface of the bowl subjects the white cells and platelets in the incoming blood to high, wall-induced shear forces. These shear forces damage white cells and platelets and initiate the process of deposit formation on the centrifuge bowl wall.

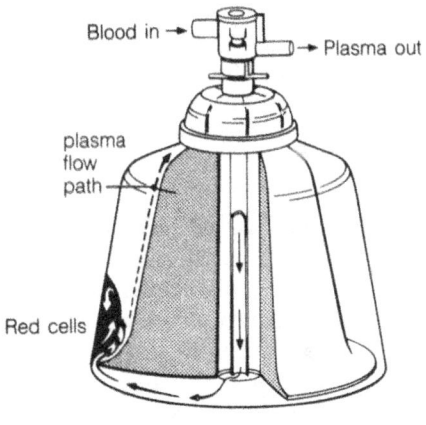

Figure 1. Normal centrifuge bowl hydraulics when salvaged blood (hematocrit ≥ 0.25) is processed. Red cells remain in the lower outer corner, plasma floats inward and upward, platelets and leucocytes travel to the inner surface of the red cell layer.

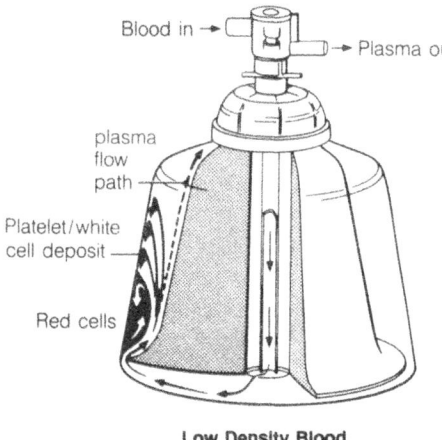

Blood in → → Plasma out

plasma
flow
path

Platelet/white
cell deposit

Red cells

Low Density Blood

Figure 2. Abnormal centrifuge bowl hydraulics when salvaged blood (hematocrit ≤ 0.20) is processed. White cells and platelets entrained in the plasma/dilutent stream strike the bowl wall above the cushioning red cell layer; they are activated and adhere to form a deposit.

CELLULAR DEPOSITS ON THE CENTRIFUGE BOWL WALL

The normal sequence of events as salvaged blood enters the spinning bowl is depicted in Figure 1. Diluted blood behaves differently, the cells in the entering plume are carried much further up into the bowl than usual. While they eventually curl outward to strike the bowl wall, they do so at a level above the cushioning layer of red cells, as illustrated in Figure 2. Lacking the normal cushioning effects of a red cell layer, the platelets strike the unprotected polycarbonate bowl wall and become activated by the high shear forces there present.

Shear activated platelets discharge the contents of their granules and become sticky. They adhere to the inside of the bowl and build up a cellular deposit. This cellular deposit accumulates white cells which increase the thickness of the deposit. The white cells also enhance the process of platelet accumulation and thus speed up the growth of the deposit. Because the deposit is tightly adherent to the bowl wall it cannot be displaced by the rising red cell layer and becomes covered by salvaged red cells as the bowl fills to capacity. An experimental deposit is shown in Figure 3. This deposit was produced by simply diluting the incoming blood with saline so as to lower its hematocrit from 44 to 15 (one part blood, two parts saline). Because the deposit is tightly adherent to the bowl wall and is covered by a deep layer of red cells it usually survives the wash cycle. It is thus in a position to spall off and contaminate the washed red cell suspensions from current or future salvage episodes. {9}

PATHOPHYSIOLOGICAL EFFECTS OF BOWL DEPOSITS

The materials known to be released by activated platelets and white cells include a variety of leukotrienes capable of impairing vascular integrity{10} as well as substances capable of activating monocytes and neutrophils. {11,12} Complement may also be activated, and other poorly characterized leukotactic and procoagulant substances released. Even if the deposit is initially firmly stuck to the bowl wall so that little of it detaches during the

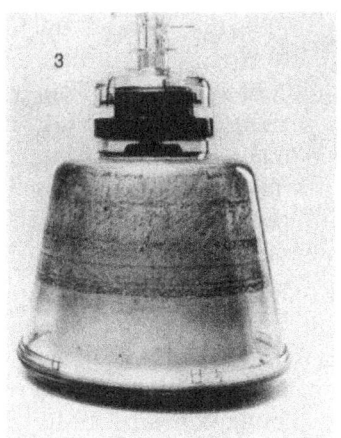 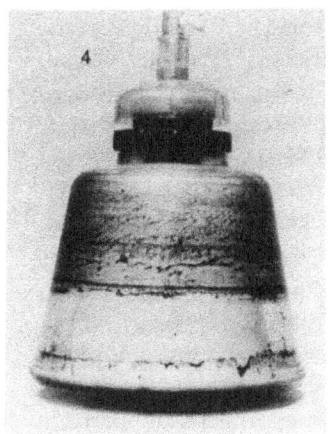

Figure 3. A platelet/leucocyte bowl deposit produced in the laboratory by diluting normal donor blood 2:1 with physiological saline prior to processing the blood.

Figure 4. A bowl recovered from the operating room after a case in which a large quantity of saline ice slush had been used to cool the heart during cardioplegia. The melted saline slush was mixed with shed bood, aspirated and processed.

bowl emptying phase, it is still in a position to contaminate subsequently processed red cell units. Indeed, the deposit contains numerous white cells rich in proteolytic enzymes and will undergo partial autodigestion with dissolution within 60–100 minutes if simply incubated in vitro. Any cellular debris that is released from the wall deposit will be retained in the bowl through subsequent concentration and cell washing steps because it will have a density similar to that of blood cells. Thus, the only opportunity such material will have to exit the bowl will be with the washed red cell suspension at the end of a processing cycle. A bowl deposit produced in the operating room as a result of aspirating saline ice-slush along with shed blood is shown in Figure 4.

As already noted, simple dilution of the blood that enters a centrifuge bowl during the fill cycle is sufficient to initiate the process of platelet/white cell deposit formation. Based upon animal models of the process, outside limits can be placed upon the dilution that will take salvaged blood into the danger zone. {13} When blood of normal hematocrit is diluted no deposit will form if the dilution is 1:1 or less. A white cell platelet deposit always forms if the dilution is 1 part blood to 2 parts saline—and the platelets and white cells are physiologically normal. For dilution with plasma, as with blood salvage from a hemodiluted patient, the limits are somewhat tighter. This is because plasma is more dense than saline and therefore the density difference between it and normal blood is less. It has already been noted that a deposit always forms if blood of normal hematocrit is diluted with 2 volumes of plasma or saline *provided the platelets and white cells are physiologically intact.* There are thus circumstances where the salvage of dilute blood fails to produce a deposit. If the blood comes from a thrombocytopenic patient, or if the platelets are nonfunctional, no deposit will form. Thus: 1) blood recovered from body cavities where clotting has taken place does not usually support deposit formation. This is because clotting followed by clot lysis renders blood thrombocytopenic. The few remaining platelets are coated by fibrin split products and are typically not able to adhere themselves much less form a substrate for the accumulation and activation of white cells. This will be true no matter how dilute the blood may be for without platelets to initiate deposit formation the process cannot get started; and 2) for similar reasons blood recovered from an extracorporeal circuit will usually not support deposit formation because most platelets in such blood are nonfunctional. They will have been rendered nonfunctional by exposure to multiple artificial surfaces.

Just as active platelets are necessary to initiate deposit formation, active or activatable white cells must be present if the full range of SBS pathophysiology is to occur. If a layer of platelets fails to attract white cells or if the white cells which accumulate are not capable of full activation of the respiratory burst enzymes, then a deposit may form which is not harmful to the patient. Although not all bowl deposits are harmful to the patient, a deposit free bowl is a guarantee that there is no risk of SBS. Since deposit free bowls can be routinely achieved on a cardiac surgery unit with relatively minor precautions, this should be the goal whenever autologous blood salvage is underway.

PRACTICAL RECOMMENDATIONS

1. All blood that is contaminated with any particulate matter should be discarded. The operating surgeons should be reminded of this precaution and a second sucker provided. *A second sucker should always be present in the operative field whenever blood salvage is underway.* The very nature of the cell washing devices precludes any subsequent removal of material that is at least as dense as blood cells. Included under this heading are such contaminants as malignant cells, bone chips and all tissue debris.

2. Each bowl should be carefully examined prior to discard. If there is evidence of a cellular deposit present, the protocol for red cell salvage should be examined in the light of the above precautions and changed until the bowls are uniformly deposit free.

3. Saline irrigation fluid, melted saline ice-slush, etc., should be discarded (most conveniently through the use of a second sucker) before these solutions become mixed with blood. Blood mixed with a large quantity of diluent should be discarded rather than aspirated into the cell saver unit unless there is a much larger quantity of high hematocrit blood already in the reservoir.

4. The use of the blood salvage device to concentrate low hematocrit blood from the bypass circuit should be restricted to those cases where platelet function is almost certainly compromised (pump runs of at least 35 to 45 minutes or more). Autologous blood salvage becomes increasingly risky with shorter pump runs, with higher platelet counts in the patient's blood or when platelet transfusions are employed liberally during the operative procedure.

5. Autologous blood salvage should be avoided whenever the patient's starting hematocrit is substantially below 30 percent and cardiopulmonary bypass will not be employed thus increasing the likelihood of physiologically active platelets in the salvaged blood.

REFERENCES

1. Goodnough LT, Shuck JM: Risks, options, and informed consent for blood transfusion in elective surgery. Am J Surg 1990; 159:602.

2. Stehling LS: Surgery without transfusion. The anesthesiologist's viewpoint, in NIH Consensus Conference on Perioperative Red Cell Transfusion, Bethesda, MD, 1988.

3. Wilkerson DK, Rosen AL, Seghal LR, et al: Oxygen extraction ratio: a valid indicator of myocardial metabolism in anemia. J Surg Res 1987; 42:629.

4. Greenwalt TJ, Buckwalter JA, Desforges J, et al: Perioperative red blood cell transfusion. NIH Consensus Development Conference Statement. JAMA 1988; 260:2700.

5. AuBuchon JP, Busch M, Epstein JS, et al: Increasing the safety of blood transfusions. American Red Cross, Washington, DC 1992.

6. Centers for Disease Control: Public Health Service inter-agency guidelines for screening donors of blood, plasma, organs, tissues, and semen for evidence of hepatitis B and hepatitis C. MMWR 1991; 40(RR-4):6.

7. Bull BS, Bull MH: The salvaged blood syndrome; a sequel to mechanochemical activation of platelets and leukocytes? Blood Cells 1990; 16:5.

8. Geigy Scientific Tables, Vol. 3, p 67. Ciba Geigy Ltd, Basle, 1984.

9. Bull BS, Bull MH: Enhancing the safety of intraoperative blood salvage. J Trauma 1988; 28:320.

10. Ford-Hutchinson AW, Bray MA, Doig MV, Shipley ME, Smith MJH: Leukotriene B, a potent chemokinetic and aggregating substance released from polymorphonuclear leukocytes. Nature 1980; 286:264.

11. Mulligan MS, Polley MJ, Bayer RJ, Nunn MF, Paulson JC, Ward PA: Neutrophil-dependent acute lung injury requirement for P-selectin (GMP-140). J Clin Invest 1992; 90:1600.

12. Wedmore CV, Williams TJ: Control of vascular permeability by polymorphonuclear leukocytes in inflammation. Nature 1981; 289:646.

13. Bull MH, Bull BS, Van Arsdell GS, Smith LL: Clinical implications of procoagulant and leucoattractant formation during intraoperative blood salvage. Arch Surg 1988; 123:1073.

AN OVERVIEW OF CONGENITAL HEART SURGERY

Edward L. Bove, M.D.

The University of Michigan
Ann Arbor, Michigan

This chapter will highlight three particular areas related to congenital heart disease, i.e., staged reconstruction for hypoplastic left heart syndrome, arterial repair for the neonate with transposition of the great arteries and surgery for pulmonary hypertension with Eisenmenger's Syndrome. The status of these particular problems will be reviewed with an emphasis on the results of the current therapy and the potential for innovations in these and other fields in the future.

HYPOPLASTIC LEFT HEART SYNDROME

Hypoplastic left heart syndrome (HLHS) is a complex anomaly which is uniformly fatal without treatment. In recent years, the advent of heart transplantation and the increasing success with staged reconstruction has renewed the interest of many physicians and surgeons who provide care for these infants with the hope of increasing survival. {1-6} HLHS is not one specific abnormality but rather represents a continuum of complex problems, all characterized by underdevelopment or hypoplasia of the left sided cardiac structures: the aorta, aortic valve, left ventricle and mitral valve. In its classic or most common form, the heart is characterized by both aortic and mitral atresia with essentially no left ventricular chamber. The ascending aorta is extremely diminutive in size, often less than 3 mm in diameter, and functionally represents a conduit providing retrograde blood flow to the coronary arteries. In the University of Michigan experience, over half of the patients had an ascending aorta less than 3 mm in diameter and approximately 25 percent were less than 2 mm. Staged reconstruction is currently done in three phases. The first stage operation, the Norwood procedure, is done within the first few days of life. The second stage, the bidirectional Glenn or hemifontan procedure, is then performed electively at six months. The final stage, the Fontan procedure, in which all systemic venous return is directly channeled into the pulmonary arteries is done between eighteen months and two years of age.

Cardiac Surgery: Current Issues 2. Edited by A. C. Cernaianu and A. J. DelRossi,
Plenum Press, New York, 1994

The entire procedure is done utilizing a single period of deep hypothermia with circulatory arrest. Initial cannulation is done by placing the aortic cannula into the proximal main pulmonary. The right and left branch pulmonary arteries are then snared in order to allow the systemic perfusate to reach the systemic circulation through the ductus arteriosus. Venous return is provided through a single cannula in the right atrial appendage. Cooling to a nasopharyngeal temperature of 18–20°C is performed. Once the circulation is arrested to perform the reconstruction, the head vessels are snared to prevent air form entering the cerebral circulation. The procedure is completed under circulatory arrest, generally lasting approximately 40–50 minutes. The technique of the Norwood procedure involves providing unobstructed systemic blood flow by connecting the right ventricle to the augmented ascending aorta and transverse aortic arch. Pulmonary venous return is then channeled through the right atrium into the right ventricle. The atrial septum must be completely excised to provide unobstructed pulmonary venous return. The entire ascending aorta, transverse arch and proximal descending aorta are augmented with cryopreserved allograft tissue. The ductal tissue must be completely excised in order to prevent recurrent obstruction. This augmented aorta is anastomosed to the proximal pulmonary artery with great care taken to preserve unobstructed coronary blood flow. The cannulas are then replaced to begin systemic rewarming while the systemic to pulmonary artery conduit is placed. A limited degree of pulmonary blood flow is then provided through a polytetrafluroethylene conduit placed between the innominate artery and central pulmonary artery. The diameter of the conduit is either 3.5 or 4 mm, reserving the larger size for infants larger than 3.5 kg.

Following the Norwood operation, the delicate balance between pulmonary and systemic vascular resistance must be maintained by careful use of ventilation and inotropes. Excessive pulmonary blood flow, characterized by systemic saturations in excess of 85 percent, may result in poor systemic perfusion and low cardiac output. This condition may result when pulmonary vascular resistance is low or the shunt is too large, resulting in a ventricular volume overload, low diastolic blood pressure and poor systemic perfusion. In this situation, the inspired fraction of oxygen is rapidly reduced to room air and minute ventilation is decreased in order to provide a mild respiratory acidosis and enhance an increase in pulmonary vascular resistance. Conversely, when pulmonary blood flow is inadequate, characterized by systemic saturations persistently below 70 percent, hypoxemia may then result in poor ventricular performance and systemic acidosis. In this situation, the inspired fraction of oxygen is increased to 100 percent and hyperventilation is begun to decrease pulmonary vascular resistance and increase pulmonary blood flow. The optimal systemic saturation is between 75–80 percent which generally indicates a pulmonary to systemic blood flow ratio of less than 1.5.

A retrospective multivariable analysis of risk factors was recently conducted of our entire series of patients undergoing reconstructive surgery for HLHS in order to determine predictors of mortality. [4] The following risk factors were evaluated: age, weight, year of operation (1986–1989 vs. 1990–1993), initial systemic arterial pO_2 and pH upon presentation to the hospital, morphologic subgroup, ascending aorta size, shunt size and circulatory arrest time. This analysis revealed that only the year of operation and the age at the time of first stage repair were significant predictors of survival. Between January 1986 and February 1993, 123 patients underwent first stage palliation at C. S. Mott Children's Hospital, The University of Michigan. In the latter years of our experience, between January 1990 and February 1993, 62/73 patients (85 percent) undergoing first stage palliation with a Norwood procedure survived to hospital discharge. This represents a significant improvement when compared to the earlier results achieved between 1986 and 1989, when only 21/50 patients (42 percent) survived, $p = .001$. Equally important to survival, the age of operation had a strong effect on outcome. Among 66 patients under one month of age undergoing operation between 1990 and 1993, 60 (91 percent) survived compared to only 2/7 patients (29 percent) who were beyond one month of age at the time of initial operation, $p = .001$. Those patients greater than one month of age represented only 10 percent of our patient population yet accounted for nearly 50 percent of the hospital deaths. Most of the older patients died of pulmonary hypertensive crises secondary to their labile pulmonary vascular resistance. The small shunt, which is now generally preferred, was unable to provide adequate pulmonary blood flow during those times when pulmonary vascular resistance was elevated, such as during noxious stimuli. When a larger shunt was used, this provided far too great a degree of pulmonary blood flow with low diastolic blood pressures and poor ventricular function when pulmonary vascular resistance was low. The actuarial survival for the 66 patients under one month of age at the time of the first stage operation was 81 percent, 74 percent and 74 percent at six months, one year and two years, respectively.

The second stage of the reconstruction, the bidirectional Glenn or hemifontan procedure, is performed at approximately six months of age. At this operation, the superior vena cava is anastomosed to the pulmonary artery and the polytetrafluroethylene shunt placed at stage I is divided. Although this generally does not result in significant improvements in arterial saturation, total pulmonary blood flow is reduced without decreasing effective flow and the volume load on the single right ventricle is consequently lowered. This approach is based on the objective of allowing the ventricle to gradually adjust to a diminished volume load, resulting in reduced muscle mass prior to the Fontan procedure. In our series, systemic saturations have generally remained at approximately 80–85 percent, providing adequate oxygen saturation for continued growth and development until the final repair. [5]

The final stage of reconstruction, the Fontan operation, is optimally done between eighteen months and two years of age. The technique of the Fontan operation involves placing a lateral tunnel of Gortex material within the right atrium which conducts inferior vena cava blood to the pulmonary arteries. Intra-atrial pathway is approximately 50 percent atrial tissue, allowing for future growth. At this time, the inferior vena cava blood is now channeled into the pulmonary artery, completely dividing systemic and pulmonary venous return. A recent modification, in which a small fenestration is placed in the atrial patch, has been added in order to allow a gradual adjustment to this new circulatory condition. The limited right-to-left shunt through the fenestration, which is generally 4 mm in diameter, maintains cardiac output at the expense of a decreased systemic oxygen saturation during the transient elevations pulmonary vascular resistance which commonly occur in the early hours to days after the Fontan procedure. At the University of Michigan, the fenestration is controlled by an external snare device and subsequently closed by exposing the snare in the catheterization laboratory approximately six months after the Fontan procedure, avoiding an additional operation.

Our recent experience with surgical reconstruction for neonates with hypoplastic left heart syndrome suggests that this procedure can be recommended for all patients, regardless of anatomic subtype or aortic size with an equal likelihood of success. Because older age so adversely affected survival, operation is optimally performed within the first 2 to 3 weeks of life. The subsequent risk for the hemifontan and Fontan procedures has been low, with an actuarial survival of 74 percent for all three stages.

TRANSPOSITION OF THE GREAT ARTERIES

Dramatic and exciting changes have been made in the surgical repair of infants born with transposition of the great arteries (TGA) over the past decade. In TGA, the aorta arises from the right ventricle and the pulmonary artery rises solely, or in part, from the left ventricle. There is a concordant connection between the atria and the ventricles such that the systemic venous return circulates back to the body and the pulmonary venous return back to the lungs. Rather than having a single circulatory pattern in series, this anomaly is one in which two separate circulations exist in parallel. As such, it is incompatible in life unless a sufficient degree of mixing of the two circulations at either atrial, ventricular or great vessel level exists. Thus, some desaturated blood returning from the body must reach the lungs and an equal amount of highly saturated blood returning from the lungs must reach the body. The degree of mixing will determine the systemic saturation and the clinical condition of the infant. In the majority of newborns, mixing is largely dependent on an atrial septal defect which is often restrictive. This can be enlarged to improve mixing by a procedure known as balloon atrial septostomy. Additionally, approximately 25 percent of patients will have a ventricular septal defect which may further improve mixing and systemic saturation. Finally, a patent ductus arteriosus may be present and maintained by an infusion of prostaglandin to improve mixing at the great vessel level.

For many years, repair of infants with TGA was done by redirecting the atrial return utilizing the Mustard and Senning procedures. These operations, devised in the late 1950's and early 1960's, resulted in a functionally normal circulation be redirecting systemic venous return across a complex atrial patch to the mitral valve, left ventricle and pulmonary artery in order to reach the lungs. Pulmonary venous return was then directed to the tricuspid valve, right ventricle and aorta. Although these procedures were done at low risk, numerous late problems resulted including atrial dysrhythmias, baffle obstructions and right ventricular dysfunction. Superior vena caval obstruction was noted in 25 percent in some series with 10 percent of these patients requiring reoperation for this complication. Although less common, pulmonary venous and inferior vena caval obstruction were also noted. Atrial arrhythmias occurred in as many as 50 percent of patients at late followup and as many as 10 percent of these required pacemakers. Because the Mustard and Senning procedures do not alter ventricular or great vessel anatomy, the right ventricle remains as the systemic ventricular chamber and late right ventricular failure, particularly in those infants with associated ventricular septal defects was common. In the 1970's, renewed interest in direct arterial repair for infants with TGA was stimulated by the early efforts of Jatene working in Brazil. His pioneering efforts as well as those of Yacoub and Castaneda were instrumental in reducing the operative risk to one that was equal to or even lower than that of the Mustard or Senning repair.

The operative technique is straightforward for most patients with TGA and begins with transection of both great vessels above the semilunar valves. The distal aorta is then brought posterior to the pulmonary artery bifurcation and anastomosed to the proximal pulmonary artery to reconstruct the left ventricular outflow tract. The coronary arteries are excised with wide buttons of adjacent arterial wall and reimplanted into the posterior great vessel. Finally, the original aortic root (neopulmonary artery) is reconstructed with a patch of pericardium to augment the posterior sinuses of Valsalva where the coronary arteries were excised and subsequently anastomosed to the pulmonary artery bifurcation to reconstruct the right ventricular outflow tract. Associated atrial and ventricular septal defects are closed completing a true anatomic repair.

The operative mortality has decreased dramatically in recent years and the arterial switch procedure can now be done with a 2–3 percent mortality in experienced centers. In our own experience of approximately 200 infants undergoing arterial repair, hospital mortality is now approximately 2 percent. Although this risk was not increased by the presence of a ventricular septal defect or the specific coronary artery arrangement, it has been our impression that certain coronary patterns have been more difficult to repair and are probably associated with a higher risk. Specifically, those patients with the rare intramural left coronary artery and those with a single right coronary artery and side-by-side great vessels have posed a greater technical challenge.

The timing of operative intervention in those infants with TGA and intact ventricular septum in whom left ventricular pressure rapidly falls to low levels and left ventricular mass regresses soon after birth, is important to the ultimate outcome. The data from large multicenter studies indicate that the operative risk begins to increase in those patients beyond the age of two weeks and repair should therefore be done before this age. Although it is uncommon for patients to present with TGA beyond the first few days or weeks of life because of the significant degree of cyanosis that is generally easily apparent, an occasional patient will present beyond the neonatal period. In these patients, who may have satisfactory systemic oxygen saturation due to a naturally occurring atrial septal defect or small ventricular septal defect, repair when left ventricular pressure is low carries an increased risk as the left ventricle is poorly prepared to accommodate the increased afterload imposed by the systemic vascular resistance. In these situations, a preliminary pulmonary artery banding combined with placement of a systemic to pulmonary artery shunt will serve to provide both a pressure and volume overload in order to "redevelop" the left ventricle allowing for a safer arterial repair usually within a few week interval.

Long-term studies support the durability of the arterial repair. [7–10] Late mortality has been negligible and left ventricular function in those studies in which it has been specifically examined has generally been normal. Encouragingly, the neoaortic valve remains competent although in some series, particularly in those in which preliminary pulmonary artery banding was performed, progressive aortic regurgitation has been noted, possibly as a result of valve distortion from the proximity of the band. Late left ventricular outflow tract obstruction has been exceedingly rare and coronary obstructions uncommon.

The development of supravalvar pulmonary stenosis, however, was an important source of late morbidity and the need for reoperation in the early experience with arterial repair. Although its cause was multifactorial, obstruction at the level of the pulmonary artery anastomosis was due to tension on the branch pulmonary arteries secondary to insufficient distal mobilization as well as the failure to adequately reconstruct the defects in the neopulmonary root resulting from coronary artery excision. Changes in the technique have included wide mobilization of the peripheral pulmonary arteries beyond the lobar branches in addition to autologous pericardial reconstruction of the proximal pulmonary root and have dramatically reduced the need for reoperation. In our own series, these technique changes have resulted in a dramatic fall in the incidence of supravalvar pulmonary stenosis to less than 2 percent. [9] Although long-term data must still be carefully examined, the results of the arterial switch repair for patients with TGA are extremely encouraging and suggest that a truly corrective operation is now available for this complex anomaly.

SINGLE LUNG TRANSPLANTATION FOR EISENMENGER'S SYNDROME

Advanced pulmonary vascular disease has been considered a contraindication to correction of associated intracardiac defects. Surgical repair in this condition has had an excessive mortality and morbidity with little chance of clinical improvement. Cardiopulmonary transplantation has offered a major break through in the treatment of these patients, however. [11,12] Although combined transplantation of the heart and lungs has been successfully performed for patients with Eisenmenger's Syndrome, the scarcity of donor organs has severely limited this treatment option. A certain subsegment of patients with advanced pulmonary vascular disease secondary to congenital heart defects, however, may be considered for single lung transplantation with correction of the associated cardiac defect. This may allow re–establishment of normal pulmonary hemodynamics in many of these patients.

Between February, 1991 and April, 1992, 7 patients with end-stage pulmonary vascular disease secondary to a congenital cardiac defect underwent single lung transplantation and correction of the cardiovascular anomaly at the University of Michigan. [11] All patients had advanced symptoms and were New York Heart Association class 4. None of the patients treated under this protocol was estimated to have a one-year life expectancy exceeding 50 percent. The patients were selected because of their anatomic suitability for intracardiac correction and the procedure was reserved for those patients with atrial, ventricular or arterial septation anomalies with well preserved ventricular function. Combined heart and lung transplantation was reserved for those patients with more complex anatomic defects not amenable to reconstructive operation.

With few exceptions, the techniques utilized followed previously well established guidelines for combined heart and lung transplantation. The single lung transplants with cardiac repair were performed via a midline sternotomy in most cases, although a right thoracotomy was found optimal for the patient with an isolated atrial septal defect. Cardiopulmonary bypass was established and elective cardioplegic induced myocardial arrest was used. The intracardiac correction was performed first followed by the lung transplant during a continuous period of cardiopulmonary bypass. The bronchial anastomoses were not buttressed with omentum or other tissues.

The diagnoses of the patients included atrial septal defect in one patient, ventricular septal defect in two, complete AV septal defect in one and aortopulmonary window in one patient. During this same time frame, one patient with tricuspid atresia underwent en block transplantation of the heart and both lungs and another patient with a previous Mustard repair of transposition of the great arteries underwent a heart and single left lung transplantation. The right lung was transplanted in the 5 patients undergoing single lung transplant and intracardiac repair.

There was one perioperative death in an 18 year-old female with a ventricular septal defect. This patient died because of donor lung dysfunction despite support with extracorporeal membrane oxygenation for four weeks. Of the four surviving patients undergoing single lung transplant and cardiac repair, all have survived at least one year after operation. Two reoperations were performed, mitral valve replacement in the patient with aortopulmonary window and left upper lobectomy for fungus ball in the left "nontransplanted" lung in the surviving patient with ventricular septal defect. Both patients survived these procedures and have resumed their previous level of activity.

Less severe complications included at least one episode of acute rejection requiring therapy within the first 30 days following transplant in all patients. Only two patients had a single episode each of rejection subsequent to the post transplant month, however. Infectious complications included cytomegalovirus pneumonia in two patients, herpes pneumonia in one patient and pneumonia from multiple organisms in a third patient, each of whom responded well to antimicrobial therapy. There were no bronchial anastomotic complications in this series.

The late results in these patients, however, have not been as encouraging. Three of the four patients surviving single lung transplantation and cardiac repair developed obliterative bronchiolitis and died at 13, 17 and 22 months following transplant. Only the patient with a ventricular septal defect remains alive and improved nearly two years after transplantation. Both patients receiving heart and single or double lung transplants remain well at 15 and 18 months after operation.

Although this limited experience with single lung transplantation and repair of associated intracardiac defects for patients with Eisenmenger's Syndrome has demonstrated satisfactory early results, the late results would seriously call into question the suitability of this treatment for this high risk group of patients. The reasons for the late deterioration in this group are not immediately apparent but may be due to the sudden large increase in blood flow going to the donor lung following transplantation as virtually the entire cardiac output enters the lung with normal pulmonary vascular resistance. Although there may be a certain limitation to this new physiology, it is not inherently clear why this should be different from the patient following pneumonectomy. However, this experience has led us to discontinue the use of single lung transplantation for patients with pulmonary hypertension, regardless of etiology.

FUTURE DEVELOPMENTS

Repair of complex congenital heart disease continues with the development of novel approaches in many areas. The use of endovascular stents for coronary artery and peripheral vascular problems has also been applied in the field of congenital heart disease. Percutaneous or intraoperative placement of stents has enabled the relief of complex pulmonary arterial and pulmonary venous stenoses which have formally been in inaccessible to surgical repair. At the University of Michigan, a large experience with the use of endovascular stents for complex congenital heart problems has been accumulated. When used in the operating room and combined with other reparative procedures, the operative exposure and procedures have been significantly simplified. Although these stents have had excellent and durable results for pulmonary arterial stenoses, the usefulness in patients with pulmonary vein stenoses remains in doubt. Early results have been encouraging, but recurrence of pulmonary vein stenoses proximally within the hilum of the lung has been the general rule, particularly for those patients in whom this procedure has been applied for recurrent pulmonary vein obstruction following repair of total anomalous pulmonary venous return.

The search for the ideal valve substitute continues. Widespread use of cryopreserved allografts has provided excellent, durable valve replacements for many young children, avoiding the need for anticoagulant therapy. Aortic valve replacement with an autologous pulmonary valve (the Ross procedure) may provide the most ideal procedure yet. In this procedure, the patients own pulmonary valve is transplanted into the aortic position providing a viable tissue replacement of a permanent nature. The pulmonary valve is then replaced with a cryopreserved allograft where minor functional imperfections are much better tolerated in the low pressure pulmonary circulation.

Increased use of prenatal testing and intrauterine echocardiography is now able to provide accurate prenatal diagnoses of many congenital cardiac defects. In particular, the diagnosis of hypoplastic left heart syndrome is one that can be made with a high degree of certainty in utero. This provides the opportunity for ample prenatal discussion of various treatment options as well as the ability to deliver the infant in a center equipped to deal with these complex congenital heart anomalies. It has been well established for many lesions that poor preoperative condition is a risk factor for survival. The prenatal diagnosis of hypoplastic left heart syndrome will allow proper resuscitative measures to be promptly instituted, including the use of prostaglandin therapy to maintain ductal patency, and avoid the often harmful effects of acidosis and cardiovascular collapse which may occur when the diagnosis is made late.

REFERENCES

1. Norwood WI Jr: Hypoplastic left heart syndrome. Ann Thorac Surg 1990; 52:688–695.

2. Meliones JN, Snider AR, Bove EL, Rosenthal A, Rosen DA: Longitudinal results after first-stage palliation for hypoplastic left heart syndrome. Circulation 1990; 82(suppl IV):151–156.

3. Norwood WI Jr, Jacobs ML, Murphy JD: Fontan procedure for hypoplastic left heart syndrome. Ann Thorac Surg 1992; 54:1025–1030.

4. Iannettoni MD, Bove EL, Mosca RS, et al: Improving results with first stage palliation for hypoplastic left heart syndrome. J Thorac Cardiovasc Surg, In press.

5. Pridjian AK, Mendelsohn AM, Lupinetti FM, et al: Usefulness of the bidirectional Glenn procedure as staged reconstruction for the functional single ventricle. Am J Cardiol 1993; 71:959–962.

6. Bove EL: Transplantation after first-stage reconstruction for hypoplastic left heart syndrome. Ann Thorac Surg 1991; 52:701–707.

7. Bove EL, Beekman RH III, Snider AR, et al: Arterial repair for transposition of the great arteries and large ventricular septal defect in early infancy. Circulation 1988; 78(suppl III):26–31.

8. Kato H, Nakano S, Matsuda H, Hirose H, Shimazaki Y, Kawashima Y: Right ventricular myocardial function after atrial switch operation for transposition of the great arteries. Am J Cardiol 1989; 63:226–230.

9. Lupinetti FM, Bove EL, Minich LL, et al: Intermediate-term survival and functional results after arterial repair for transposition of the great arteries. J Thorac Cardiovasc Surg 1992; 103:421–427.

10. Kirklin JW, Blackstone EH, Tchervenkov CI, Castaneda AR, Congenital Heart Surgeons Society: Clinical outcomes after the arterial switch operation for transposition. Circulation 1992; 86:1501–1515.

11. Lupinetti FM, Bolling SF, Bove EL, et al: Selective lung or heart-lung transplant for pulmonary hypertension associated with congenital cardiac anomalies. Circulation, In press.

12. Spray TL, Mallory GB, Canter CE, Huddleston CB, Kaiser LR: Pediatric lung transplantation for pulmonary hypertension and congenital heart disease. Ann Thorac Surg 1992; 54:216–225.

ANESTHESIA FOR CORONARY ARTERY BYPASS SURGERY

The Nursing Prospective

Margaret M. Burgoyne, R.N., M.S., C.R.N.A.

University of Medicine and Dentistry of New Jersey
Robert Wood Johnson Medical School
Cooper Hospital/University Medical Center
Camden, New Jersey

The anesthetic management of patients undergoing cardiac surgery is still controversial. The most appropriate anesthetic, narcotic or inhalation agent as well as the best muscle relaxant for each particular patient remains an open question. The use of advanced monitoring technologies such as the pulmonary artery catheterization and the transesophageal echocardiography (TEE) and the manipulation of myocardial oxygen parameters during cardiac surgery is still under much debate and most of these issues are presently under investigation. Ultimately, the perioperative management and the understanding of these issues rely upon the elucidation of the underlying disease.

In the United States, there are over 500,000 deaths per year resulting from myocardial infarction. Moreover, approximately 5 million patients are treated for ischemic heart disease each year. Some of these patients will eventually undergo general surgery or surgical myocardial revascularization (CABG).

The majority of these patients have a number of common characteristics that are of concern to the anesthesia care team. Frequently associated medical conditions such as hypertension, smoking, diabetes, and peripheral vascular disease including carotid artery stenosis may be present in the cardiac surgical patient and should be of concern during patient's management. Moreover, an increased number of patients presenting for CABG surgery are middle-aged and older. CABG in septuagenarians and octogenarians becomes frequent at many institutions. Table 1. outlines some of the functional cardiovascular changes associated with aging.

The advanced age is generally characterized by a less efficient heart with deminished reserves, particularly if subjected to additional stress. The presence of serious medical conditions such as hypertension, diabetes, pulmonary disease, gout, etc., can further precipitate cardiac decompensation. The

Cardiac Surgery: Current Issues 2, Edited by A. C. Cernaianu and A. J. DelRossi,
Plenum Press, New York, 1994

Table 1. Cardiovascular Changes Seen in the Elderly

Maximal coroanry blood flow	↓
Cardiac index	↓
Resting heart rate	↓
Maximal heart rate	↓
Arterial distensibility	↓
Peripheral vascular resistance	↑
Impedance to left ventricular output	↑
Maximal coronary blood flow	↑
Stroke volume	↑

characteristics of a patient with ischemic heart disease, presenting for either CABG surgery or for any surgical intervention are presented in Table 2.

The pre-operative assessment is essential for the evaluation of the patients presenting for surgery. Table 3 presents some of the elements to be considered during the preoperative evaluation.

It is important to assess the vital signs, current values and prior ranges, while hospitalized, and the patient's height and weight (for calculation of drug regimens and the patient's body surface area)

Jugular venous distension and the presence of carotid bruit may alert for either congestive heart failure or cerebrovascular disease. The landmarks for jugular vein cannulation should also be established. The examination should also include the heart (murmurs, clicks, abnormal sounds), lungs (rales, rhonchi, wheezes), vasculature (sites for venous and arterial access; peripheral pulses), abdomen (pulsatile liver as seen in congestive heart failure or tricuspid regurgitation), extremities (peripheral edema), and the nervous system (motor or sensory deficits).

After accumulating as much information on the patient as possible, a decision is made towards the anesthetic technique that will best serve the patient's needs.

Table 2. Ideal Cardiovascular Parameters during Cardiac Surgery

Preload	keep the heart small; decrease wall tension; increase perfusion pressure
Afterload	maintain pressure; hypertension is better than hypotension
Contractility	if left ventricular function is adequate, depression can be beneficial
Rate	slow
Rhythm	sinus rhythm if possible
Myocardial oxygen balance	control of oxygen demand is frequently not enough: monitor for and treat "supply" ischemia
Post-CPB	elevated ventricular filling pressure is usually not needed after CABG surgery

CPB = cardiopulmonary bypass.

Table 3. Preoperative Evaluation

Medical History	
Electrocardiogram	Ischemia and/or infarction, type of rhythm and conduction abnormalities
Chest roentgenogram	Cardiomegaly, pulmonary vascular congesion, pulmonary edema, pleural effusion
CBC with differential	
Platelet count	
Chemistry (7 and 12)	
Coagulation profile	
Cardiac catheterization	LVEDP >18, EF < 0.4, C.I. < 2 mL/min.
Ventriculography	Low EF, hypo, and/or dyskinesis
TEE	Low EF, wall motion abnormalities
Pulmonary function test	History of pulmonary disease
Typing and crossing of homologous blood according to the institution standards	

LVEDP= left ventricular end–diastolic pressure; EF= ejection fraction; CI= cardiac index; TEE= transesophageal echocardiography

Maintaining myocardial oxygen balance is an essential step toward ensuring proper management of the cardiac surgical patient. The elements which contribute to the myocardial oxygen balance are presented in Table 4.

PREPARATION FOR SURGERY:

Patient's premedication in preparation for anesthesia and surgery is very important. Preoperative medication consists of administration of oral benzodiazepines (usually 2 mg of valium) followed by an i.m. injection of morphine sulfate (0.1 to 0.15 mg/kg) depending on the patient's physical and pulmonary status and the administration of an antimuscarinic drug (scopolamine 0.4 mg). Transportation is performed on 3 to 4 liters nasal oxygen (2 liters in the case of CO_2 retainers). If the patient is already on a cardiac monitor in the hospital room, the transport to the operating room should include cardiac monitoring. Generally, the patient arrives in the holding and anesthesia preparation room approximately 2 hours prior to the scheduled surgery. The patient is placed on oxygen and connected to the EKG, blood pressure and

Table 4. Elements of Myocardial Oxygen Balance

Demand	Supply
Wall tension	Coronary blood flow
ventricular radius	driving pressure
pressure generation	diastolic time
Contractility	arteriolar tone
Heart rate	Arterial O_2 content
	Myocardial O_2 extraction

pulse oximetry monitors. The patient is quickly re-evaluated, shaved and the chart is reviewed again. During preparation for surgery in the holding area, a critical care nurse is assigned to monitor the patient. The same cautions are taken during the patient's transfer into the operating room. The patient is immediately connected to the end-tidal CO_2 monitor, pulse oximetry and automatic blood pressure cuff. Blood pressures are measured in both arms. The blood pressure cuff should be placed on the arm which is used for placement of the arterial line. EKG monitoring (lead II and V_5) which captures approximately 75 to 85 percent of all possible ischemic changes during surgery is used. In addition, leads for the intra-aortic balloon pump are applied in case cardiac assistance is needed later. Upon local i.v. infiltration of lidocaine either 14 or 16 Jelcos are placed in each arm for administration of Ringer's solution at a slow rate.

Sedation is obtained with 0.5 mg increments of i.v. midazolam to the desired effect. An i.v. nitroglycerine drip solution is started at 50 μg/minute under careful monitoring. Usually the left radial artery is prepared for cannulation for arterial pressure monitoring unless the right arm is deemed more appropriate.

The right side of the neck is prepared aseptically for cannulation of the right internal jugular with the cordis kit. The technique is straightforward, and is generally associated with a lower incidence of pneumothorax than the subclavian route.

After comparing the blood color sampled from the jugular vein to the blood sampled from the radial artery to check for inadvertent carotid artery cannulation, the cordis line is threaded and the pulmonary artery catheter is placed. If the patient presents with decreased left ventricular function, an Oximetrix® pulmonary artery catheter (Abbott Critical Care, Mountain View, CA) may be used because of its ability to monitor mixed venous oxygen saturation (SvO_2) and oxygen transport variables. The increased cost of this type of catheter may be offset during the treatment of heart failure.

INDUCTION OF ANESTHESIA

The two most common opioids used for induction of anesthesia for cardiac surgery are (fentanyl citrate) sublimaze and sufenta (sufentanil).

Fentanyl citrate is a potent narcotic analgesic. Each mL of solution contains 50 μg. A 100 μg dose (2 mL) is equipotent to 10 mg morphine or 75 mg demerol as analgesic dose. Fentanyl citrate preserves cardiac stability, and decreases stress-related hormonal changes at higher doses. Usual doses for cardiac surgery in the presence of oxygen and muscle relaxant are 50 to 100 μg/kg. Doses up to 150 μg/kg may also be used safely when necessary. The elimination half-life of the drug is 219 minutes (approximately 4 hours). Weaning of the patient postoperatively from the ventilator must be performed carefully, keeping in mind that the respiratory depression may outlast the analgesia from the drug. The drug is primarily metabolized in the liver and excreted in the urine (75 percent) and in the feces (9 percent).

Sufentanil is a potent opioid analgesic. It is reported to be as much as 10 times as potent as fentanyl. Usual dose range for sufentanil is 10 to 15 μg/kg. Doses can be increased up to 30 μg/kg during the case if necessary to block stress responses and provide potent anesthesia. Elimination half-life of the drug is 164 minutes (approximately 3 hours). Postoperative ventilation is necessary and weaning and extubation should be performed under careful monitoring. The liver and small intestine are the major sites of biotransformation. Approximately 80 percent of the drug is excreted in 24 hours.

The most commonly used muscle relaxants for cardiac anesthesia are vecuronium bromide and pancuronium bromide.

Vecuronium bromide is a nondepolarizing neuromuscular blocking agent of intermediate duration. It acts by competing for cholinergic receptors at the motor end-plate. The dosage for intubation during the induction of anesthesia is 0.08 to 0.10 mg/kg. The patient is ventilated by mask for approximately 3 to 5 minutes for maximal effect of muscular relaxation and then is carefully intubated. Repeated boluses of vencuronium bromide can be administered throughout the case while the patient is being monitored with a peripheral nerve stimulator applied to the face. A continuous infusion of vencuronium bromide can also be employed (1 μg/kg/min, average maintenance dose for a 100 kg person would be 6 mg/hr). The elimination half-time of this drug in this dose range is 65 to 75 minutes. The use of this type of drug facilitates earlier weaning and extubation of the postoperative CABG patient in the ICU. The drug is eliminated by both renal and biliary route.

Pancuronium bromide is a long-acting nondepolarizing neuromuscular blocking agent. The drug increases heart rate and arterial blood pressure without causing a fall in stroke volume. It appears also to have an inotropic effect. The intubating dose is 0.06 to 0.1 mg/kg (i.e., 6 to 10 mg i.v. for induction in a 100 kg person. Most practitioners use the larger dose. Three to 5 minutes ventilation is performed to attain maximal relaxation for intubation. Monitoring with a peripheral nerve stimulator is usually indicated, particularly when incremental doses of pancuronium bromide (0.03 to 0.06 mg/kg per hour) are necessary to achieve desired relaxation.

Biotransformation of the drug is accomplished by renal and hepatobiliary routes. Elimination half-time is longer than that of vencuronium bromide and the return to normal of the muscle function is delayed, thus weaning from the ventilator and extubation may take longer.

Our institutional preference is the combination of fentanyl citrate and vencuronium bromide for sleep and relaxation. The disadvantages of pure narcotic anesthesia relate to the fact that the patient may remain aware (i.e., somewhat awake and recall operative experience). Because of the anti-recall properties, drugs such as scopolamine and benzodiazepines (midazolam) may resolve the problem if the patient presents with good ventricular function. The addition of small quantities of isoflurane (up to approximately 0.5 percent titrate to clinical response) may also produce retrograde amnesia. The use of isoflurane allows to increase the depth of anesthesia at times of increased stimulation with rapid reversibility as needed. When the vaporizer is turned off, the isoflurane is quickly eliminated. Some patients may tolerate concentrations of up to 1 percent without hemodynamic decompensation.

Once the patient is asleep, ventilated by mask with 100 percent oxygen and maximally relaxed (as maintained with peripheral nerve stimulator), 50 to 100 mg i.v. lidocaine may be administered for protection of tracheal intubation-induced stimulation. The vocal cords are visualized, and the appropriate size endotracheal tube is placed. The cuff is inflated and auscultatory and monitoring methods (end-tidal CO_2 and peak inspiratory pressure) are used for control of correctness of tube placement. Ventilation is started at an approximate volume of about 10 mL/kg/b.w. and a rate of 10 to 12 per minute and is adjusted depending upon blood gases and end-tidal CO_2. A nasogastric tube is placed for emptying the stomach. Suction is used intermittently throughout the case. An esophageal temperature probe and a Foley catheter also are placed. During this phase, avoidance of tachycardia, hypotension and myocardial ischemia is mandatory. Before sternal incision, administration of an additional dose of fentanyl citrate (50 mcg/kg) may be necessary. Cardiac output is measured more frequently before cannulation and the establishment of cardiopulmonary bypass (CPB). TEE may be required for valve replacement cases or when left ventricular dysfunctions is present or is expected during the procedure.

Before cannulation for CPB, heparin (3 to 4 mg/kg or 300 to 400 U/kg is administered. Activated clotting time (ACT) is assessed after approximately 3 minutes. When the ACT reaches 480 sec, CPB can be instituted. If the ACT is a lower, an additional 10,000 U of heparin is administered and followed by another ACT measurement in approximately 3 minutes. During cannulas placement for bypass, careful observation is necessary. Discoloration or swelling of the patient's face may be the result from poor drainage or kinked tubing. Proper drainage is mandatory throughout the case. Arterial blood gas, hemoglobin, Hct and electrolytes are monitored throughout the bypass, as necessary. ACT and urinary output measurements are repeated every 15 minutes.

Once the patient is onto full CPB, the ventilation is discontinued, however, the anesthesia machine remains on with the pop-off valve open delivering one liter of oxygen. When the aortic is cross-clamp (AXC), the nitroglycerine infusion is stopped and cardioplegia is infused into the patient's coronary system. The patient's mean arterial pressure is maintained between 50 and 75 mg Hg with phenylephrine hydrochloride (Neosynephrine) or trimethophan camsylate (Arfonad) or sodium nitroprusside titrated to clinical response. Muscle relaxants and fentanyl citrate are added as needed. Upon the removal of the AXC, restarting the nitroglycerine drip at 50 µg/min may be necessary. As the warming process continues, most patients' hearts start to beat on their own. Sometimes, defibrillation with direct low-voltage shocks is necessary. Laboratory parameters are carefully checked again. Ventilation is restarted, the venous cannula are partially occluded and circulation of blood to the right ventricle is reinstituted under careful observation of the blood pressure. If inotropic support is needed, an epinephrine drip will be employed (1 to 2 mcg/min). In most patients, this may not be necessary. The use of TEE may help in establishing when the patient can be weaned off inotropic support. TEE may be used to determine the heart's wall motion, blood flow, valve function, and diagnose the presence of air bubbles in the cardiac circulation. Upon decannulation and careful evacuation of air from the heart, the reversal of heparin with protamine sulphate (1 mg of protamine for every mg of heparin given) is started. Protamine sulphate is administered slowly (no more than 50 mg/minute) along with 300 to 500 mg i.v. calcium chloride. The patient is monitored carefully for any reaction to protamine, which is relatively rare. During this period of time, more laboratory studies and cardiac output determinations are being performed. Three to 5 minutes after the total amount of protamine sulphate has been administered, another ACT is determined. If the ACT has not returned to pre-heparinization levels, an additional 50 mg protamine sulphate is administred and a Hep-Con test is performed to establish how much heparin is left in the system. Patients on chronic long-term aspirin regimens may sometimes require pharmacologic manipulation of the coagulation cascade with either desmopressin acetate (DDAVP) or epsilon-amino caproic acid (Amicar) post-bypass. Fresh-frozen plasma (FFP) and/or platelet therapy may be necessary. The administration of postoperative blood products is presently under a great deal of controversy and scrutiny. The methods of blood conservation with autologous donation, the use of the cell saver and the technique of sequestering autologous blood before CPB, have been discussed in another chapter in this book.

Occasionally, patients may need more support to come off CPB and to remain hemodynamically stable. Inotropic support and afterload reduction to maintain normal cardiac output and myocardial oxygen balance are titrated to clinical response.

Patients undergoing valve replacement in the presence of a recent myocardial infarction, or chronic or intermittent congestive heart failure and poor left ventricular function are more prone to develop low cardiac output syndrome post CPB and to be weaned with difficulty off bypass. The IABP may be needed for postoperative cardiac support.

At the time of sternal closure, the ICU is contacted and a detailed report about the patient's status is given. The report should describe the infusion lines and their location, present cardiac output values pre- and post-CPB, significant preoperative history, drug allergy and the surgical procedure. The patient's transfer to the ICU is performed under strict monitoring with displays of electrocardiogram and arterial pressure. The patient is transported under 100 percent oxygen ventilation and all drips and pumps to provide support drugs such as lidocaine, calcium chloride, neosynephrine, atropine, etc. are taken with us.

Upon the patient's arrival in the ICU, EKG is connected first while the attachement to the blood pressure monitor is maintained. In the presence of an acceptable EKG tracing, the arterial line is disconnected from the portable monitor and connected to the ICU monitor. This sequence allows continued observation of vital signs.

The care of the patient undergoing cardiac anesthesia is a team effort. Everyone plays an important, intricate part to produce a good outcome. Clear, concise and friendly communication between all members of the team should help accomplish this goal.

Selected Bibilography

Barash PG, Cullen BF, Stoelting RK: Clinical Anesthesia. J. B. Lippincott Co., 1989.

Benumof JL, Saidman LJ: Anesthesia and Perioperative Complications. Mosby Year Book, Chicago, 1992.

Duncan PG, (ed): Problems in Anesthesia, Anesthetic Risk and Complications: J. B. Lippincott Co., 1992.

Kaplan JA (ed): Cardiac Anesthesia, Cardiovascular Pharmacology. Grune and Stratton, 1988.

Katz RL, (ed): Seminars in Anesthesia. W. B. Saunders, in Philadelphia, 1990.

Moreno-Cabral CE, Mitchell RS, Miller DC: Manual of postoperative management in adult cardiac surgery. Wilkins and Wilkins, 1988.

Rogers MC, Tinker JH, Covino BG, Longnecker DE: Principles and Practice of Anesthesiology.
    Mosby Year Book. Chicago, 1993.
Tuman KJ, McCarthy RJ, Ivankovich AD: Cardiothoracic and Vascular Anesthesia Update.
    W. B. Saunders Co., Philadelpia, 1991.

PERIOPERATIVE MYOCARDIAL ISCHEMIA AND INFARCTION

The Nursing Perspective

Kathleen C. Tully, R. N., MSN, CCRN

Our Lady of Lourdes Medical Center
Camden, New Jersey

Myocardial infarction is a frequent complication of coronary artery bypass surgery and is associated with increased mortality and morbidity. [1,2] It accounts for most deaths which occur postoperatively and within the first month after the operation. [1] In the cardiac surgical patient population, the estimated morbidity and mortality related to myocardial infarction ranges between 4 and 40 percent. [3-9]

Infarction is the result of ischemia which represents an imbalance between myocardial oxygen supply and oxygen demand. Myocardial ischemia initiates a continuum of progressively more serious cellular changes which may lead to irreversible injury, cellular death and myocardial necrosis. [10] This process is time dependent; the longer the myocardium remains ischemic, the greater the chances are that infarction may occur. Additionally, the size of the infarct is related to the ischemic time. [11] Therefore, patient outcomes are directly dependent upon early identification and treatment of ischemia. When ischemia is identified, interventions to balance oxygen supply-demand can be instrumental in averting myocardial infarction. It is, therefore, incumbent upon the nurse caring for the cardiac surgical patient, at risk for ischemia and infarction, to recognize and be prepared to manage signs of myocardial ischemia which may be a precursor to myocardial infarction.

PATHOPHYSIOLOGY OF MYOCARDIAL ISCHEMIA

Ischemia can be defined as the reversible injury which results when the demand for oxygen exceeds the available supply. The consequences of ischemia to the myocardium are tissue hypoxia, accumulation of metabolic waste products, acidosis and impaired myocardial contractility. When allowed to continue, cellular changes occur and irreversible damage ensues. The end result of prolonged ischemia is infarction, which can be defined as

Cardiac Surgery: Current Issues 2, Edited by A. C. Cernaianu and A. J. DelRossi,
Plenum Press, New York, 1994

the irreversible injury and tissue necrosis resulting from the cessation of blood to a specific area of the myocardium. Infarcted or necrotic myocardium is unable to properly contract. The extent of myocardial dysfunction correlates with the size of the infarction and the consequences to the patient may range from mildly decreased ventricular function to extensive myocardial necrosis, with pump failure and death.

The oxygen supply-demand ratio is of paramount importance in the discussion of myocardial ischemia and infarction. As long as oxygen supply is able to balance the oxygen requirements, ischemia and thus, infarction does not occur.

Oxygen demand is directly proportional to the preload, afterload, myocardial contractility and heart rate. {12,13} *Preload* is defined as the left ventricular end-diastolic pressure and corresponds to the pulmonary artery occlusion pressure (wedge pressure). A high end-diastolic pressure will be correlated to an increased myocardial oxygen demand.

Afterload is the resistance that the left ventricle must overcome to open the aortic valve and eject the blood into the systemic circulation. Afterload is a function of arterial pressure and vessel diameter. When afterload is increased as in hypertension or elevated systemic vascular resistance, myocardial work is increased, as is oxygen demand.

Contractility is the ability of cardiac muscle fibers to shorten when stimulated. The oxygen demand is directly proportional to the force of myocardial contraction.

Heart rate influences both the oxygen demand and supply. The heart requires more energy and oxygen to beat 120 times than it needs to beat 60 times per minute. Moreover, during tachycardia, diastole is shorter, resulting in less ventricular filling time and decreased cardiac output. Since most coronary blood flow occurs during diastole, a shortened diastolic filling time results in a reduction of coronary blood flow and myocardial oxygen supply.

Coronary blood flow is the primary factor responsible for supplying oxygen to the myocardium. Coronary blood flow is dependent upon cardiac output and the amount of oxygen available to be delivered to the tissue. It is directly proportional to the aortic pressure and inversely proportional to the resistance of the coronary vessel. Thus, an increase in pressure will cause an increase in flow whereas, an increase in resistance will cause a decrease in flow. Through a mechanism known as autoregulation, coronary blood flow is adjusted to the metabolic demand. Blood vessels, including those of the coronary circulation dilate in the presence of increased metabolic activity and constrict with decreased activity. The healthy coronary vasculature has the intrinsic ability to alter its resistance so that coronary blood flow will meet oxygen demand. {13,14}

Resistance to coronary blood flow is also influenced by the intra-myocardial pressure. During ventricular systole, the contracting myocardium exerts a pressure on the coronary blood vessels, increasing vascular resistance and limiting blood flow to the coronary arteries. As a result, most coronary blood flow occurs during diastole when resistance is diminished. {14} The vascular resistance is also dependent on the caliber of the vessels. Small diameter vessels may be a factor of genetic makeup, or they may result from pathological conditions such as atherosclerosis, thrombosis or vasoconstriction.

On the supply side of the equation, another mechanism of ischemia and possible infarction is coronary artery spasm. Coronary vasospasm is a transient contraction of coronary artery smooth muscle that decreases coronary blood flow (CBF). It occurs in both the normal and atherosclerotic coronary artery. {12} Prostaglandins and platelets appear to play a major role in the generation of coronary artery spasm and ischemia. {12,13}

Prostaglandins are by-products of arachidonic acid, which is synthesized by the phospholipids in the cell membrane. In the presence of the enzyme cyclooxyegnase, arachidonic acid is converted to prostaglandin G2 which is then converted, by peroxidase, to prostaglandin H_2. Prostaglandin H_2 is further converted into prostaglandins D, E and F, thromboxane A_2 and prostacyclin. Prostaglandin E promotes vasodilation. Thromboxane causes vasoconstriction and platelet aggregation, while prostacyclin opposes the results of thromboxane by promoting vaso-dilation and decreasing platelet aggregation. {12,13}

Platelets also play a role in the generation of vasospasm. Platelets have a tendency to aggregate on the endothelial lining of blood vessels where they secrete vasoactive substances, including prostaglandins. Some of these substances, specifically, thromboxane, serotonin and adenosine diphosphate (ADP) promote further platelet aggregation and smooth muscle contraction. ADP also stimulates healthy endothelial cells to release additional substances which oppose these effects. One, "endothelium derived relaxing factor" (EDRF), limits vessel contraction. The other substance, prostacyclin, promotes vasodilation and prevents further platelet aggregation. Presently, it is believed that the balance between aggregation and vasoconstriction is upset in the presence of a disrupted, or atherosclerotic, endothelium. In this case, platelets may continue to secrete thromboxane, serotonin and ADP. However, in the damaged endothelium ADP is unable to stimulate the release of EDRF and prostacyclin. As a result vasoconstriction and platelet aggregation occur unopposed, thus promoting spasm and creating an internal environment conducive to the pathogenesis of ischemia. There is current experimental and clinical evidence to support the fact that an imbalance between thromboxane and prostacyclin exists in the setting of myocardial ischemia and infarction. {12,15,16}

Of interest also, particularly in the anesthetized surgical patient, is the phenomenon of silent ischemia. *Silent ischemia* may be defined as objective evidence of ischemia without chest pain or other anginal symptoms. {17} In recent years, there has been substantial evidence indicating that a significant number of people who experience myocardial ischemia are asymptomatic. {16–18} It appears that pain may be a very late indicator of coronary artery occlusion and that myocardial wall motion abnormalities are frequently the first indicators of ischemia. {16} Wall motion changes precede electrocardiographic signs of ischemia, which often occur before the perception of pain. Silent ischemia may represent an early stage of ischemia, possibly the vasoactive component. There is also support for the theory that painless episodes are shorter in duration and involve less myocardium than those events which are painful. It has also been suggested that higher levels of endogenous morphine-like substances, (endorphins) are present in people who experience silent ischemia. {19} Some investigators relate this phenomenon simply to the fact that pain threshold and perception vary among individuals. {16,17,20}

The term *stunned myocardium* has appeared with increasing frequency in the literature and it bears some discussion here since its clinical symptoms can mimic myocardial infarction. Additionally, this entity is believed to be associated with myocardial ischemia and/or reperfusion of the ischemic tissue. {13} Stunned myocardium can be defined as a reversible injury which results in myocardial dysfunction without evidence of necrosis. {21} Although contractility is impaired, it returns to normal within a period of time. The reduction in pump function may be significant and it may last for a week or longer. {22} The exact mechanism responsible for myocardial stunning is unknown. Myocardial stunning may result from ischemia and occur because ischemic cells are unable to produce sufficient amounts of adenosine triphosphate (ATP). {23} Without adequate ATP, there is insufficient energy for contraction. Stunned myocardium may also result from the damaging effects of oxygen derived-free radicals which are intermediates of oxygen metabolism. They are toxic substances which normally have catalytic pathways to neutralize them soon after their production. {13,21} In the presence of ischemia, these pathways may no longer be functional. As a result, the free radicals remain and may have a damaging effect on the myocardial cells. {13} Other possible mechanisms of myocardial stunning include calcium overload, which results in contractile dysfunction; {24} collagenous tissue dysfunction; {22} and increased catecholamine levels which may further enhance the production of oxygen free radicals. {24} Research is currently underway to identify interventions for prevention and treatment of the stunned myocardium.

RISK FACTORS

Myocardial infarction can have devastating effects for the patient. If ischemia is promptly identified and treated, myocardium may be salvaged and infarction may be prevented. It, therefore, becomes important to identify patients at risk for the development of ischemia, during the perioperative period, in order to prevent its deleterious consequences.

Many cardiac surgical patients experience pre-, intra- and postoperative electrocardiographic changes suggestive of ischemia. These episodes have been identified by ST segment changes and hemodynamic alterations. Although the exact significance of these episodes is not known, studies suggest that there is a correlation between the amount of preoperative ischemia and the development of perioperative infarction. {2,6,9} It can be surmised, then, that those patients who come to the operating room for emergency bypass, as well as those experiencing ECG changes and/or chest pain on arrival in the holding area, are at high risk for the development of perioperative infarction and need to be closely monitored for signs of ischemia. {6}

The risk of perioperative infarction appears to increase proportionately with the age of the patient and the existence of co-morbidities, especially insulin-dependent diabetes mellitus, previous myocardial infarction, and low left ventricular ejection fraction. In spite of advances made in myocardial preservation and surgical techniques, there is a trend toward increasing postoperative complications, including myocardial infarction, due to the changing population of patients who undergo the procedure. Today, all centers are reporting that patients undergoing myocardial revascularization are older and sicker than they were just a few years ago. {25} The patients of the 90's are more often diabetic, have a higher incidence of triple vessel disease and have more left ventricular dysfunction than did their counterparts of the 80's. It becomes clear then the problem of perioperative myocardial ischemia and infarction is of greater concern today, and probably will become even more so, as larger numbers of elderly and high-risk patients undergo the procedure. {5,26}

Another important risk factor for CABG surgery is the female gender. {9} In almost all reports, operative morbidity and mortality is significantly higher for women than for men. {27,28} Several factors seem to contribute to the poorer outcomes for women. These include later referrals for surgery in females than in males, and the fact that woman are frequently older and have more concomitant illnesses than their male counterparts at the time of referral for surgery. In addition, the operative mortality is inversely proportional to height and vessel size; therefore a woman's smaller body size, and smaller vessels for grafting, put her at higher risk for incomplete revascularization, difficult anastomoses and earlier re-occlusion. {28} All these factors combine to place women at risk for perioperative myocardial ischemia and infarction.

The ischemic (aortic cross-clamp) time has also been positively correlated with perioperative infarction. Patients requiring technically difficult surgical procedures and, thus, longer aortic cross-clamp time, have an increase in incidence of perioperative myocardial infarction. {2,8,9}

Re-operation is also frequently mentioned as a factor which places the patient at high risk for adverse surgical outcomes. Re-operation has been associated with longer anesthetic time, and an extended stress of the surgical procedure. {5}

The use of the internal mammary artery as a conduit has also been associated with higher risk for perioperative myocardial infarction. The internal mammary artery is longer and has a smaller diameter than most vein grafts. As a result, it may provide greater resistance to coronary blood flow. Additionally, internal mammary arteries have increased vascular tone, as compared with vein grafts, which may also predispose them to vasospasm during the perioperative period. Some studies have suggested that, initially, there is a decreased flow in the internal mammary artery, as compared with vein grafts, making these conduits more susceptible to complications related to hypovolemia and hypotension.

Perioperative infarction may also occur secondary to disrupted activity of the fibrinolytic system, in the immediate hours following cardiac surgery. It has been proposed that surgery enhances secretion of an inhibitor of tissue plasminogen activator (t-PA) which further depresses an already depressed fibrinolytic system. Low levels of protein C, a regulatory agent in the coagulation process, coupled with a poor endothelial fibrinolytic response to surgery, prompt the release of this t-PA inhibitor, which may then predispose to thrombus formation in the surgically manipulated artery. {8}

While these categories represent the patients at highest risk for morbidity and mortality associated with ischemia and/or myocardial infarction, all patients must be closely monitored for the development of these adverse outcomes. Even patients, considered to be at low-risk for complications, can experience myocardial ischemia as a result of circulating catecholamines, hypovolemia, dysrhythmias, cardiac tamponade, early graft closure, technical failure, embolization, or inadequate myocardial protection. Aneurysectomy and unrepaired lesions also predispose to myocardial infarction. [1,9] The use of vasoactive medication may also mediate adverse hemodynamic effects which, if prolonged, may initiate the appearance of ischemic changes and ultimately result in myocardial infarction.

DIAGNOSIS OF ISCHEMIA AND INFARCTION

Recognition of ischemic events becomes a nursing responsibility during all phases of the patient's hospitalization. Ongoing nursing assessment, utilizing clinical skills and judgement, along with specific diagnostic tests, will allow for early identification and treatment of this potentially life-threatening complication of cardiac surgery. Ischemia, like infarction, is identified through the utilization of hemodynamic parameters and electrocardiographic monitoring. In addition, laboratory tests may be used to diagnose myocardial infarction. Although, poor hemodynamics may result from a multitude of causes including bleeding, fluid shifts and hypothermia, once these have been ruled out, ischemia must be considered. A decrease in cardiac output and arterial pressure, coupled with elevated pulmonary artery occlusion pressure (PAOP) and/or right atrial pressure, should trigger the performance of 12-lead electrocardiogram to rule out myocardial ischemia.

While the ultimate goal is to identify ischemia and prevent infarction, in reality, infarction does occur. Usually the initial indicators are hemodynamic changes. Often the problem is recognized for the first time within the setting of the operating room when impaired left ventricular function makes it difficult to wean the patient from bypass. Frequently, some form of ventricular assistance is required. The assistance may consist of either pharmacological support and/or some type of ventricular assist device.

In the postoperative recovery room, hemodynamic alterations, associated with left ventricular impairment, result in decreased cardiac output and index, accompanied by increases in systemic vascular resistance, and left atrial and pulmonary artery occlusion pressures. When the infarction involves a papillary muscle, the murmur of mitral regurgitation may be evident and associated with a concomitant rise in the PAOP. Right atrial pressures may be elevated if the right ventricle is involved in the infarction process. These hemodynamic alterations may be transitory if the patient is experiencing ischemia, or they may be persistent if myocardial necrosis has occurred.

Recent technological advances have allowed for the early identification of electrocardiographic changes which may reflect ischemic conditions. Today, the state-of-the-art equipment utilizes continuous ST segment monitoring, pre- intra-, and postoperatively to identify episodes of ischemia with the goal of treatment, resolution and prevention of infarction.

Those who are monitoring for ischemia must be knowledgeable about the anatomy of the coronary circulation and the perspective of the leads of the 12-lead electrocardiogram. It is also important to remember that the bedside monitor has the ability to detect dysrhythmias, however, it is limited in its ability to detect ischemic changes. At the present time, the 12-lead ECG is the only way to view electrical activity in all areas of the heart. The commonly used diagnostic criteria for ischemia is ST segment displacement, equal to or greater than 1 mm at 60 ms after the J-point of the electrocardiogram tracing. In the setting of ischemia, this displacement is reflected as ST depression. ST segment elevation reflects a more advanced state of ischemia and is indicative of actual tissue injury. ST elevations of 2 mm ·or more are considered significant for myocardial injury and require immediate treatment. {6}

Electrocardiographic diagnosis of myocardial infarction can be difficult in the perioperative setting. Because of the trauma to the surgically manipulated heart, conventional electrocardiographic diagnostic criteria may be unreliable. The development of Q-waves on the electrocardiogram has generally been regarded as a positive diagnostic indicator of myocardial infarction, however, in the setting of coronary artery surgery, one must further investigate the Q-waves. Following cardiac surgery, transient Q-waves may occur with or without any other evidence of myocardial infarction. It is believed that these Q-waves may be caused by subendocardial surgical damage or they may represent the unmasking of a previous infarction during the reperfusion of the ischemic contralateral wall. {8,30} For example, an old inferior wall myocardial infarction may become evident after the anterior wall is revascularized. A Q-wave can be considered significant if it is equal to or greater than one third of the R-wave in one lead, or equal to or greater than one quarter of the R-wave in two leads, or greater than 0.04 seconds, or if a pre-existing Q-wave is further prolonged by an additional 0.02 seconds. {1,30}

Another electrocardiographic marker used to diagnose perioperative infarction is the presence of a new bundle branch block. The interpretation of this finding must be made cautiously, particularly in the presence of cardiac edema and volume overload. Bundle branch block can actually mask or mimic a myocardial infarction. {30} It may also be transient with no clinical significance. If it is associated with other diagnostic indicators, such as low cardiac output and/or an increase in the isoenzyme activity, bundle branch block may have clinical significance. {30,31}

Laboratory testing, specifically the measurement of creatine kinase (CK) and CK-MB, can also support the establishment of the diagnosis of perioperative myocardial infarction. The test is not as specific in the surgical population as it is in the medical counterpart. All coronary artery bypass patients will have elevated CK levels as a result of the surgical procedure. {4} Additionally false-positive levels may result from aneurysectomy, prolonged aortic cross-clamp (AXC) time or repeated defibrillations. {31} CK activity normally attains its peak in 24 hours in the medical patient with myocardial infarction, however, in the cardiac surgical patient, CK achieves peak earlier, usually within 4 hours after the discontinuation of bypass. {4,30} This phenomenon is considered to be associated with wash-out seen during the reperfusion phase. Normal CK levels have also been reported in the presence of myocardial infarction, particularly in the presence of bleeding, massive transfusion or other special conditions. {30} Additionally, changes in plasma volume make enzymatic quantification of myocardial infarction uncertain. {31} In this circumstance, it becomes important to correlate CK activity with other associated findings.

Other diagnostic tests which may be utilized to detect post-CABG myocardial infarction are technetium pyrophosphate scanning and single photon emission computed tomography (SPECT). [3] Both techniques are available and accurate for detecting myocardial infarction, however, their use is frequently limited in the perioperative period due to their unavailability in the operating room or ICU and the need to transport the patient to the nuclear medicine area of the hospital.

Echocardiography can be used to detect ventricular wall motion abnormalities which are frequently the first indicator of myocardial ischemia. Transthoracic echocardiography cannot be utilized in the operating room. Moreover, its use in the immediate postoperative period is also limited because of the presence of chest tubes, pacemaker wires and dressings, all of which can obscure structural visibility. [32] Of increasing interest today is the use of transesophageal echocardiography (TEE). This technique can be performed during the surgical procedure to identify ventricular wall motion abnormalities associated with ischemia. It can also be performed postoperatively, in the cardiac recovery room or intensive care unit, to evaluate possible structural defects and left ventricular function. A detailed description of this technique and its applications is outlined in another chapter in this book.

MEDICAL AND NURSING INTERVENTIONS

Once ischemia and infarction have been identified, treatment consists of interventions to balance myocardial oxygen supply and demand. The therapeutic goal is to increase the supply and/or to reduce the demand by manipulating the preload, afterload, heart rate and contractility. [14] The issue of myocardial oxygen supply/demand has been discussed in detail in another chapter of this book.

To ensure the adequacy of oxygen supply, both arterial blood gasses and hemoglobin must be closely monitored. Ventilator adjustments must be made as necessary and, if indicated, blood must be administered to ensure adequate oxygenation.

The mechanism for supplying oxygen to the myocardium is coronary blood flow which is a factor of aortic pressure and vascular resistance. Both are influenced by cardiac output. Inadequate cardiac output results in low aortic pressure. In order to maintain perfusion to vital organs, compensatory vasoconstriction will occur, resulting in increased vascular resistance and increased oxygen demand. Because the determinants of cardiac output are the stroke volume and heart rate these factors must be manipulated to provide optimal output.

In the cardiac surgical patient, the optimal heart rate has been defined to be between 80 and 100 beats per minute. [33] Bradycardia or tachycardia compromises cardiac output and worsens ischemic conditions. Since the cardiac surgical patient has epicardial pacemaker wires in place, slow rates are easily corrected by temporary pacing. Rapid rates are more difficult to treat. Postoperative tachycardia may represent a compensatory response to hypovolemia, fever or anemia. All these conditions must be ruled out, or corrected, prior to pharmacological treatment of the tachycardia. It is important to be aware of the detrimental effects of tachycardia in the presence of myocardial ischemia. Some investigators have defined a heart rate threshold for ischemia to be about 110 beats per minute, above which, the incidence of myocardial ischemia can actually double. Digitalis, beta-blockers or calcium channel blockers are often used to correct a tachycardia. However, in the presence of myocardial ischemia, the inotropic effects of digitalis may further increase myocardial oxygen demand and actually worsen the ischemic state. Both beta-blockers and calcium channel blockers have negative inotropic effects which may further depress the ischemic or stunned myocardium.

Stroke volume is influenced by preload, afterload and contractility. Fluid shifts in the early postoperative period, coupled with rewarming and vasodilation, may produce relative hypovolemia and a decreased preload. Infusion of colloids and crystalloids should be initiated to maintain adequate filling pressures. It is important to recognize that a patient who has sustained a myocardial infarction requires a much higher filling pressure, in order to induce the appropriate amount of stretch, for effective contraction. In the presence of a myocardial infarction, the optimal wedge pressure may be approximately 15 to 20 mm Hg, depending upon the extent of the infarction. Stroke volume may also be reduced by increased afterload. In most institutions, nitroprusside is the drug of choice for afterload reduction. Nitroprusside should be administered only after establishing an adequate preload. The administration of nitroprusside may precipitate a rapid fall in the mean arterial pressure, thus, further compromising the coronary blood flow and worsening, or causing, an ischemic condition.

Another factor which contributes to the optimization of cardiac output is contractility. As previously discussed, an ischemic or necrotic myocardium is unable to generate contractions sufficient to maintain cardiac output. Optimizing preload and decreasing afterload is sometimes sufficient to promote increases in cardiac output, however, when it is not, inotropic agents must be used to directly influence contractility. Again, in the presence of ischemia one must use these drugs with caution, as increasing contractility may also increase myocardial oxygen demand and consumption. The choice of agents is usually specific to each institution and, most commonly, includes drugs such as epinephrine, dopamine, dobutamine or amrinone.

Myocardial oxygen supply can also be increased through the use of vasodilator agents, which have a direct effect on the smooth muscle of the coronary arteries. These agents include i.v. nitroglycerine and calcium channel blockers specifically, nifedipine. {34,35} The intra-aortic balloon pump is also utilized to both increase supply and reduce oxygen demand. Balloon inflation, at the beginning of diastole, promotes blood flow into the coronary arteries. Balloon deflation, just prior to systole, reduces the afterload and allows the aortic valve to open against a lower pressure, thus, decreasing left ventricular work and oxygen demand. Beta-blockers and calcium channel blockers can also be utilized to reduce oxygen demand by decreasing both heart rate and contractility.

Nurses can play a major role in reducing the demand placed on the sick ventricle. Ongoing nursing assessment, with attention to modification of those factors which increase oxygen demand, may be instrumental in preventing and/or limiting ischemia. Close control of blood pressure and hemodynamics is imperative in order to minimize cardiac work. Relief of shivering and pain, assistance with positioning and activities, and provision of a quiet, stress-free environment are nursing interventions which can be instrumental in reducing oxygen demand. The fiberoptic pulmonary artery catheter, Opticath® (Abbott Critical Care Mountain View, CA) allows for the continuous monitoring of mixed venous oxygen saturation (SvO_2), which is an excellent indicator of oxygen utilization. SvO_2 monitoring allows the nurse to continuously evaluate the patient's oxygenation status and to apply nursing interventions so that oxygen balance is optimized.

ON THE HORIZON

Newer concepts related to the treatment of perioperative ischemia and infarction are evolving daily. The use of beta-blockers and calcium channel blockers in the pre- and intraoperative periods show promise for reducing and treating myocardial ischemia. The prophylactic use of nifedipine, in some centers, has shown a reduction in the incidence of myocardial infarction when compared with i.v. nitroglycerine. Perioperative internal mammary artery spasm, which may cause myocardial infarction, could be prevented by prophylactic use of nifedipine. Intracoronary papaverine has also been successfully used for this purpose. {36}

The cardiac effects of magnesium are receiving much attention in the literature these days. High levels of magnesium have been found to have a depressant effect on the myocardium, although, concurring vasodilation appears to help maintain cardiac output. Magnesium reduces calcium re-entry into the vascular smooth muscle, blunting the contractile response of vascular tissue to vasoconstrictors. {37} It is known to interfere with the vasoconstrictive but not the inotropic effects of epinephrine. {37}

The use of prostaglandins in the perioperative period may also prove to be useful in preventing ischemia. Prostaglandin E_1 has anti-platelet aggregation properties. It may also be used as a potent vasodilator to increase cardiac index and oxygen delivery. {38} Attempts to prevent irreversible injury secondary to ischemia are important. There has been some renewed interest in the idea that metabolic support with glucose, insulin, and potassium may improve left ventricular function in the stunned myocardium, following hypothermic ischemic arrest. {39}

Also, limitation of the production of oxygen-free radicals during ischemia and reperfusion has been attempted experimentally and clinically. Since the formation of the hydroxyl radical, during ischemia, appears to be associated with the release of iron, an iron-chelator (deferoxamine) has been successfully used to limit post-ischemic dysfunction and to reduce oxygen-free radical production. {40} Another free radical, superoxide anion, is normally neutralized by the enzyme superoxide dismutase (SOD). Myocardial ischemia is known to be associated with decreased levels of SOD. Additionally, reperfusion of ischemic myocardium results in increased levels of free radical production. It has been suggested that the formation of superoxide anion can be eliminated by administration of SOD, just prior to myocardial reperfusion. {41}

The use of antioxidants for improving myocardial protection has also been suggested. {41} Some clinicians are presently including administration of vitamin C and vitamin E, both with antidoxidation properties as part of their routine preoperative orders.

Continuous infusion of blood cardioplegia during the cardiac surgical procedure has shown promise as a mechanism for reducing both the ischemic time and reperfusion injury. Since the heart is being continuously perfused, it becomes unnecessary to induce a state of profound hypothermia.

Other interventions being investigated include the use of intraoperative ultrasound which is being tested and will soon become widely available. This technology will allow the surgical team to identify the best sites for graft anastomosis and may help to evaluate, and correct, graft-related problems in the operating room. {42} Likewise, electrocardiogram computer analysis is an evolving technique which allows the physician and the nurse to detect subtle, but significant, changes in cardiac function. The ultimate goal is early identification and treatment of ischemia and prevention of myocardial infarction. {43}

Because myocardial ischemia and infarction present such disastrous consequences for the cardiac surgical patient, medical research related to prevention and treatment is ongoing. Likewise, nursing research must also be directed to this arena. In today's outcome oriented environment, it is imperative that nursing identify interventions which prevent and/or correct ischemic episodes. In so doing, nurses can make a difference for their patients. If the downward spiral of ischemia is averted, or promptly identified and treated, myocardial infarction and its devastating consequences can be averted.

REFERENCES

1. McGregor CGA, Muri AL, Smith AF, Miller HC, Hannan WJ, Cameron EWJ, Wheatley DJ: Myocardial infarction related to coronary artery bypass graft surgery. Br Heart J 1984; 51:399–406.

2. Slogoff S, Keats AS: Does perioperative myocardial ischemia lead to postoperative myocardial infarction? Anes 1985; 62:107–114.

3. Burns RJ, Gladstone PJ, Tremblay PC, Feindel CM, Salter DR, Lipton IH, Ogilvie RR, Tirone DE: Myocardial infarction determined by technetium-99 pyrophosphate single-photon tomography complicating elective coronary artery bypass grafting for angina patients. Am J Card 1989; 63:1429–1434.

4. Devine JE, Wiens RD, Halstead JM, Codd JE: Quantitation of CK-MB release: diagnostic utility in coronary artery bypass grafting. Clin Chimica Acta 1986; 156:145–149.

5. Jones EL, Weintraub WS, Craver JM, Guyton RA, Cohen CL: Coronary bypass surgery: is the operation different today? J Thor CV Surg 1991; 101:108–115.

6. Knight AA, Hollenberg M, London MJ, Tubau J, Verrier E, Browner W, Managano DT & the S. P. I. Research Group: Perioperative myocardial ischemia: importance of preoperative ischemic pattern. Anes 1988; 68:681–688.

7. Naunheim KS, Fiore AC, Arango DC, Pennington DG, Barner HB, McBride LR, Harris HH, Willman VL, Kaiser GC: Coronary artery bypass grafting for unstable angina pectoris: risk analysis. Ann Thor Surg 1989; 47:569–574.

8. Oysel N, Bonnet J, Vergnes C, Benchimol D, Boisseau M-R, Moreau C, Bernadet P Baudet E, Larrue J, Bricaud H: Risk factors for myocardial infarction during coronary artery bypass graft surgery. Eur Heart J 1989; 10:806–815.

9. Yousif H, Davies G, Westaby S, Prendiville OF, Sapsford RN, Oakley CM: Preoperative myocardial ischaemia: its relation to perioperative infarction. Br Heart J 1987; 58:9–14.

10. Hearse DJ: The protection of the ischemic myocardium: surgical success vs clinical failure? Prog CV Dis 1988; 6:381–402.

11. Opie, HL: Myocardial infarct size: Part I. Basic considerations. Am Heart J 1980; 100:355–372.

12. Enger EL, Schwertz DW: Mechanisms of myocardial ischemia. J Cardiovasc Nursing 1989; 3(4):1–15.

13. Wolff PR, Nugent M: mechanisms of myocardial ischemia and infarction. Anes Clin NA 1988; 6(3):461–484.

14. Berne RM, Levy MN: Cardiovascular physiology. St. Louis: C. V. Mosby Co. 1981.

15. Grande P: Platelet aggregation in ischemia. Acute Ischemic Syndromes: Mechanisms and Future Management. Symposium Proceedings. New York: Cahners Publishing Company 1990.

16. Valle GA, Lemberg L: Silent ischemia: a clinical update. Chest 1990; 97:186-191.

17. Cohn PF: Silent ischemia. Ann Int Med 1988; 109:312–317.

18. Frishman WH, Hirsch H: Silent myocardial ischemia: emerging concepts. Coronary Acute Care 1992; 3(1):2–13.

19. Sheps DS et al: Endorphins are related to pain perception in coronary artery disease. Am J Card 1987; 59:982.

20. Droste C, Roskamm H: Experimental pain measurement in patients with a symptomatic myocardial ischemia. JACC 1983; 1:949.

21. Crisholm B: Stunned myocardium. Focus on Critical Care 1990; 17(6):458–462.

22. Zhaom J, Zhang, Robinson TF, Factor SM, Sonnenblick EH, Eng C: Profound structural alterations of the extracellular collagen matrix in postischemic dysfunctional "stunned" but viable myocardium. JACC 1987; 10:1322–1334.

23. Braunwald E, Kloner RA: The stunned myocardium. Circulation 1982; 66:1146–1148.

24. Maza SR, Frishman WH: Therapeutic options to minimize free radical damage and thrombogenicity in ischemic/reperfused myocardium. Am Heart J 1987; 114:1206-1213.

25. Naunheim KS, Fiore AC, Wadley JJ et al: The changing profile of the patient undergoing coronary artery bypass surgery. J Am Coll Card 1988; 11:494–498.

26. Gersh BJ, Califf RM, Loop FD, Akins CW, Pryor DB, Takaro TC: Coronary bypass surgery in chronic stable angina. Circulation 1989:I46-I59.

27. CASS principal investigators: Myocardial infarction and mortality in the coronary artery surgery study (CASS) randomized trial. N Engl J Med 1984; 310:751–758.

28. Fisher LD, Kennedy JW, Davis KB, Maynard C, Fritz JK, Kaiser GC, Myers WO & the participating CASS Clinics: Association of sex, physical size and operative mortality after coronary artery bypass in Coronary Artery Surgery Study (CASS). J Thor and Cardiovasc Surg 1982; 84:334–341.

29. von Segesser LK, Lehmann K, Turina M: Deleterious effects of shock in internal mammary artery anastomoses. Ann Thor Surg 1989; 47:575–579.

30. Olthof H, Middelhof D, Meijne NG, Fiolet JWT, Becker AE, Lie KI: The definition of myocardial infarction during aorto-coronary bypass surgery. Am Heart J 983; 106:631–637.

31. Hake U, Iversen S, Sadony V, Jakob, H-G, Neufang A, Oelert H: Diagnosis of perioperative myocardial necrosis following coronary artery surgery - a reappraisal of isoenzyme analysis. Eur J CT Surg 1990; 4:79–84.

32. DiLucente L, Gorcsan J: Transesophageal echocardiography: application to the postoperative cardiac surgery patient. Dimen Crit Care Nursing 1991; 10(2):75-80.

33. Moreno-Cabral CE, Mitchell Rs, Miller DC: Manual of postoperative management in adult cardiac surgery. Williams & Wilkins, Baltimore 1988.

34. Seitelberger R, Zwolfer W, Binder TM, Huber S, Peschl F, Spatt J, Schwarzacher S, Holzinger C. Coraim F, Weber H Wolner E: Infusion of nifedipine after coronary artery bypass grafting decreases the incidence of early postoperative myocardial ischemia. Ann Thor Surg 1990; 49:61–68.

35. He GW, Rosenfeldt FL, Buxton BF, Angus JA: Reactivity of human isolated internal mammary artery to constrictor and dilator agents: implications for treatment of internal mammary artery spasm. Circulation 1989:I141-I150.

36. Gurley JC, Booth DC, DeMaria AN: Circulatory collapse following coronary bypass surgery: multivessel and graft spasm reversed in the catheterization laboratory by intracoronary papaverine. Am Heart J 1990:1194–1195.

37. Zaloga G, Eisenach JC: Magnesium, anesthesia and hemodynamic control J Anes 1991; 74(1):1–2.

38. Appel PL, Shoemaker WC, Kram HB: Effects of prostaglandin E_1 in postoperative surgical patients with circulatory deficiency. Chest 1991; 99:945–950.

39. Coleman GM, Gradinac S, Taegtmeyer H, Sweeny M, Frazier H: Efficacy of metabolic support with glucose-insulin-potassium for left ventricular pump failure after aorto-coronary bypass surgery. Circulation 1989:191–196.

40. Illes RW, Silverman NA, Krukenkamp IB, del Nido PJ, Levitsky S: Amelioration of postischemic stunning by deferoximane-blood cardioplegia. Circulation 1989:III30-III35.

41. Lee RB, Stewart JR, Merril WH, Frist WH, Hammon JW, Bender HW: Pharmacokinetics of superoxide dismutase during hypothermic cardiopulmonary bypass. Circulation 1989 (suppl III):III25-III29.

42. CV NEWS: Intraoperative ultrasound for CABG. CV Nurse: Trends in Cardiovasc Care 1991; 4(1):10.

43. CV NEWS: Detecting changes in heart function. CV Nurse: Trends in Cardiovasc Care 1991; 4(1):10.

PERIOPERATIVE CARE OF THE CARDIAC SURGICAL PATIENT AND ITS IMPACT ON POSTOPERATIVE CARE

What the Operative Report Can Tell You

Patricia C. Seifert, R.N., M.S.N., C.R.N.F.A., C.N.O.R.

The Arlington Hospital
Arlington, Virginia

INTRODUCTION

The hospital record provides a wealth of information about the patient's past and present health history, the physical examination, invasive and non-invasive diagnostic tests, psychosocial factors, and therapeutic interventions. Surgical patients will have an additional report describing the operative procedure.

The operative report is a valuable but underutilized source of information for nurses in the operating room, the immediate postoperative care unit, the step-down and recuperative unit, and in cardiac rehabilitation. Perioperative nurses can use the reports retrospectively to plan care for patients undergoing similar procedures. Critical care nurses can use the reports concurrently or retrospectively depending on when the report is placed in the chart, usually within 48 hours. Computerized, voice-recognition technology is now available that allows immediate generation of written reports via spoken commands. Nurses caring for patients in the post critical care phase and during rehabilitation can benefit from the information specific to their patient. The reports are also useful for research data collection.

Reluctance or inability to utilize the information contained within the operative report may be due to a number of factors such as the time required for placement on the chart, not knowing it exists or unfamiliarity with the technical jargon of surgery.

Reimbursement agencies and credentialling bodies have fostered prompter completion of the report and its inclusion into the patient's record. Unfortunately, difficulty interpreting portions of the report continues to deprive the nurse of the benefits of this concise discussion of the indications for surgery, the pathoanatomic findings, and the surgical intervention deemed most appropriate for that particular patient.

Cardiac Surgery: Current Issues 2, Edited by A. C. Cernaianu and A. J. DelRossi,
Plenum Press, New York, 1994

213

Because the report addresses the patient's unique situation as well as standard operating practices, information contained within it can be used to facilitate decision-making during assessment, diagnosis, planning, and implementation of care that is specifically tailored to the patient's needs. Postoperative physiologic responses can be more accurately predicted, and the potential psychosocial impact on the patient and family often can be inferred from the surgical report. The collection of data for research purposes can also be facilitated through the use of information found in the report.

COMPONENTS OF THE OPERATIVE REPORT

Although each surgeon will have his or her own particular method of dictation, the following are standard components to be included in the report.

Introductory Data

The patient name, hospital record number, and date of operation are listed at the beginning of the report, followed by the preoperative and the postoperative diagnosis. Commonly, the diagnoses are the same (the purpose of the postoperative diagnosis being to confirm the preoperative diagnosis), but intraoperative findings not apparent during the preoperative assessment may alter the postoperative diagnosis. The operation performed is stated, with specific aspects of the procedure noted (e.g., mitral valve replacement with a 33 mm St. Jude Medical prosthesis). Urgent or emergent procedures are so described. The surgeon and the first assistant are listed; additional surgical assistants, if present, may be listed as well.

Indications for Operation

This section provides background information about the patient's medical history and identifies reasons for surgical intervention. Indications may be briefly summarized, or they can be more detailed to include the presenting symptoms, findings from the history and physical examination, initial treatments and the patient's response, and diagnostic data supporting operation. Determination of the need for and the timing of surgery is substantiated by the clinical signs and symptoms.

Operative Findings

This part of the report details the general and specific appearance and condition of the lesion and the surrounding structures. Occasionally, operative reports may have an additional section entitled "Operative Data" which tabulates some of the information in outline form (see Figure 1). Evidence is provided to support decisions regarding the treatment, and unusual findings are mentioned in addition to the expected ones. This section also correlates the intraoperative observations with preoperative diagnostic tests and examinations.

Associated cardiac lesions may be described and compensatory mechanisms noted, such as cardiac chamber hypertrophy or dilation. The absence of certain significant conditions may be specifically addressed as well. For example, in a patient with mitral valve disease, the presence or absence of an enlarged left atrium, intra-atrial thrombus, history of transient ischemic attacks and atrial fibrillation, and concomitant coronary artery diseases are all pertinent to the plan of operation as well as to postoperative regimens.

Procedure

In the final section of the report, the steps of the operation are detailed from the time the patient is placed on the operating table to the application of the dressing and transfer to the postoperative unit. The account is often a combination of standardized statements ("the patient was prepped in the usual manner. . ."), and patient-specific comments about the quality of the tissue, the size of the lesion(s), the diameter of blood vessels being anasto-mosed, protective measures taken, the surgical technique employed, etc. The status of the patient upon transfer to the postoperative unit is stated (e.g., stable, critical), and results of needle, instrument, and sponge counts are documented (e.g., "the counts were correct").

To illustrate some of the newer trends in the surgical management of coronary artery disease and valvular heart disease, two generic operative reports are included in this discussion. The first report describes a patient undergoing repeat coronary artery bypass grafting (CABG) using arterial conduits. The second report outlines a mitral valve repair of the posterior leaflet with ring annuloplasty in a patient with mitral regurgitation, It should be emphasized that all operative reports vary according to hospital policy and physician preference. Specific questions should be referred to the dictating surgeon.

OPERATIVE REPORT FOR CORONARY ARTERY BYPASS GRAFTING

Introductory Data

The report in Figure 1 describes a repeat CABG in a symptomatic, relatively young (47 year old), male who underwent initial myocardial revascularization with saphenous vein grafts. The presence of three-vessel disease with diffusely palpable atherosclerosis of the coronary arteries in a patient with previous surgery attests to the aggressive progression of coronary artery disease in certain subgroups. Upon review of the preoperative data, it is not unlikely that this patient may present with elevated lipid serum levels, and that the admission assessment may demonstrate a familial history of coronary disease.

The decision to use arterial bypass conduits is based on a number of factors. There may be insufficient saphenous vein remaining after its removal for the initial surgery, or it may be of poor quality. Vein graft failure requiring re-operation is considered an indication for the use of arterial grafts by some investigators. [1] Even if available, saphenous vein are less desirable than the IMA, because of the IMA's superior long-term function as a bypass conduit, especially in young patients with hyperlipidemia. Although additional venous conduits, such as lessor saphenous and cephalic veins, are available, their long-term patency has not been as good as originally anticipated. [2] More-over, because the patency rates of the IMA have been excellent, it is hoped that similar patency rates are possible with other arterial grafts such as the

GENERAL HOSPITAL
1500 MAIN STREET
ANY CITY, ANY STATE

Operative Report

PATIENT:
MEDICAL RECORD NUMBER:
DATE OF OPERATION:
PREOPERATIVE DIAGNOSIS: Coronary Artery Disease
POSTOPERATIVE DIAGNOSIS: Same
SURGEON:
ASSISTANT:
OPERATION: Redo Coronary Artery Bypass Grafts X 3:

1. Right Gastroepiploic Artery (RGEA) to the Left Anterior Descending Coronary Artery (LAD),
2. Right Internal Mammary Artery (RIMA) to the Right Coronary-Posterior Descending Coronary Artery, and
3. Left Internal Mammary Artery (LIMA)

OPERATIVE DATA:
   RGEA:Satisfactory
   LIMA:Satisfactory
   RIMA:Satisfactory
   LAD size: 1.3 mm, distal disease-severe
   RCA-PD size: 1.5 mm
   Ramus size: 1.4 mm
   Preoperative ejection fraction: 0.55
   Bypass time: 70 minutes
   Aortic occlusion time: 55 minutes
   Wean from cardiopulmonary bypass: without catechols
   Blood transfusion: No
   Sponge and needle counts: Correct
   Cardioplegia: Blood 4:1; antegrade/retrograde protocol
   Comments: Bilateral saphenous vein excised for initial CABG, no leg vein available; severe, diffuse atherosclerotic coronary plaque palpable

INDICATIONS FOR OPERATION: This forty-seven year old male underwent previous CABG at Main Hospital, and now has three vessel coronary disease and important stenosis in the only patent bypass graft to the LAD.

OPERATIVE FINDINGS: The three arterial conduits were all sufficient size and all had brisk arterial flow. Coronary measurements were as follows: LAD 1.3 mm, Ramus 1.4 mm, RCA-PD 1.5 mm. Cross clamp time was 55 minutes. The patient received no blood transfusions. There was the usual amount of dense scar presence surrounding the heart. The right mammary could not be stretched to reach the midportion of the LAD, and therefore was used as the conduit for the RCA-PD. Sponge and needle counts were reported as correct. The patient was sent to the CVICU in stable condition.

Figure 1. Operative report for coronary artery bypass grafting.

right gastroepiploic{1,3} and the inferior epigastric arteries. {4,5} It should be noted that the time required to dissect these arterial grafts could preclude their use in an emergency where expeditious revascularization is important to avoid irreversible ventricular damage.

Research into the dynamic function of the endothelial cell lining of blood vessels may provide some insights into the function of arterial conduits and

PROCEDURE: The patient was placed supine on the operating table and general anesthesia induced. Prep and drape of the chest, abdomen and legs were done. A redo sternotomy was made and the incision extended down to the umbilicus in the midline. The heart was separated from dense adhesions and prepared for cannulation. First the left internal mammary and then the right internal mammary arteries were dissected free and prepared. Next the right gastroepiploic artery was freed from its gastric attachments and prepared for use. A small slit was made in the pericardial surface of the diaphragm and the gastroepiploic artery tunnelled through this opening. Systemic Heparin was administered and cannulation performed. A retrograde cardioplegia infusion catheter was inserted into the coronary sinus via the right atrium, and cardiopulmonary bypass instituted. The aorta was cross clamped and 4-to-1 blood cardioplegia administered by standard antegrade/retrograde techniques. With the heart quiet, the right IMA was anastomosed end-to-side to the RCA-PD. Next, the Ramus was identified, opened, and the left internal mammary artery anastomosed end-to-side to it. Both the RCA-PD and the RCA were intramyocardial vessels. The LAD was opened and the gastroepiploic anastomosed end-to-side to it. Blood cardioplegia was administered between construction of each distal anastomosis. Following rewarming, a warm dose of cardioplegia was given after which time the cross clamp was released. After a period of time, the patient was weaned form cardiopulmonary bypass. Hemostasis was obtained; heparin was reversed with protamine sulfate.

The drainage tubes were placed in both pleural spaces and in the mediastinum, and brought out interiorly. Pacing wires were placed on the atrium and brought out interiorly. The sternum was closed with interrupted wire, and the abdomen and fascia closed with running 2-0 polypropylene. Subcutaneous tissue and skin were closed with absorbable suture.

---

their high patency rates. For example, responses to vasoactive substances differ between arteries and veins (and among different arteries as well). When the endothelium is intact, arteries and veins both contract in the presence of norepinephrine, but there is significantly more relaxation in arteries compared to veins. This relaxation is mediated by endothelium-derived relaxing factor (EDRF) which is present in large amounts in the gastroepiploic artery (GEA) and the IMA, but minimally present in the saphenous vein. {6,7} In addition to its vasodilating effects, EDRF inhibits platelet adhesion and aggregation, making it an important antithrombotic agent in the circulation. {7}

As mentioned above, vasoreactivity varies among arteries and it has been found that the GEA contracts more forcefully than the IMA (although both dilate in response to EDRF). It has been suggested that this contraction is related to the greater muscular mass of the GEA compared to the more elastic properties of the IMA. Thus, the GEA may be more prone to vasospasm in the presence of high circulating levels of catecholamines. However, the artery vasodilates in response to nitrates which can be an effective pharmacologic tool in preventing ischemia due to vasospasm. {7}

Other arterial grafts have been investigated such as the splenic artery and the radial artery. There is renewed interest in the radial artery with the publication of improved results using this graft. {8} Homograft saphenous and umbilical vein, and synthetic grafts have shown variable results, necessitating further research. {2}

Operative Data

Although the information in this section may be incorporated into the "operative findings", it can be more succinctly presented in this form. Tabulating these data is particularly useful in CABG patients. Shown here, the operative data lists the arterial grafts and comments on their quality as conduits. The surgeon is especially interested in the briskness of blood flow through the vessel. A dilator (1–1.5 mm) may be used to enlarge the vessel and papaverine is frequently used intraluminally or externally to reduce arterial spasm and enlarge the lumen (commonly 1 to 2 mm). Also listed are the size of the native vessels (measured at the anastomotic site), bypass and cross-clamp times, and whether catecholamines or inotropes were required to wean the patient from cardiopulmonary bypass and maintain an adequate cardiac output. Noting that catecholamines were not used is important in that it implies that ventricular function was adequate and that myocardial protection was maintained during the period of cardiac arrest.

The fact that no allogeneic transfusion was used is an indication that the hematocrit was maintained within an acceptable range. Additionally, the patient was not placed at risk for blood-borne diseases or transfusion reactions.

Indications for Operation

Although not specifically stated, patients with new onset of ischemic symptoms are referred for cardiac catheterization to determine progression of the disease within the native coronary arteries and the bypass grafts. In this case, cardiac catheterization demonstrated progressive three-vessel coronary artery disease with obstruction in all of the original vein grafts except for the one supplying the left anterior descending (LAD) coronary artery (which showed significant stenosis).

Operative Findings

The decision to use arterial grafts in situ or as free grafts is often dependent on the length of the artery that can be mobilized and how far it must reach for anastomosis to the coronary artery. Stretching of the artery is avoided to reduce tension on the suture line postoperatively. Thus, if the GEA pedicle is not long enough to reach the desired location on the heart, it is excised and one end attached to the aorta and the other end anastomosed to the coronary artery. Unlike venous conduits, there are no intraluminal valves to consider during placement to the graft.

Surgical Procedure

Vein grafts to the LAD are often placed proximally on the anterior wall of the ascending aorta. During repeat operations, this poses an increased risk of hemorrhage from transection of the graft during opening of the sternum and division of the adhesions between the heart and the thoracic wall. Manipulation of the existing vein grafts shall be avoided to prevent dislodging intraluminal clot and atheroma (which tends to be more diffuse and friable than in the native vessel disease). Obstructed grafts may be ligated to prevent downstream migration of internal debris.

When the report states that the body and legs were prepped and draped in the "usual manner", it refers to the application of an antimicrobial solution to the chest, abdomen and both legs. Sterile drapes are then placed to cover the head and feet, and both sides of the body (as well as the operating table). The chest, abdomen and legs are exposed to allow access to the underlying structures. It is important to retain access to both femoral arteries in the event that an alternative arterial pressure line or the use of intra-aortic balloon is required. The legs are exposed in case the arterial grafts are unsuitable, and lesser saphenous vein is needed. For similar reasons, some surgeons routinely prepare the arms to retrieve cephalic vein.

Bilateral IMA dissection can cause considerable pain due to the sternal retraction necessary to expose each artery. The GEA requires entry into the peritoneum, thereby creating abdominal pain and the likelihood of a postoperative ileus.

Heparin is used to prevent clotting of the blood during cardiopulmonary bypass. It is given before the arterial conduits are divided in order to prevent vessel thrombosis. The cut end of the conduit is trimmed in preparation for anastomosis to the coronary artery.

Protection of the myocardium is achieved with systemic and topical hypothermia and the infusion of cardioplegia. The introduction of retrograde cardioplegia delivery via the coronary sinus has enhanced myocardial preservation of those areas distal to the obstructive lesions, and in particular the subendocardium which is at high risk for intraoperative ischemic injury. {9,10} This combination of antegrade and retrograde cardioplegia provides more global protection of the heart. The addition of blood to the cardioplegic solution (rather than using purely crystalloid solutions) enhances myocardial substrate replenishment. A final warm dose of cardioplegia is infused to minimize reperfusion injury.

Although the main coronary arteries lie close to the epicardial surface of the heart, occasionally they are located within the muscle. The dissection of these intramyocardial vessels may be more difficult and can cause increased bleeding.

At the completion of surgery, pericardial chest tubes are placed to drain blood and prevent tamponade. The pleura is often entered during IMA dissection, and chest tubes are placed in each pleural space to drain fluid and promote lung expansion postoperatively. Dissection of the GEA does not usually require insertion of a drainage tube if adequate hemostasis has been achieved. When the inferior epigastric artery (IEA) is used as a conduit, a small drain is commonly inserted. {4}

Nursing Considerations in the Surgical Intensive Care Unit

Repeat Sternotomy. Reoperative median sternotomy is associated with a higher morbidity and mortality than initial cardiac surgery. {11} Complications include increased postoperative bleeding due to dissection of sternal and mediastinal adhesions, increased risk of blood-borne pathogens from transfusion, sternal infection, and perioperative myocardial infarction due to intraluminal atheromatous debris within pre–existing grafts. During sternal reentry, traumatic injury can occur to retrosternal structures such as the right ventricle, ascending aorta, innominate vein, and existing bypass grafts. {12}

Standard nursing care for CABG patients is instituted, with special attention to signs of excessive bleeding and electrocardiographic changes indicating myocardial ischemia or infarction.

Bilateral Internal Mammary Artery Grafts. Heye {13} has noted that pain is a special problem in patients with IMA grafts. This is attributed to the additional sternal retraction required to expose and dissect the artery and the use of electrosurgery to cauterize bleeding vessels. In order to decrease tension on the graft from inflating lungs, the pleura and pericardium may be incised where the IMA crosses over to the heart, and this may contribute to postoperative discomfort. Patients receiving bilateral mammary artery grafts can anticipate additional pain.

Galbut and his colleagues{14} compared the use of bilateral IMA's in patients undergoing initial and repeat sternotomy. In addition to an increase in mortality in the reoperation group, they found that this group had an increase in respiratory insufficiency with intubation for more that 48 hours (Galbut, 1990), a higher incidence of perioperative myocardial infarction, and prolonged hospitalization. The combination of increased pain and a tendency toward respiratory insufficiency supports the use of additional interventions to control the patient's discomfort which can further impair gas exchange.

Other potential complication are associated with IMA grafts. There is a statistically significant higher incidence of sternal infection reported in diabetic patients receiving bilateral IMA's. IMA grafts may be hypoperfused with subsequent coronary ischemia. Because IMA blood flow is pressure–dependent, the nurse should monitor the blood pressure and try to maintain a mean arterial pressure (MAP) of 90 to 100 mm HG. The pleural drainage tubes are monitored for excessive drainage due to either frank bleeding (usually from the IMA pedicle), or sequestered (old) blood within the pleural cavities.

Gastroepiploic Artery Graft. Surgery on the upper abdomen is required to expose the GEA, causing additional pain, a more severe inflammatory response from the surgery, and compromised pulmonary function. Associated morbidity includes immobility, hypercoagulability, venous thrombosis, and increased myocardial oxygen consumption when pain causes increased blood pressure or heart rate. Intravenous pain management may be necessary for a longer period of time than that needed for other cardiac procedures. Oral analgesia may not be feasible for 3 or 4 days after surgery. {15}

Gastric manipulation may produce protracted paralytic ileus. The nasogastric tube is often maintained for 48 to 72 hours after surgery. Patients will be unable to receive food by mouth until bowel sounds are evident. Clear liquids are given first, then full liquids and solid food.

Deep breathing and coughing, use of the incentive spirometer, and interventions to avoid the potential respiratory depression associated with narcotic analgesia, may help to improve the patient's respiratory function.

These interventions are also applicable to the patient receiving an IEA graft. When this conduit is used, the nurse should monitor the drain exit site for signs of infection.

Recuperation. After, the patient is transferred to the step-down unit, nursing care is focussed toward continued monitoring of the respiratory and cardiac function. The patient is encouraged to ambulate and perform breathing exercises. Pain medication is switched to oral routes once the IV's are discontinued. This period may be slightly prolonged (1 to 3 days) compared to the length of stay for patients with vein grafts, due to the laparotomy incision. {1} Suma and his co-workers{16} showed no significant increase in postoperative complications with the GEA graft.

All incisions should be assessed for signs of infection. Abdominal incisions may become infected, dehisce, or develop hernias. These observations are also pertinent in patients with IEA grafts whose dissection from the abdominal muscle may pose a risk for rectus muscle necrosis, Dietary considerations are those described above with the patient progressing from a liquid to a solid diet.

Antiplatelet regimens may be started during this period, or in the intensive care unit. Aspirin is often given to patients with arterial as well as venous grafts to retard progression of the disease in the native coronary artery and for its beneficial antiembolic protection of the central nervous system. Dipyridamole is generally used only in patients with vein grafts.

Patient education is begun in the preoperative period and focuses on short-term and long-term objectives for achieving risk factor modification and behavioral changes. During the inpatient period, emphasis is placed on those skills necessary during the first 6 weeks postdischarge. {17} In addition to the standard teaching employed for CABG patients, information can be provided on the benefits (long-term patency, no leg incision) and drawbacks (increased pain) of arterial grafts.

Few research studies have distinguished between the effects of venous grafts and arterial grafts on recovery and rehabilitation. Studies by Gortner and colleagues{18} on self-efficacy have shown that in addition to preoperative functional status, patients' perceptions of their ability to undertake an activity can enhance recovery. Building the patient's confidence may be as important as attending to the physiologic aspects of recovery. The long-term patency rate seen with arterial grafts and improved survival compared to venous grafts, and the possible relationship to perceived efficacy might be a topic for further investigation.

Rehabilitation.   Although there is a great deal of literature describing general principles for rehabilitation of patients with coronary artery disease, specific references to patients with CABG using arterial grafts are relatively sparse. It is anticipated that the excellent patency rates of the IMA will be similar in the GEA and other arterial grafts, although this has not yet been confirmed. It is unclear whether arterial revascularization is much different than CABG with venous conduits on exercise performance or risk factor modification. Moreover, it is unclear whether atherosclerosis of the abdominal aorta can invade the celiac system and affect GEA patency.

One advantage of arterial grafts is the avoidance of leg incisions and the persistent swelling found in patients with saphenous vein removal. This may produce less discomfort for the patient performing leg exercises, although the abdominal incisions may neutralize a potential advantage. Progression of the underlying disease is not halted, so efforts to retard coronary atherosclerosis continue to be important aspects of the rehabilitative process.

OPERATIVE REPORT FOR MITRAL VALVE REPAIR

Mitral valve repair is most feasible in patients with pure mitral regurgitation (MR). The best long-term results have been seen with the so-called prolapsed "floppy" mitral valve. Rheumatic valves have shown less successful outcomes due to the effects of scarring and distortion of the valve. Mixed regurgitant/stenotic lesions have demonstrated the least successful results after repair.

Alain Carpentier, in France, was one of the first to advocate the use of reparative techniques for the mitral valve. The excellent results obtained by salvaging the native valve, and the avoidance of prosthetic-related complications (notably, anticoagulation-related hemorrhage), have made reparative procedures increasingly popular. Repair is especially attractive in children, females of child-bearing age, sportsmen, and adults with an active lifestyle. Repair may not be as advantageous in the older patient with long standing atrial fibrillation necessitating chronic coumadin prophylaxis. [19]

Although most of the techniques have been developed for the mitral valve, techniques to repair the aortic valve are beginning to appear in the literature. [20] Because the closing mechanism of the aortic valve is more precise than the mitral valve and less tolerant of inadequate repair, reparative surgery for this valve is less commonly performed.

Introductory Data

The report in Figure 2, describes a mitral valve repair of the posterior leaflet by quadrangular excision and plication, and insertion of a prosthetic ring to reduce the circumference of the annulus, thereby producing coaptation of the leaflets and valvular competence. The patient has severe (non-acute) mitral regurgitation, unrelated to coronary artery disease (which if present, would be noted in the diagnosis).

Indications for Operation

This section of the report describes the course of the disease and the diagnostic studies performed. The diagnosis of mitral regurgitation can be made with echocardiography, however, cardiac catheterization is routinely performed in adults to detect the presence of coronary artery disease. The attached report demonstrates that coronary angiography was normal, thereby removing ischemic heart disease as a major etiologic factor in the development of mitral regurgitation. The feasibility of valve repair can be determined only after inspection of the valve lesion and surrounding anatomy. In the case of severe destruction of the valve, replacement may be required. Therefore the report notes that the patient has been referred for repair or replacement.

Operative Findings

The description of the heart and the left atrium is consistent with the preoperative studies. The valve lesion did not appear to be rheumatic (no history of rheumatic fever was not elicited during the history and physical examination). There was no evidence suggesting active or old endocarditis which is the usual cause of the ruptured posterior chordae tendineae.

Elongation of the chordae, thinning of the leaflets, and dilation of the valve annulus (in the absence of rheumatic changes, severe calcification, or infection) are typical of myxomatous ("floppy") mitral valve prolapse. According to Roberts, [21] this is the major cause of pure, severe, isolated mitral regurgitation.

The pathologic features of this lesion include excessive proliferation within the valve of the spongiosa layer, which contains mucopolysaccharide material, and a relative reduction in the fibrosa layer. These changes are thought to account for the stretching and thinning of segments of the mitral apparatus. [21] Valves demonstrating these changes are often amenable to surgical repair.

Surgical Procedure

Many aspects of the procedure (such as skin preparation, groin exposure, incision and closure) are similar to those used for CABG. Transesophageal echocardiography (TEE) is commonly performed before the incision is made in order to establish a baseline for ventricular function and valve performance.

Double venous cannulation (instead of the single venous cannulation used in CABG) is employed to decompress the right atrium and to prevent systemic venous return from entering the heart and causing a temperature gradient. When the relatively warmer blood from the systemic circulation enters the atrium, it can compromise myocardial protection. In the absence of obstructive coronary artery lesions, antegrade cardioplegia infusion is adequate for global myocardial protection. If coronary artery disease or left ventricular hypertrophy were present, retrograde infusion would be instituted as well. Suction catheters are used to clear the field of blood, particularly when the left atrium is open.

The description of the mitral valve repair reflects the technique developed by Carpentier. [22] Excess posterior leaflet tissue is excised and the edges reapproximated, thereby reducing the leaflet size. The dilated annulus is reduced with a prosthetic ring designed to reduce the excess annular tissue. The reduction in annular circumference allows the attached leaflets to coapt along their free edges. The competency of the repaired valve is tested with normal saline injected through the valve orifice into the left ventricle with a bulb syringe. Minimal or no fluid should regurgitate into the left atrium. TEE is also used to assess the repair once the heart has resumed beating.

Removal of air from the left atrium and the left ventricle is vital to protect the patient from air embolus. A number of maneuvers are employed, including needle aspiration of the left ventricular apex and right superior pulmonary vein, insertion of venting catheters in the left side of the heart and the aorta, lowering the patient's head (to allow rising air to escape through the aortic venting needle rather than being directed toward the brain), moving the table from side to side, and jiggling the heart to mobilize air trapped within the left ventricular trabeculations.

In order to avoid lifting the ventricular apex which could cause injury to the endocardium from a rigid mitral prosthesis, the surgeon can aspirate the left ventricular apex transseptally with a long (spinal) needle inserted via the right ventricle. TEE can also be employed as an important tool for detecting air.

GENERAL HOSPITAL
1500 MAIN STREET
ANY CITY, ANY STATE

Operative Report

PATIENT:
MEDICAL RECORD NUMBER:
DATE OF OPERATION:

PREOPERATIVE DIAGNOSIS: Severe Mitral Regurgitation
POSTOPERATIVE DIAGNOSIS: Severe Mitral Regurgitation

SURGEON:
ASSISTANT:

OPERATION: 1. Mitral valvuloplasty
                2. Mitral annuloplasty using a 30 mm Carpentier-Edwards prosthetic ring

INDICATIONS FOR OPERATION: This 53 year old male was found to have a mitral valve murmur in 1984. He did well until January of 1990 when he developed endocarditis with subsequent severe dyspnea on exertion. In the summer of 1991, he developed wheezing and was started on bronchodilators. He again seemed to stabilize for several months, but over the past several months, experienced more symptoms of progressive congestive heart failure, aggravated by intermittent atrial fibrillation. He was placed on quinidine with a subsequent development of a high fever which resolved with discontinuation of quinidine. Cardiac catheterization performed on 10/22/92 at General Hospital by ___ revealed a dilated left ventricle with an ejection fraction of 0.52. There was severe mitral valvular insufficiency and enlargement of the left atrium. Coronary angiography was normal. The patient was referred for elective valve repair of replacement.

OPERATIVE FINDINGS: At operation, the heart was dilated. The left atrium was considerably enlarged as was the mitral valve annulus. The findings at operation was consistent with transesophageal echocardiography findings preoperatively. Multiple chordae supplying the entire central 2/4ths of the posterior mitral leaflet were ruptured and the posterior leaflet was flail. The anterior leaflet was somewhat enlarged with elongation of the chordae tendineae, but no rupture was present. There was no evidence of active or old endocarditis on the valve. There was no thrombus within the left atrium. Coronary arteries were normal to palpation. Transesophageal echocardiography was performed by ___and will be reported separately.

Figure 2. Operative report for mitral valve repair.

Both atrial and ventricular temporary pacing wires are attached to the heart to provide postoperative sequential pacing Supraventricular rhythm disturbances are common after mitral valve surgery, and the ability to pace both chambers helps to maintain appropriate cardiac rate and rhythm.

Closing procedures are similar to those described for CABG. Unless the pleura was entered during sternotomy, drainage tubes within the pericardium are sufficient for removing blood from the chest.

Nursing Considerations in the Surgical Intensive Unit

Ventricular Function.   As in most cardiac surgical procedures, preoperative left ventricular function (as determined by ejection fraction) is an important determinant of left ventricular systolic performance after surgery. [23] Patients with mitral regurgitation and normal preoperative ejection

PROCEDURE: The patient was taken to the operating room and placed supine upon the operating table. Following the induction of adequate general anesthesia, the chest and both groins were prepped and draped in a sterile fashion. Baseline transesophageal echocardiography was performed. Median sternotomy incision was made and the pericardium opened and sewn to wound towels. Systemic heparin was administered and the right atrium cannulated with 38 and 40 French superior and inferior vena cavae cannulae. The aorta was cannulated through a side-biting clamp with a 24 French infusion catheter. An antegrade cardioplegia/venting catheter was placed in the anterior aorta proximal to the aortic infusion cannula. Venous and arterial lines were connected to cardiopulmonary bypass and the patient cooled to 25°C. The aorta was cross clamped and 122 cc of cold cardioplegic solution infused into the aortic root while the pericardial well was washed with cold saline. A left arteriotomy was performed parallel to the interatrial groove and the mitral valve inspected with findings as noted above.

A quadrangular excision of the central portion of the posterior leaflet of the mitral valve was then performed and sewn to and including a shallow rim of annulus which was subsequently repaired with a figure-of-eight suture of 2-0 polyester suture. The edges of the excised posterior leaflet were then reapproximated with multiple closely spaced 5-0 polypropylene sutures. One thousand cc of cold cardioplegic solution was infused into the aortic root. A 30 mm Carpentier-Edwards mitral ring was then brought into the operative field and 10 horizontal pledgetted mattress sutures of 2-0 polyester were taken circumferentially about the mitral annulus and placed so as to provide tightening of the commissures. The sutures were then passed throughout the prosthetic ring. One thousand cc of cold cardioplegic solution was reinfused into the aortic root. The prosthetic ring was then lowered into place and all sutures securely tied and cut. The valve was tested by injecting saline through the valve orifice and the valve was noted to be competent. The patient was placed in deep Trendelenburg's position with the fight side up, Valsalva maneuvers employed, and transseptal needle aspiration performed to vent the left ventricular apex. The left atrium was then closed with running 3-0 polypropylene as the patient was rewarmed. Prior to tying the last suture, the aortic root needle catheter was placed on pump suction and under a Valsalva maneuver, the aortic cross clamp removed. The heart was noted to be fibrillating, and was defibrillated with two shocks of 10 watt seconds.

The table was brought to the level position. The heart was allowed to fill and eject blood. Intraoperative transesophageal echocardiography demonstrated a competent mitral valve; no residual air was noted. The aortic venting needle was then removed and the venting site controlled with as purse-string suture of 4-0 polypropylene. Temporary atrial and ventricular pacing wires were attached, and following complete rewarming, the patient was weaned from cardiopulmonary bypass without difficulty. The atrial cannula was removed and purse-string sutures secured. The aortic cannula was removed through a side-biting clamp and the aortotomy oversewn with a back-and-forth running suture of 4-0 polypropylene. Two retrosternal chest tubes were passed through stab wounds in the epigastrium and secured with 0 silk sutures. Midline abdominal fascia was closed with interrupted 2-0 polyester suture, and the sternum reapproximated with six interrupted crimped #5 wires. Presternal fascia was closed with running 0 absorbable suture, subcutaneous tissue with 2-0 absorbable suture, and the skin with a running subcuticular 3-0 absorbable suture. Dry sterile dressings were applied and patient transported to the Cardiac Surgical Intensive Care Unit in stable condition. Sponge, instrument, and needle counts were noted to be correct.

---

fraction, may often present with a reduction in ejection fraction after mitral valve replacement. This is commonly attributed to the increased afterload that results from closure of the low impedance pathway provided by the regurgitant valve. After mitral valve repair (which also closes the low impedance pathway), it has been noted that ejection fraction does not always drop to below preoperative levels. Moreover, the use of inotropes may not be necessary, and the cardiac index is often better that preoperative levels. This may be associated with the function of the subvalvular apparatus, e.g., the chordae tendineae and the papillary muscles, and not be solely related to afterload changes.

During early systole in the normal heart, the longitudinal axis of the ventricle decreases as the papillary muscles and the chordae, acting through the mitral leaflets, pull the atrioventricular ring toward the apex. Simultaneously, left ventricular circumference increases, allowing greater fiber length in the mid-left ventricle and greater force of contraction by the Frank–Starling mechanism. Lillehei and his colleagues[24] first suggested that excision of the mitral apparatus would disrupt this sequence and decrease left ventricular performance. Their studies demonstrated no low cardiac output in the early postoperative period. Unfortunately, no tests were available at that time to confirm the theory.

More recent studies shave been able to demonstrate that retaining the subvalvular apparatus retains left ventricular geometry, thereby enhancing contractility. This phenomenon has been seen both after valve replacement as well as after valve repair where chordal continuity is maintained. When increased afterload remains a problem, intra-aortic balloon counterpulsation may be instituted.

Hemodynamic studies performed 1 week postoperatively have shown an increase in the cardiac index, and reduction in pulmonary pressures and left ventricular end-systolic and end–diastolic indices. Ejection fraction may change day-to-day, but the average remains unaffected. For this reason it has been suggested that retention of the chordae preserves left ventricular geometry, resulting in improved left ventricular function. [25,26]

Renal Function.   Impaired renal function is often related to inadequate perfusion of the kidneys during bypass. In valve patients, additional factors may warrant close monitoring of renal function. Patients with severe pulmonary hypertension may have increased intraoperative bronchial collateral return to the left ventricle. This often necessitates high suction (with the cardiotomy suction) to keep the operative field clear of blood. Low bypass flow rates also may be necessary to reduce blood return. Constant and prolonged use of the cardiotomy suction at high negative pressures can create substantial hemolysis and lead to acute tubular necrosis. The institution of dialysis for the ensuing renal failure can place the patient at increased risk for pneumonia, sepsis, and possibly death within a few weeks. [25] Interventions to maintain adequate renal perfusion may be required to protect the kidneys.

Integrity of Valve Repair.   Severe systemic hypertension (greater than 200 mm Hg) can disrupt the valve repair. Uncontrollable, chronic hypertension may be a contraindication to valve repair. Propranolol may be administered to some patients postoperatively for a few weeks to reduce the stress on the sutured valve leaflets. The blood pressure should not be allowed to reach the hypertensive range. Trivial regurgitation may persist, however it should be distinguished from significant regurgitation due to valvular dehiscence.

Recuperation.   Prevention of infection, maintaining optimum left ventricular function, and avoiding the complications of anticoagulation remain issues of concern for patients undergoing valvular surgery. Although long-term coumadin therapy may not be necessary in patients with mitral valve repair, they are routinely placed on a short-term prophylactic anticoagulation regimen a few days after surgery. This helps to prevent the development of acute thrombosis while healing occurs. Unless chronic anticoagulation is indicated (e.g., chronic atrial fibrillation), coumadin will be discontinued at approximately 3 months. While the patient is receiving anticoagulants, teaching should focus on techniques to avoid bleeding complications and signs and symptoms that should be reported to a health care professional.

Prevention of infection is crucial to achieve for invasive procedures and is as important for patients undergoing repair as it for those who have valve replacement. Although it may produce normal function, valve repair does result in some distortion of the mitral apparatus and this provides increased risk for bacterial invasion. In addition, the nurse should be alert to the development of fungal endocarditis with peripheral embolus.

Rehabilitation. There is scarce information available related to the rehabilitative aspects of valvular heart disease(27) as well as to the physiologic effects of exercise on the preoperative patient with mitral regurgitation or on the person who has had reparative surgery. Of significance, it should be noted, that monetary reimbursement for these patients has only recently been made available through Medicare. Patients with papillary muscle dysfunction attributed to ischemic heart disease may be considered eligible for reimbursement more easily.

The exercise standards of the American Heart Association {28} briefly describe the use of exercise tests for patients with mitral regurgitation, and refer to valvular heart disease in the risk stratification for designing exercise protocols. Signs and symptoms such as elevated pulmonary pressures, murmurs, and left ventricular dysfunction, common to a number of patients with valvular heart disease, are often important contraindications for exercise.

It may be possible, however, to make some inferences related to the surgical patient. Since exercise increases afterload, limited exercise may be advisable in the patient with a repaired or replaced valve; it should be performed in such manner as not to aggravate the already increased afterload seen after surgery. A regular exercise protocol may not have to be delayed for too long with a repaired valve; a rapid resumption of activity and a prompt decline in heart size has been seen by some investigators. {25} David noted that repaired valves show improvement in ejection fraction, especially with exercise. He also found that preoperative pulmonary hypertension is alleviated in most patients, and this would further promote increased exercise tolerance.{26}

Patients who have long-standing pulmonary hypertension may have right ventricular dysfunction secondary to the pressure load placed on the right ventricle by the elevated pulmonary pressures. Signs and symptoms of right ventricular failure (e.g., venous engorgement, peripheral edema, abdominal pain) as well as left ventricular failure (e.g., hypotension, elevated pulmonary pressures, oliguria, changes in mentation) should be monitored.

Preoperative left ventricular function is predictive of postoperative outcome, and the trend to perform reparative surgery before the patient becomes severely functionally compromised (functional Class IV) may enhance rehabilitation efforts. Patients often complain of fatigue preoperatively and are likely to be deconditioned. If the preoperative left ventricular function is adequate (e.g., ejection fraction greater that 50 percent), it can be expected to recover by the second postoperative week. If preoperative left ventricular function and ejection fraction are reduced, the patient may show more signs of postoperative fatigue and mental depression. Unfortunately, improvement in physical condition is not necessarily accompanied by an analogous improvement in the psychosocial condition. {29}

Patients on anticoagulants either temporarily or permanently are at risk for bleeding. High impact exercises may induce bleeding complications, and this should be considered in designing an exercise protocol.

A few articles{29,30} have been published on the psychosocial aspects of valvular heart disease, and an increasing number of recent papers are reflecting quality of life issues. Recently Starr and Grunkmeier {31} wrote an editorial addressing the impact of customer demands on the postoperative functional status of patients undergoing mitral valve replacement. Although the mentioned studies{32,33} did not include patients with mitral valve repair, they should provide further impetus for the study of this patient population. Building confidence may be especially important in the valve patient undergoing valve surgery. Unlike many coronary patients, the person with a history of valvular hear disease has been chronically debilitated and deconditioned. Life style adjustments may include taking on a "sick role", which may be difficult to abandon once the physiologic derangement has been corrected. Building the patient's self confidence during the in-hospital phase I of rehabilitation, as well as during the post-discharge program, may be important in achieving maximal functional capacity. Decreasing the fear of normal activities by engaging the patient in early mobilization and exercise, and providing education and counselling soon after surgery, has been recommended. {34}

Further research is warranted, and the following questions may serve as topics for discussion:

- What considerations are important in designing an exercise prescription for a deconditioned patient with surgical valve repair for mitral regurgitation, with and without concomitant coronary artery disease?

- What preoperative factors are significant for cardiac rehabilitation in a patient with mitral valve repair for mitral regurgitation? Ejection fraction? Left ventricular function? Pulmonary function?

- Are there differences between patients with mitral valve repair and mitral valve replacement?

- Are psychosocial considerations for the patient with valvular heart disease similar or different from patients with coronary heart disease?

- What are the potential risks and associated educational needs of patients requiring temporary (3 months) anticoagulation?

- Is self efficacy a significant determinant of successful rehabilitation in a patient with mitral valve repair?

CONCLUSION

The operative report provides supplemental information for the nurse during the patient's postoperative and rehabilitation phases. The report is usually placed on the chart within 48 hours after surgery; rehabilitation nurses can request the old chart from the medical record department. A collection of operative reports may be a helpful resource, especially when accompanied by a glossary to define technical terms. The reports can be requested from the surgeon and kept on file (with precautions to protect patient confidentially), or the surgeon can dictate a generic report typical of the kind of operation performed. Perioperative nurses and surgeons can assist nurses in interpreting the technical aspects of the operative report.

In addition to being a useful clinical resource, the operative record can serve as an impetus for greater communication between all members of a cardiac service. This promotes collaborative efforts which can only enhance patient's outcome.

The author is grateful to Ursula Anderson, CNP; John Garrett, MD; Quentin Macmanus, MD; John Sandiford, MD; and Sue Wingate, DNSc, for their expert advice and guidance.

REFERENCES

1. Lytle BW, Cosgrove DM, Ratliff NB, et al: Coronary artery bypass grafting with the right gastroepiploic artery. J Thorac Cardiovas Surg 1989; 97(6):826.

2. Glick D, Liddicoat J, Karp R: Alternative conduits for coronary artery bypass grafting. In: Karp R (ed): Adv Cardiac Surg, 1990; 2:191.

3. Mills N, Everson C: Right gastroepiploic artery: A third arterial conduit for coronary artery bypass. Ann Thorac Surg 1989; 47:706.

4. Mills N, Everson C: Technique and use of the inferior epigastric artery as a coronary bypass graft. Ann Thorac Surg 1989; 47:706.

5. Buche M, Schoevaerdts J, Louagie Y, et al: Use of the inferior epigastric artery for coronary bypass. J Thorac Cardiovasc Surg 1992; 103(4):665.

6. Ochiai M, Ohno M, Taguchi J, et al: Responses of human gastro-epiploic arteries to vasoactive substances: Comparison with responses of internal mammary arteries and saphenous veins. J Thorac Cardiovasc Surg 1992; 104(2):453,1992.

7. Yang Z, Wiebenmann R, Studer M, et al: Similar endothelium-dependent relaxation, but enhanced contractility, of the right gastroepiploic artery as compared with the internal mammary artery. J Thorac Cardiovasc Surg 1992; 104(2):459.

8. Acar C, Jebara V, Portoghese M, et al: Revival of the radial artery for coronary artery by[ass grafting. Ann Thorac Surg 1992; 54:652.

9. Partington MT, Acar C, Buckberg GD, et al: Studies of retrograde cardioplegia. Part I. Capillary blood flow distribution to myocardium supplied by open and occluded arteriels. J Thorac Cardiovasc Surg 1989; 97:605–612.

10. Partington MT, Acar C, Buckberg GD, et al: Studies of retrograde cardioplegia. Part II. Advantages of antegrade/retrograde cardioplegia to optimize distribution in jeopardized myocardium. J Thorac Cardiovasc Surg 1989; 97:613–622.

11. Schaff H, Orzulak T, Gersh B, et al: The morbidity and mortality of re-operation for coronary artery disease and analysis of late results with the use of actuarial estimate of event-free interval. J. Thorac Cardiovasc Surg 1983; 85(4):508.

12. Grondin C: Re-operation in patients with coronary graft disease. In McGoon D, (ed): Cardiac Surgery, ed 2. Cardiovascular Clinics. Philadelphia: FA Davis, 1987:31–39.

13. Heye ML: Pain and discomfort after coronary artery bypass surgery. Cardiovasc Nurs 1991; 27(4):19.

14. Galbut D, Traad E, Dorman M, et al: Bilateral internal mammary artery grafts in reoperative and primary coronary bypass surgery. Ann Thorac Surg 1991; 52:20.

15. Agency for Health Care Policy and Research (AHCPR): Acute pain management: operative or medical procedures and trauma. Clinical Practice Guideline. Rockville, MD: AHCPR Pub. No. 92–0032, 1992.

16. Suma H, Wanibuchi Y, Furuta S, et al: Does use of gastroepiploic artery graft increase surgical risk? J Thorac Cardiovasc Surg 1991; 101:121.

17. Hoeymans G: Coronary heart disease: surgical therapy. In Wingate S, (ed): Cardiac Nursing: A Clinical Management and Patient Care Resource. Gaithersburg, MD: Aspen Publishers, Inc. 1991.

18. Gortner S, Miller N, Jenkins L: Self-efficacy: a key to recovery. In Jillings C (ed): Cardiac Rehabilitation Nursing. Rockville, MD, 1988.

19. Antunes M: Mitral Valve Repair. Berger Strasse: R. S Schulz, 1989.

20. Cosgrove DM, Rosenkranz ER, Hendren WG, et al: Valvuloplasty for aortic insufficiency. J Thorac Cardiovasc Surg 1991; 102(4):571.

21. Roberts W: Congenital cardiovascular abnormalities usually silent until adulthood. In Roberts W: Adult Congenital Heart Disease. F. A. Davis Company, Philadelphia, 1987.

22. Carpentier A: Cardiac valve surgery: The "French Correction". J Thorac Cardiovas Surg 1983; 86(3):323.

23. Crawford M, Souchek J, Oprian C, et al: Determinants of survival and left ventricular performance after mitral valve replacement. Circulation 1990; 81(4):1173.

24. Lillehei C, Levy M, Bonnabeau R: Mitral valve replacement with preservation of papillary muscles and chordae tendinea. J Thorac Cardiovas Surg 1964; 47(4):532.

25. Bonchek L, Olinger G, Siegal R, et al: Left ventricular performance after mitral reconstruction for mitral regurgitation. J Thorac Cardiovasc Surg 1984; 88(1):122.

26. David T: A rational approach to the surgical management of mitral valve disease. In Karp R, (ed): Advances in Cardiac Surgery, Vol 2. St. Louis: Mosby Year Book, 1990.

27. Wingate S: Rehabilitation of the patient with valvular heart disease. J Cardiovasc Nurs 1987; 1(3):52.

28. Fletcher G, Froelicher V, Hartley L, et al: American Heart Association Medical/Scientific Statement. Special Report. Exercise Standards: A Statement for Health Professionals from the American Heart Association. Circulation 1990; 82(6):2286.

29. Magni G, Unger HP, Valfre C, et al: Psychosocial outcome one year after heart surgery. Arch Intern Med 1987; 147:473.

30. Jenkins CD, Stanton B, Savageau J, et al: Physical, psychologic, social, and economic outcomes after cardiac valve surgery. Arch Intern Med 1983; 143:2107.

31. Starr A and Grunkemeier G: An artificial valve-A real life (editorial). J Heart Valve Dis 1992; 1(1):32.

32. Phillips RC, Lansky DJ: Outcomes management in heart valve replacement surgery: Early experience. J Heart Valve Dis 1992; 1(1):42.

33. Walter PJ, Mohan R, Amsel B: Quality of life after heart valve replacement. J Heart Valve Dis 1992; 1(1):35.

34. Agency for Health Care Policy and Research (AHCPR): Cardiac Rehabilitation Programs, Number 3: Heart transplant, percutaneous transluminal coronary angioplasty, and heart valve surgery patients. (Prepared by S. Hotta.) Rockville, MD:AHCPR Pub. No. PB92–120690, 1991.

THE CRITICAL BALANCE

Streamlining Cardiovascular Care while Maintaining Quality Excellence

Cynthia P. Arnold, M.B.A.

University of Medicine and Dentistry of New Jersey
Robert Wood Johnson Medical School
Cooper Hospital/University Medical Center
Camden, New Jersey

The demands that are placed on our health care system, as well as the complexity of our organizational structures, make it necessary to continuously strive to reach the "critical balance" between streamlined cardiovascular care and service excellence. The "critical balance" is a dynamic equilibrium that can be approached through a consistent use of various management techniques.

This article reviews the environmental factors impacting the health care delivery system and discusses several management techniques currently being utilized in cardiovascular programs.

ENVIRONMENTAL FACTORS

The United States spends approximately 733 billion dollars per year for health care which amounts to 23,000 dollars per second. Due to the magnitude and growth of this expense, a number of efforts have been made to limit further growth. Almost ten years ago, the Prospective Payment System for inpatient Medicare hospital services was enacted. [1] Under this system, Medicare charges are paid prospectively based on set rates which are classified according to diagnostic related grouping (DRG). This was a radical departure from the "reasonable cost basis" by which hospitals were previously paid. Hospitals are now being paid, not on their retrospective costs per case, but on a budget for a diagnostic grouping. Within the same diagnostic grouping, patients who require more hospital resources are reimbursed the same as patients requiring fewer resources. One example of a cardiovascular grouping is DRG 106, which represents coronary artery bypass graft with cardiac catheterization, which pays the same rate for a patient who has had both procedures, regardless of the hospital length of stay.

Cardiac Surgery: Current Issues 2, Edited by A. C. Cernaianu and A. J. DelRossi.
Plenum Press, New York, 1994

To compensate the difference in reimbursement, hospitals started to charge unregulated payers higher rates, establishing an actual "cost shifting" to private payers. Predictably, other payers have responded by demanding special rates, and adding complexity to a fragmented health care market.

Additionally, a number of environmental factors relating to the concept of quality have impacted the health care delivery system.

The Health Care Financing Administration's (HCFA) Coronary Artery Bypass Graft Surgery Demonstration Project is a pilot project that includes four hospitals in various regions of the country that have packaged a combined hospital/physician case pricing. Hospitals were chosen for the pilot based on quality, costs, program size and age. HCFA has negotiated a five to twenty percent charge reduction from each participating facility. Michael D. Blaszyk, Executive Vice President of University Hospital at Boston University Medical Center, one of the participating centers, was quoted as stating: "We're going to work very hard to try to find ways we can minimize unnecessary testing and unnecessary delays so we can find the greatest amount of efficiency."[2] Packaged pricing will be discussed in detail later in this article.

Health care spending reached 13 percent of the gross national product (GNP) in 1991, and is predicted to increase 14 percent in 1993. Health care insurance averages $3,161.00 per employee, and private business are reporting to spend as much on health care as they earned in after-tax income. If unchecked, health care expenses could eliminate profits for these companies, and make it very difficult for small companies to even offer health insurance to their employees. Correspondingly there has been a change in the expectations of our patients and our payers. Dr. Paul M. Elwood, an expert in outcomes management, stated that "Patients, payers and executives of health care organizations now have high expectations and greater power and this crisis is disabling the vast machinery of medicine. . . Our divergent, even conflicting view points cause everyone to lose perspective."[3]

In the managed care arena, US Healthcare, the largest HMO in the United States, has recently developed a program called "CapTainer". [4] In this program, a portion of the agreed upon hospital and physician fees, approximately 10 to 15 percent, is held aside by US Healthcare. If the service quality is at an acceptable level, the hospitals and physicians receive the percentage portion held by US Healthcare.

Prudential Insurance is marketing the "centers of excellence" concept, whereby they include hospitals in their care network that meet demonstrated levels of quality. Prudential customers are directed to the "centers of excellence" for their patient care needs.

Hospitals are also actively seeking direct contracting relationships with employers. Elimination of the "middle man" (insurance or managed care company) provides some savings to the employer, and allows the employer to work directly with the health care provider in customizing a health care package for their employees that includes preventative care. At present, these arrangements are more prevalent in the West Coast, in part because the employer size is large enough to merit offering specific packages. The incidence of cardiovascular disease requiring CABG surgery in the general population is only a few cases per thousand, thus only very large employers have the need to develop cardiovascular surgery packages.) Some medical centers have even hired salespersons to work directly with employers. [5]

The cardiovascular marketplace has matured, and competition between hospitals has increased. Traditional competition is being supplemented by competition from alternative delivery models such as mobile cardiac catheter labs, outpatient settings, etc.

The Joint Commission on Accredation on Healthcare Oranizations (JCAHO) has also launched its own quality initiative, i.e., "The Agenda for Change". Their program, with approximately 100 hospitals participating as beta sites, is committed to measuring performance variations in numerous areas such as cardiovascular programs. True management requires specific measurable attributes. In the past, without any agreement upon standards, measurement of quality was difficult.

The Total Quality Management (TQM) movement that has impacted many industries has changed how the nation's process of delivering goods and services. Awareness and successful participation in TQM efforts, has generally raised businesses' expectations of what can be delivered by health care providers. The techniques of TQM are discussed later in this article as tools that can be applied to health care.

As a nation, we pride ourselves as providers of the best health care in the world. There is no dispute that technologically, the United States provides the most advanced care, however, when you examine some of the other indicators of overall health care status, such as infant mortality or longevity, the United States is not providing the best health care system.

As these environmental factors impact and change how providers deliver care, several basic questions arise: 1) Will cost containment reduce the quality of healthcare? 2) Will a two-tier health system evolve with small segments of the population receiving a lower quality of care? 3) Will the public accept a rationing of healthcare as an alternative to high costs?

CARDIOVASCULAR PROGRAMS

The 1980's represented a period of tremendous growth for cardiovascular programs. Figure 1 illustrates annual growth in cardiovascular procedures

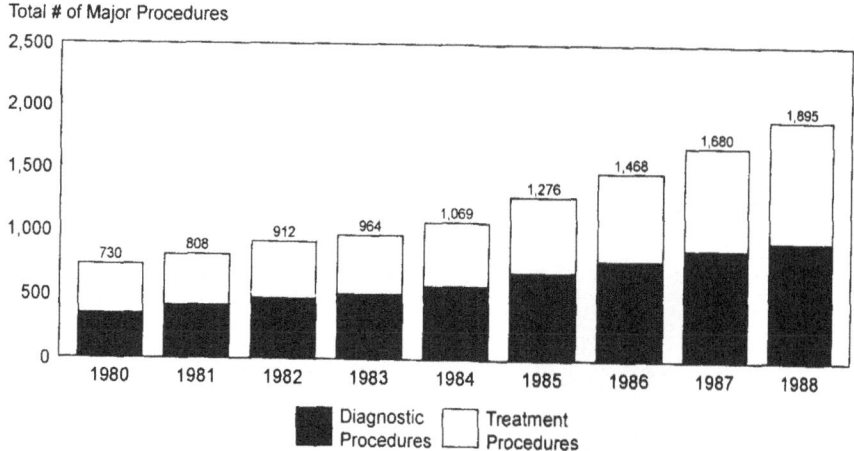

Figure 1. 13% annual growth in cardiac procedures. Note: Treatment procedures include bypass surgery, angioplasty, valve surgery, pacemaker procedures, atrial ventricular septal procedures.

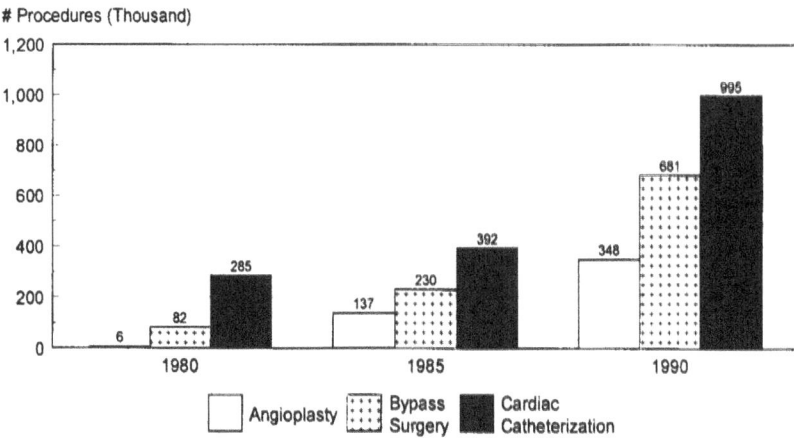

Figure 2. Growth in cardiac procedures.

from 1980 through 1988. Nationally we spend 46.7 billion dollars per year just for cardiovascular care, which accounts for approximatelly 34 percent of all hospital discharges. [6] Only ten years ago, cardiology programs were primarily located in tertiary care medical centers with cardiac surgery programs. [2] Due to the profitability of cardiovascular care (net margin of $4,000 to $5,000 per case) and technological advancement, hospital cardiovascular programs have proliferated. [7] As a result, there are over 1400 hospitals in the USA with a recognizable cardiovascular program.

Primarily, angioplasty, bypass surgery and cardiac catheterization, account for the most of this growth, as illustrated in the Figure 2.

The number of bypass surgery programs and cardiac catheterization labs has grown more rapidly (Figure 3), than the total volume of procedures, thus limiting volume growth for individual programs Figure 4).

The cardiovascular market is very attractive to hospitals, however it has few barriers to overcome. Program components include attracting qualified physicians, purchasing equipment and obtaining appropriate state permission and certification. Since the volume of procedures is increasing, hospitals are competing aggressively for each patient undergoing cardiac surgery. The

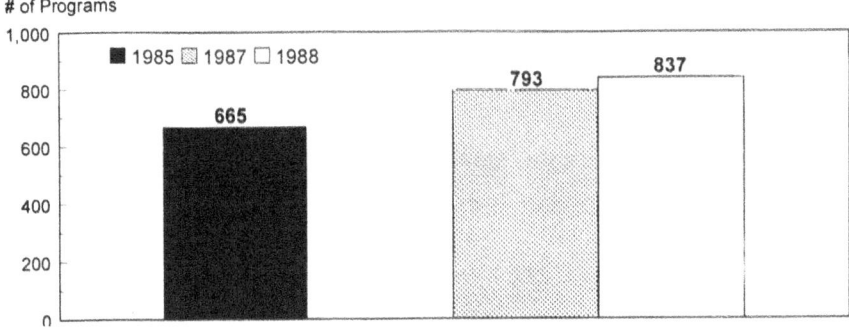

Figure 3. Growth in cardiac surgery programs: 26% growth in 3 years.

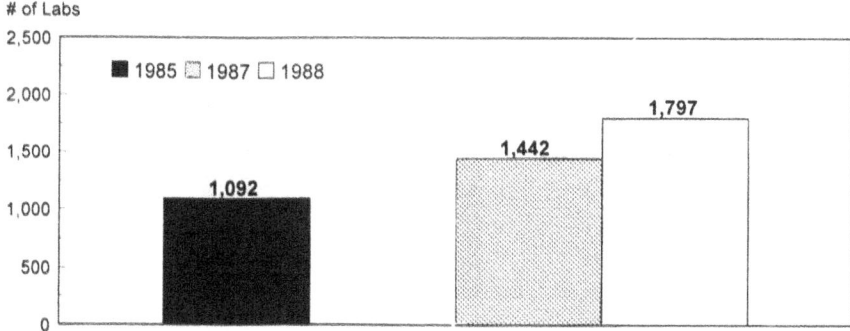

Figure 4. Growth in cardiac surgery catheterization laboratories: 65% growth in 3 years.

continued growth of the cardiovascular market appears positive, due to the aging of our population (Table 1).

Despite these favorable demographics, many experts predict a decline in heart disease due to a number of contributing breakthroughs (Figure 5).

Contributing factors to the eventual decline in heart disease include: lifestyle alterations (people are decreasing their risk factors by quitting smoking, lowering cholesterol, increasing exercise, etc.), medical advances (refinement of PTCA techniques, and new therapeutic electrophysiology procedures), advances in pharmacological and genetics (thrombolytic drugs providing the patient a "life preserver" until therapeutic procedures can be performed, or even removal of the genetic predisposition for cardiovascular disease in the next twenty years).

Indeed, annually, there are approximately 10,000 bypass procedures due to patients living long enough to receive this type of care. [6]

It appears that forces impacting the cardiac surgical market by the year 2000 are divergent. Limitation is related to the fact that the federal government is more selective and reimburses less, uncompensated care is increasing, patients and payers are more demanding, physicians are requiring more high-technology tools, and regulatory agencies have more requirements. Conversely, demographics show an increase in the need for cardiovascular care, and innovative technology has created new procedures.

In general, the cardiovascular market has matured in three directions: 1) There are many product providers. 2) Buyers of care are more knowledgeable and selective. 3) Health care providers differentiate themselves based on quality and/or price.

Considering all of these factors, one could envision that in the future, cardiovascular care will become a retail business with everyone participating

Table 1.

Age	% Total Population	% All Heart Cases	Age Related Risk (%)
Under 40	62	32	1.2
40–59	21	24	2.9
60+	17	44	6.5

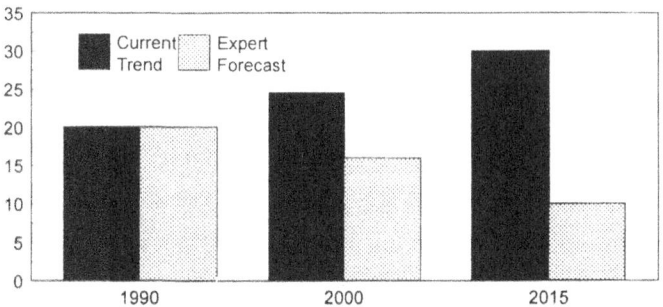

Figure 5. Projection of coronary artery disease.

and competing. In contrast, cardiovascular care may well become a wholesale business. Since payers will be more selective, they will define quality. More medical centers will develop networks, with one tertiary magnet hospital and a number of smaller hospitals. Patients will be routed to the facility offering the level of care needed. Both scenarios may present difficulty in managing these changes.

MANAGEMENT TECHNIQUES

There are a number of different approaches that are being utilized to manage cost and the quality of care. However, anyone who has embarked on a project designed to evoke "change" knows how difficult it is to implement that change and then sustain that change over time.

Total Quality Management (TQM)

Total Quality Management (TQM), also known as Continuous Quality Improvement (CQI), is a strategy or philosophy used to improve every aspect of the daily activity, in order to create more customer satisfaction. Many health care organizations have already, or are planning to implement, TQM programs.

Although there have been a number of leaders in this movement such as Deming, Juran, and Crosby, all programs share the same basic elements in their philosophy of TQM.

1. TQM involves the entire organization. Everyone from CEO to front-line worker is involved in creating the right quality atmosphere.
2. TQM uses statistical tools and techniques to resolve problems. Anecdotes of patient care experiences are not utilized to solve problems. Rather, problems are examined through objective data collection and statistical analysis. Systematically, root causes of the greatest magnitude are addressed first.
3. TQM empowers employees. The employees who actually perform the work know best how to improve it. This is an old, approach based on common sense which is not customary in the hierarchical business

structure of America, which is accustomed to directives from the CEO and having reluctant employees to suggest alternative methods.

4. TQM involves training and development, so that the entire work force understands how change will take place, not just the management staff.
5. TQM focuses on customer orientation and satisfaction. Our customers obviously include patients, but also other people encountered in the process such as family members, insurance companies, physicians, and quality auditing organizations. There is a need to understand all of their expectations.
6. TQM is process oriented. A consistent process for approaching situations produces predictable results and is positively accepted by the people involved. Focusing only on outcomes, is the "end justifies the means" approach. This kind of approach encourages quick fixes that cannot be sustained and ultimately requires "fixing" again.
7. TQM looks at the organization as a system, and within that system, additional smaller systems. This is particularly well illustrated in hospitals where each department is dependent upon interaction with other departments. As an example, the nursing units are dependent upon food service to provide meals, and food service is dependent upon nursing to supply the patient's dietary orders.
8. TQM seeks to minimize variation. When processes are consistent, work flow is smooth. However, when exceptions occur, additional time is required to resolve the situations, which in turn slows the entire process.

The relationship between cost and quality has been widely documented, and is referred to as the "cost-quality cycle". If work is done correctly the first time, it is less expensive than work that has to be repeated due to errors. Quality work is rewarded by customer loyalty and attraction of new customers. The customer market is captured, and your business prospers. Defective work in industry can be discarded. In health care we are working with patient's lives, and cannot accept defective work. It has been proven that hospitals and surgical teams, that perform greater than 200 CABG's per year, have better outcomes in terms of mortality, length of stay, charges and costs. [9]

During the application of TQM, traditional roles which are compartmentalized and comfortable, need to be discarded. There is a need to look beyond the current methods of working and become facilitators of change. As the work barriers diminish and every person performs the job, people will focus on the customer needs. When there is a change in focus to the customer, barriers will be lifted and the work will be more naturally performed.

Physicians have compared the TQM to the scientific process, which has three phases: 1) plan to improve, 2) implement, and 3) innovate. Once the process is started, implementation and innovation become an ongoing cycle, as one may constantly strive to develop new ideas and implement them.

The first phase of this strategy (plan to improve) comprises of identification of the customers, and data collection on focus areas. Patient billing summaries, length of stay, and reimbursement data should be collected. Additionally, interviewing people involved in the cardiovascular process, and asking more questions such as "What is the path of the typical post-operative

CABG patient?", or "What percentage of cases are physicians late for in the catheterization lab?", may give you information related to the areas to be improved.

After collecting these data, an expert panel is assembled (steering committee and an implementation task force) to address specific issues. Representation on the committees should include physicians, managers, nurses and other representatives of the entire process.

Several consultative sessions should be held to prioritize specific issues. As the solutions are implemented, the baseline data are used to determine the impact.

Hospitals are marketing high service quality product lines as "Centers of Excellence". Payers are now attempting to identify hospitals which can be labeled as "centers of excellence" in order to provide better service for their patients.

Standard Treatment Protocols

The standard treatment protocol (STP) is a reference document which establishes the consensus of what should happen to a patient given certain levels of patient response have been achieved. STPs provide standards for a patient care unit, and create more efficiency, both from the resource perspective and from the clinical perspective. Patient care is improved by applying more attention to patients experiencing true clinical variations. The potential benefits of STPs include:

1. Enhanced profit margins through both, decreased costs and selectively decreased charges. In hospitals, although we are paid primarily on DRG or capitated rates, we still place charges to track individual patient utilization. Auditing groups often look at charges and use them as a proxy for costs, since cost measurement is very difficult for hospitals.
2. Increased resource efficiency through standardization. As discussed earlier, standardization creates a smoother work flow resulting in reduced costs and decreased length of stay.
3. STPs provide an opportunity to enhance quality, and implement creative ideas.
4. Establishment of multi-disciplinary communications forum that empowers clinical personnel to make changes in the way patients are treated. A formalized committee allows the group to reflect and plan care.

CRITICAL PATH METHOD

The STP focuses on patient care delivery for a specific point in the course of a patient's stay, whereas, the Critical Path Method (CPM) examines the entire patient hospital visit, from admission through discharge.

The CPM and Program Evaluation and Review Technique (PERT) were developed in the late 1950's as business tools to control time, cost and resource availability. The CPM was originated in 1957, by J. E. Kelley of Remington-Rand and M. R. Walker of duPont to aid in scheduling shut downs of chemical processing plants. {10} PERT was developed in 1958 by the United States Navy Special Projects Office as a management tool for scheduling and controlling the Polaris missile project. Since that time there have been a number of variations of this program.

The purpose of the CPM is to find the longest time consuming path through a network of tasks, and streamline that path. CPM has been successfully used as a project management tool to control time and cost, since it is based on the premise that there is a relationship between activity completion time and the cost of a project. The characteristics of the CPM include:

1. Well defined tasks whose completion marks the end of the project.
2. Tasks are independent, they may be started, stopped, and conducted separately within a sequence.
3. Tasks are ordered within a given sequence.
4. Tasks, once started, must continue until completion.

The New England Medical Center Nursing Department was the first to adapt this program for patient care. The purpose of tracking a patient's stay on a critical pathway is to objectively review the most time-intensive pathway components, and develop ways of shortening the critical pathway, which decreases the overall length of stay. The clinical path is a combination of medical practices that result in the most resource efficient, clinically appropriate and shortest length of stay for a specific medical condition or procedure. For example, DRG 106, "coronary artery bypass graft with cardiac catheterization" has a standard critical path diagram. As the patient progresses during the stay, he/she experiences a unique set of events that may vary from the standard clinical pathway. These variances may be positive (more efficient than the standard pathway) or negative (less efficient).

The variances may also signal the need for a patient consultation to "get the patient back on the standard path". At the unit team meetings the variances are discussed, aggregated, analyzed and addressed to continuously improve patient care. The Clinical Path concept implies: 1) Clinical appropriateness, 2) Efficiency and 3) Quality.

There are a number of different opinions as to the value of CPM use:

1. **PRO:** Adapts to any care delivery system and motivates staff;
   CON: Creates additional responsibilities for nurse managers and case managers.
2. **PRO:** Conceptually bridges nursing and medical models thus creating truly collaborative practice;
   CON: Each discipline may have political and philosophical reasons to be hesitant.
3. **PRO:** Establishes and empowers nurses as the managers of the acute care business;
   CON: Requires major mindset changes and additional training.
4. **PRO:** Decrease prejudicial barriers between units, smooth patient transitions and more equally distribute work;
   CON: Requires facilitation to get the group off the ground and adds another piece of paper to the shift.

A number of refinements need to occur before CPM are universally accepted. CPM are paper intensive, thus automated tools are needed for daily pathway tracking as well as aggregation of variations. Bedside Computer Charting Systems are in their infancy and will require future integration with CPM. Finally, standard CPM will need to allow bridging from one pathway to another when a patient's variances lead to a completely different medical experience. Presently the patient "falls off the pathway" and is not tracked.

The future promises a new focus on the patient care stay. Medical centers are scrutinizing length of stay and patient outcomes. Multi-disciplinary teams are actively problem solving quality and cost issues. These efforts will lead to a sophisticated case utilization approach with internal bench marking, credible data and easy access to protocol costs for ongoing review and revision.

OUTCOMES MANAGEMENT

Presently, outcomes management is primarily a physician driven activity. Outcomes management, according to Paul Elwood, is the "technology of patient experience designed to help patients, payers and providers make rational, medical care related choices based on better insight into the effects of these choices based on the patient's life". {11} Currently we examine a number of health care statistical indicators such as mortality, morbidity, financial class, and patient satisfaction. These statistics only begin to describe the quality of patient care. Additional data is obviously available from our critical pathways, severity of illness indicators, and other sources. However, little agreement exists as to which data should be consistently collected at all medical centers, how that information should be compared, and what decisions should be made.

A number of pioneers are developing data collection tools such as the short-form health survey by John Ware at the New England Medical Center. {1} This particular health survey lets the patient evaluate his/her health care based on physical functioning, role limitations resulting from illness and duress, or role limitations due to emotional adjustments. The patient then scales the responses and can quantitatively evaluate the quality of care that they received. The Cooperative Cardiovascular Project is another example of coordinated review of the quality of patient care. This project is designed to involve PROs, hospitals, and physicians in improving the processes and outcomes of care, by reviewing Medicare beneficiaries hospitalized for myocardial infarction, coronary artery bypass grafting, or percutaneous coronary angioplasty. The project was initiated in 1992. {12}

As discussed earlier, the HCFA CABG Demonstration Program is an example of a packaged program that is monitoring outcomes. At four participating medical centers, the bundled package has increased physician-hospital communication and provided an incentive to physicians to be more cost effective. The project has been operational for over a year, and thus far the patient volume has not increased at these medical centers. However, the surgeons are now preparing packages and actively marketing their services to businesses in their region.

SUMMARY

"In attempting to arrive at the truth, I've applied everywhere for information but, in scarcely an instance, have I been able to obtain hospital records fit for any purpose of comparison. If they could be obtained, they would enable us to decide many other questions besides the ones alluded to. They would show subscribers how their money was being spent, what amount of good was really being done with it and whether the money was not doing mischief rather than good." Florence Nightingale (1863)

Many of our problems in assessing health care are not new. Environmental factors will continuously impact our organizations, challenging us to find and maintain the "Critical Balance" between cost and quality.

REFERENCES

1. Unger WJ: Medicare prospective payment system for inpatient hospital services, J Cardiovasc Manage 1992; 3(4):31–40.
2. Franc CW: Facing the challenge of providing cardiac care in the 1990's: Part One. J Cardiovasc Manage 1991; 2(5):20–22.
3. Unger WJ: The interdependence of outcomes management. Decisions in Imaging Economics 1992; 5(4):4–11.
4. George J: Keying on quality, carrots and a stick? Phil Bus J 1992:5B.
5. Johnsson J: Direct contracting: employers look to hospital-physician partnerships to control costs. Hospitals 1992:56–60.
6. Health Care Advisory Board, Hospital Cardiology, Volume 1 Major Business Strategies. The Advisory Board Company, Washington, D. C., 1990:7–54.
7. Souhrada L: Hospitals pursue heart programs despite pitfalls. Hospitals 1989; 63(20):40–46.
8. Walton M: The Deming Management Method. Dodd, Mead & Company, New York, Chapter 18: Point fourteen; Take action to accomplish the transformation. 1986:87.
9. McGregor M, Pelletier G: Planning of specialized health facilities: size versus cost and effectiveness in cardiac surgery. N Engl J Med 1978; 299:179–81.
10. Chase RB, Aquilano NJ: Production and operations management. A life cycle approach. Third edition, Richard B Irwin, Inc., Homewood, IL, 1981:553–578.
11. Elwood PM: Outcomes Management: A technology of patient experience. New Engl J Med 1988; 318:1549–1556.

FURTHER SUGGESTED READING

American Heart Association, 1992 Heart and Stroke Facts, 1991.
Coile RC Jr: Forecast of Cardiac Care "Megatrends" for the 1990's. J Cardiovasc Manage 1990; 1(6).
James BC: Quality management for health care delivery. The Hospital Research and Educational Trust of the American Hospital Association, Chicago, 1989.
Koska MT: HCFA's bundled CABG payment project yields results, insights. Hospitals 1992:46–50.
Koska MT: PROs, providers, and physicians to collaborate on cardiac outcomes. Hospitals 1992:36–37.
Kralovec JO III, Huttner CA, Dixon MD: The application of total quality management concepts in a service-line cardiovascular program. J Cardiovasc Manage 1991; 2(4):22–29.
Kritchevshy S, Simmons MD, Bryan P: Continuous quality improvement concepts and applications for physician care. JAMA 1991; 266(15): 1817–1823.

Kyes K: The outcomes management model: appropriate sequencing and channeling. Decisions in Imaging Economics. 1990; 3(6):16–28.

Merry MD, Martin D: Commentary: Total quality management for physicians: translating the new paradigm. QRB 1990.

Roby C: Give everyone keys to the asylum. Information Week August 1992:60.

Schaffer RH, Thomson HA: Successful change programs begin with results. Harvard Business Review 1991:80–89.

Zander K: Nursing case management: strategic management of cost and quality outcomes. JONA 1988; 18(5):23–30.

CONTRIBUTORS

James B. Alexander, M.D.
Associate Professor of Clinical Surgery
UMDNJ-Robert Wood Johnson Medical
  School at Camden
Cooper Hospital/University Medical Center
Camden, New Jersey

Cynthia P. Arnold, MBA
Administrative Director, Cardiology
  Services
UMDNJ-Robert Wood Johnson Medical
  School at Camden
Cooper Hospital/University Medical Center
Camden, New Jersey

Edward L. Bove, M.D.
Professor of Surgery
Director, Pediatric Cardiac Surgery
University of Michigan
Ann Arbor, Michigan

Brian S. Bull, M.D.
Professor and Chairman
Department of Pathology and Laboratory
  Medicine
Loma Linda University Medical Center and
Loma Linda University School of Medicine
Loma Linda, California

**Margaret M. Burgoyne, R.N., M.S.,
  C.R.N.A.**
Staff Nurse Anesthetist
Department of Anesthesiology
UMDNJ-Robert Wood Johnson Medical
  School at Camden
Cooper Hospital/University Medical Center
Camden, New Jersey

Rudolph C. Camishion, M.D.
Professor of Surgery
UMDNJ-Robert Wood Johnson Medical
  School at Camden
Head, Division of General Surgery
Cooper Hospital/University Medical Center
Camden, New Jersey

Aurel C. Cernaianu, M.D.
Associate Professor of Surgery
UMDNJ-Robert Wood Johnson Medical
  School at Camden
Director, Research Programs
Division of Cardiothoracic Surgery
Cooper Hospital/University Medical Center
Camden, New Jersey

Ray C.-J. Chiu, M.D., Ph.D.
Professor and Chairman
Division of Cardiovascular & Thoracic
  Surgery
McGill University
Montreal, Quebec, Canada

Dipak K. Das, Ph.D.
Professor of Surgery
Director of Cardiovascular Research
University of Connecticut School of
  Medicine
Farmington, Connecticut

Laurie K. Davies, M.D.
Assistant Professor of Anesthesiology
University of Florida College of Medicine
Gainesville, Florida

Richard F. Davis, M.D.
Professor of Anesthesiology
Oregon Health Sciences University and
  Anesthesiology Service
Portland Department of Veterans Affairs
  Medical Center
Portland, Oregon

David W. Deaton, M.D.
Assistant Professor of Surgery
University of Connecticut Medical School
Farmington, Connecticut
Attending Surgeon
Division of Cardiac Surgery
Baystate Medical Center
Springfield, Massachusetts

Anthony J. DelRossi, M.D.
Professor of Surgery
UMDNJ-Robert Wood Johnson Medical
    School at Camden
Chairman, Department of Surgery
Head, Division of Cardiothoracic Surgery
Cooper Hospital/University Medical Center
Camden, New Jersey

L. Henry Edmunds, Jr., M.D.
W.M. Measey Professor
Department of Surgery
University of Pennsylvania School of
    Medicine
Philadelphia, Pennsylvania

Richard M. Engelman, M.D.
Chief, Division of Cardiac Surgery
Baystate Medical Center
Springfield, Massachusetts
Clinical Professor of Cardiothoracic
    Surgery
Tufts University School of Medicine
Boston, Massachusetts

N. Simon Faithfull, M.D., Ph.D.
Vice President, Medical Research
Alliance Pharmaceutical Corporation
San Diego, California

Joseph E. Flack, III, M.D.
Assistant Professor of Surgery
University of Connecticut Medical School
Farmington, Connecticut.
Attending Surgeon
Baystate Medical Center
Springfield, Massachusetts

Robert L. Kormos, M.D.
Associate Professor
University of Pittsburgh School of Medicine
Director, Artificial Heart Program
University of Pittsburgh Medical Center
Pittsburgh, Pennsylvania

Gerald M. Lemole, M.D.
Chief, Cardiovascular Surgery
The Medical Center of Delaware
Wilmington, Delaware

William H. O'Connor, M.D.
Associate Professor of Clinical Medicine
UMDNJ-Robert Wood Johnson Medical
    School at Camden
Director, Echocardiography Laboratories
Cooper Hospital/University Medical School
Camden, New Jersey

A. Bernard Pleet, M.D.
Professor of Neurology
Tufts University School of Medicine
Boston, Massachusetts
Chief, Department of Neurology
Baystate Medical Center
Springfield, Massachusetts

John A. Rousou, M.D.
Assistant Professor of Surgery
Tufts University School of Medicine
Boston, Massachusetts
Division of Cardiac Surgery
Attending Surgeon
Baystate Medical Center
Springfield, Massachusetts

**Patricia C. Seifert, R.N., MSN, RNFA,
    CNOR**
Operating Room Coordinator
Cardiac Surgery
The Arlington Hospital
Arlington, Virginia

Norman E. Shumway, M.D.
Professor and Chairman
Department of Cardiothoracic Surgery
Stanford University School of Medicine
Stanford, California

Richard K. Spence, M.D.
Professor of Surgery
UMDNJ-Robert Wood Johnson Medical
    School at Camden
Head, Section of General Vascular Surgery
Cooper Hospital/University Medical Center
Camden, New Jersey

Paul I. Tartter, M.D.
Associate Professor
Department of Surgery
Mount Sinai Medical Center
New York, New York

Kathleen C. Tully, R.N., MSN, CCRN
Nurse Manager
Cardiovascular Unit
Our Lady of Lourdes Medical Center
Camden, New Jersey

Roger A. Vertrees, B.A., C.C.P.
Perfusionist, Department of Surgery
University of Texas Medical Branch
Galveston, Texas

INDEX

The manufacturer's authorised representative in the EU is Springer
Nature Customer Service Centre GmbH, Europaplatz 3, 69115 Heidelberg,
Germany. If you have any concerns regarding our products, please
contact ProductSafety@springernature.com

Printed and bound by CPI Group (UK) Ltd, Croydon, CR0 4YY
23/04/2026
02095607-0013